Critical Review for the MRCPsych

'The ability to critically appraise scientific evidence is a foundational skill for ALL clinicians. This guide, while aimed at the MRCPsych exam candidate, is an essential companion for all clinicians to help them embed evidence-based scientific practice in their daily work. Dr Suleman has a knack for making complex concepts easily comprehensible – often with brilliant analogies and illustrations.'

Professor Subodh Dave, President, Royal College of Psychiatrists, Consultant Psychiatrist and Deputy Director of Undergraduate Medical Education, Derbyshire Healthcare Foundation Trust; Professor of Psychiatry, University of Greater Manchester

Critical Review for the MRCPsych

Sajid Suleman
Chair of the MRCPsych Critical Review Examination Writing Panel

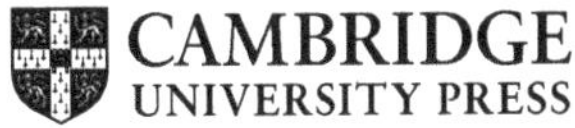
CAMBRIDGE
UNIVERSITY PRESS

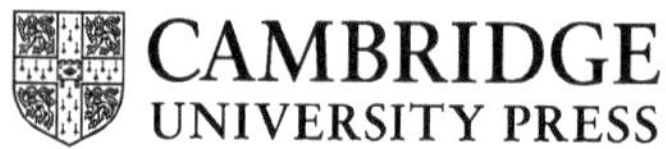

Shaftesbury Road, Cambridge CB2 8EA, United Kingdom

One Liberty Plaza, 20th Floor, New York, NY 10006, USA

477 Williamstown Road, Port Melbourne, VIC 3207, Australia

314–321, 3rd Floor, Plot 3, Splendor Forum, Jasola District Centre, New Delhi – 110025, India

Cambridge University Press is part of Cambridge University Press & Assessment, a department of the University of Cambridge.

We share the University's mission to contribute to society through the pursuit of education, learning and research at the highest international levels of excellence.

www.cambridge.org
Information on this title: www.cambridge.org/9781009182522

DOI: 10.1017/9781009182539

When citing this work, please include a reference to the DOI 10.1017/9781009182539

First published 2026

Cover image: filo / DigitalVision Vectors

A catalogue record for this publication is available from the British Library

A Cataloging-in-Publication data record for this book is available from the Library of Congress

ISBN 978-1-009-18252-2 Paperback

Contents

Foreword vii
Dr Vivek Agarwal

1 **Introduction to Epidemiology** 1
2 **Cross-Sectional and Ecological Studies** 8
3 **Case–Control Studies** 17
4 **Diagnostic Studies** 34
5 **Cohort Studies** 64
6 **Self-Controlled Case Series Studies** 77
7 **Causation in Epidemiological Studies** 83
8 **Clinical Trials** 92
9 **Systematic Review** 117
10 **Network Analysis** 147
11 **Descriptive Statistics** 158
12 **Analytic or Inferential Statistics** 185
13 **Economic Analysis** 233
14 **Qualitative Studies** 252
15 **Audit and Quality Improvement** 281
16 **Research Ethics, Ethical Approval, and Reporting Standards in Research Studies** 293

Glossary 303
Index 324

Foreword

Carl Sagan, in his book *The Demon Haunted World*, talks about the 'baloney detection kit', which can be roughly summarized as developing a set of skills that encourage sceptical thinking. He encourages people to avoid automatic belief and to question things before deciding whether a piece of information is factual or needs to be treated with doubt.

Medical professionals need to apply the same principles of doubt and scepticism in their practice. The ability to critically appraise research is essential to maintain a healthy level of scepticism, prior to judging the veracity of evidence, in the pursuit of effective evidence-based practice. While anyone can look at the results of published research as the basis for their clinical decision-making, lack of ability to critically appraise the research evidence can lead to unsafe or poor-quality decision-making, to the detriment of patients and/or efficient resource use.

This issue is particularly important in psychiatry, where outcomes are not always clear or quantifiable. Psychiatrists need to have good critical appraisal skills to judge the quality and applicability of the evidence. This is the reason that critical appraisal forms a significant proportion of the syllabus for medical postgraduate examinations.

I would like to commend Dr Sajid Suleman and colleagues for producing a text that is comprehensive and pragmatic. It reflects not only expertise in the subject matter, but also a clear understanding of the needs of future psychiatrists and other doctors. This is a resource that will serve as a valuable reference for clinicians seeking to strengthen their research literacy and fulfil essential competency requirements during training.

From the outset, and throughout the text, the book is helpful in demystifying epidemiology, research methodology, and statistics – domains that may seem complex and challenging to most people without research experience or training. There is a structured progression in the book, from core concepts such as study design and measures of association, through to more advanced topics, including statistical terms and tests and measures of significance and errors, which reflects both pedagogical thoughtfulness and practical insight.

The distinguishing features of this work are its considered layout, clarity of explanation, and efforts to focus on applied understanding. Complex research terms and statistical tests are presented in an accessible and clinically meaningful way, helping to bridge the gap between theory and practice. The use of examples, summary boxes, and practice questions encourages active learning, as well as developing transferrable analytical skills that can aid everyday clinical decision-making.

This book will undoubtedly become an essential companion for resident doctors and experienced clinicians navigating the complexities of critical appraisal, and it will contribute meaningfully to the development of reflective, evidence-based psychiatric practice.

Dr Vivek Agarwal, Chief Examiner, The Royal College of Psychiatrists

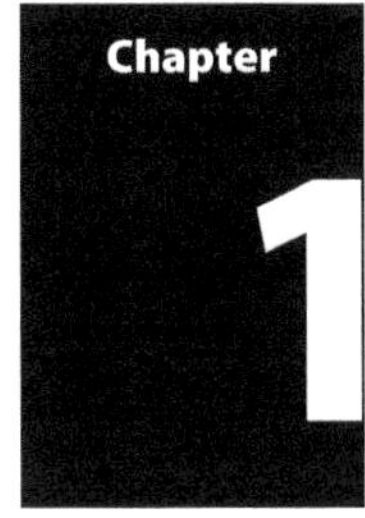

Introduction to Epidemiology

Epidemiological Study Designs

Epidemiological studies are scientific investigations that examine the patterns, causes, and effects of health conditions in populations. Analytical epidemiological studies, which are commonly used, operate on the simple and intuitive principle that if two factors frequently or repeatedly occur together, they are likely to be related. For example, if fish consistently appear whenever fish food is thrown into a river, it suggests there is a link between fish food and fish responding. Similarly, if a disease occurs more frequently when a particular risk factor is present, it indicates a possible association between the two.

The key difference between various epidemiological study designs lies in how and where the study begins.

- **Cohort study:** starts with a risk factor and follows participants over time to observe the outcome (disease).
- **Case–control study:** begins with the outcome (disease) and looks backwards to identify potential risk factors.
- **Cross-sectional study (survey):** examines both the risk factor and the outcome at a single point in time.
- **Experimental study:** actively manipulates the exposure, determining who is exposed to a risk factor rather than merely observing naturally occurring exposures.

Epidemiological studies are broadly classified into observational and experimental studies:

1. Observational studies are separated into descriptive and analytical studies:
    - Descriptive studies describe the distribution of diseases or health conditions in a population. They focus on 'who, what, when, and where'. Examples include:
        - Case reports: detailed descriptions of individual cases.
        - Case series: collections of case reports.
        - Cross-sectional studies: studies that examine data from a population at a single point in time.
    - Analytical studies aim to identify and evaluate the causes and risk factors of diseases or health conditions in a natural setting without intentionally manipulating the exposure. They focus on 'why and how'. Examples include:

  - Cohort studies: studies that follow a group of people over time to see who develops a disease.
  - Case–control studies: studies that compare people with a disease (cases) to people without the disease (controls) to identify potential risk factors.
  - Ecological studies: studies that use group-level data to assess relationships between exposures and health outcomes.

2. Experimental studies (interventional studies) involve intentionally changing one or more factors (an intervention/exposure) in a population and observing the effect on outcome.

Measurements in Epidemiological Studies

Prevalence

Prevalence is the proportion of a population that has a particular disease or condition at a given time:

$$\text{Prevalence} = \frac{\text{Total number of cases (new + old)}}{\text{Population at risk during the specified period of time}}.$$

Types of prevalence:

- **Point prevalence:** the proportion of a population that has a disease at a specific point in time.
- **Period prevalence:** the proportion of a population that had the disease at any time during a specified period (e.g. a month or a year), including both existing and new cases.
- **Lifetime prevalence:** the proportion of a population that has ever had the disease or condition at any point in their life, up to the time of the survey.

Incidence

Incidence is the number of new cases of a disease over a specified period of time:

$$\text{Incidence} = \frac{\text{New cases during a period}}{\text{Population at risk during the specified period of time}}.$$

Prevalence Bathtub Model

The difference between prevalence and incidence is best understood through the prevalence bathtub analogy (Figure 1.1), where:

- inflow is incidence (new cases entering the tub)
- water in the tub is prevalence (existing cases)
- outflow is recovery, death, or change in diagnosis (cases leaving the tub).

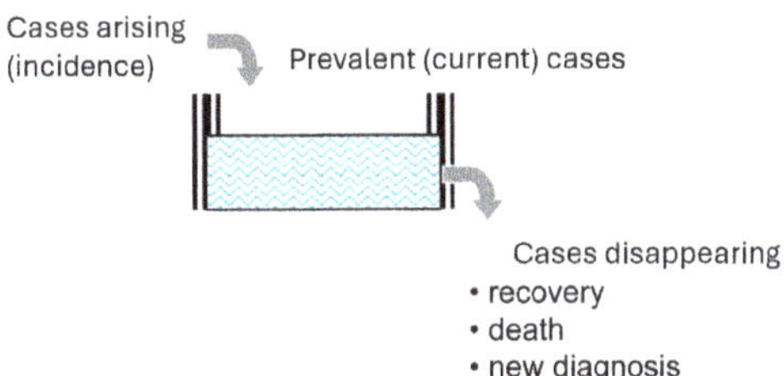

Figure 1.1 The prevalence bathtub model.

Risk

Risk is the proportion of subjects initially at risk who experience an event during a study period. The correct denominator for risk measurement can sometimes be difficult to determine.

Rate

Rate is the frequency of events occurring over a defined time period, divided by the total person-time at risk during that period. Rates are often used to estimate risk and are adjusted using multipliers (e.g. per 100,000) for easier interpretation.

Crude Death Rate

The crude death rate is the total number of deaths occurring in a population during a specific period (usually one year), divided by the total population. It does not account for population characteristics such as age or gender:

$$\text{Crude death rate} = \frac{\text{Number of deaths due to a particular cause}}{\text{Total population, usually midpoint (same place and time)}} \times 1{,}000.$$

Cause-Specific Death Rate

The cause-specific death rate measures the death rate due to a specific cause in the total population:

$$\text{Cause-specific death rate} = \frac{\text{Number of deaths due to a particular cause}}{\text{Total population, usually midpoint (same place and time)}} \times 100{,}000.$$

For example, if 200 people die from heart disease in a population of 500,000:

$$\frac{200}{500{,}000} \times 100{,}000 = 40 \text{ deaths per 100,000 population}$$

Standardized (Adjusted) Rates

Standardized rates compare disease or mortality rates across different populations by accounting for differences in demographic factors such as age and sex. These rates help remove the effect of confounding variables, ensuring a fair comparison.

Direct Standardization

A standard population is chosen as a reference and used when age-specific rates are available:

$$\text{Standardized rate} = \frac{\sum(\text{age-specific rate} \times \text{standard population for that age group})}{\text{Total standard population}},$$

where:

- Σ means *the sum of*
- age-specific rate is the death (or disease) rate for a particular age group in the population
- standard population for that age group is the population of that same age group in the standard population
- total standard population is the total number in the standard population.

Standardized Mortality Rate

The standardized mortality rate (SMR) is used when age-specific rates are unknown or unstable (e.g. due to small numbers). It is calculated as:

$$\text{SMR} = \frac{\text{Observed cases (or deaths)}}{\text{Expected cases (or deaths)}}.$$

For example, if a mining workforce has 150 observed lung cancer deaths, but the expected deaths based on a standard population is 100, then:

$$\text{SMR} = \frac{150}{100} = 1.5 \text{ SMR}.$$

This means the miners have a 50% higher mortality rate than expected.

Chapter Summary

Epidemiology is the study of the distribution and determinants of health conditions in populations. Epidemiological study designs differ in their starting point and how exposures and outcomes are assessed. Cohort studies begin with a risk factor and follow participants over time, whereas case–control studies start with disease status and look backwards for exposures. Cross-sectional studies measure exposure and outcome at a single point in time, while experimental studies involve active manipulation of an intervention.

Key epidemiological measurements include prevalence and incidence. Prevalence describes the proportion of individuals with a disease at a given time and may be classified as point, period, or lifetime prevalence. It is calculated as:

$$\text{Prevalence} = \frac{\text{Existing cases of disease}}{\text{Total population}}.$$

Incidence refers to the number of new cases occurring over a specified period and is calculated as:

$$\text{Incidence} = \frac{\text{New cases during a time period}}{\text{Population at risk during that period}}.$$

Risk represents the probability of developing an outcome during follow-up and is expressed as:

$$\text{Risk} = \frac{\text{Number of individuals who develop the outcome}}{\text{Number initially at risk}}.$$

Rates measure the frequency of events over time and incorporate person-time:

$$\text{Rate} = \frac{\text{Number of events}}{\text{Total person-time at risk}}.$$

Mortality can be described using crude death rates, which measure overall deaths in a population:

$$\text{Crude death rate} = \frac{\text{Total deaths in a year}}{\text{Total population}} \times 1000.$$

Cause-specific death rates focus on deaths attributable to a particular condition:

$$\text{Cause-specific death rate} = \frac{\text{Deaths from a specific cause}}{\text{Total population}} \times 100{,}000.$$

Comparisons between populations often require standardized (adjusted) rates. Direct standardization adjusts for differences in age structure when age-specific rates are available:

$$\text{Age-standardised rate} = \frac{\sum (a_i \times N_i)}{\sum N_i}.$$

When age-specific rates are unavailable or unstable, the standardized mortality ratio (SMR) is used. SMR compares observed deaths with expected deaths:

$$\text{SMR} = \frac{\text{Observed deaths}}{\text{Expected deaths}}.$$

An SMR greater than 1 indicates higher mortality than expected, while an SMR less than 1 indicates lower mortality than expected.

Together, these study designs and measurements form the foundation for describing disease patterns, assessing risk factors, and comparing health outcomes across populations.

Practice Questions

Q1. Which of the following is best described as a cohort study?

A. Start with the disease and control and look backwards for risk factors.
B. Examine risk factors and outcomes at a single point in time.
C. Begin with a risk factor and control and follow participants over time.
D. Actively manipulate exposure to a risk factor and look for outcomes.
E. Use group-level data to assess relationships.

Q2. Which of the following is an example of a descriptive observational study?

A. Cohort study
B. Case–control study
C. Cross-sectional study
D. Experimental study
E. Interventional study

Q3. Which of the following studies uses group-level data to assess relationships between exposures and health outcomes?

A. Cohort studies
B. Case–control studies
C. Cross-sectional studies
D. Experimental studies
E. Ecological studies

Q4. Choose the appropriate measurement rate for the definitions given below.

A. Age-specific death rate
B. Case fatality rate
C. Cause-specific death rate
D. Crude death rate
E. Incidence
F. Standardized mortality ratio
G. Prevalence
H. Standardized (age-adjusted) rate

1. The number of existing cases of a disease in a population at a particular time, expressed as a proportion of the total population.
2. The number of deaths per 1,000 people in a population over a specific period, without adjusting for age or other factors.
3. The proportion of new cases of a disease occurring over a specified period, relative to the at-risk population.
4. A mortality rate that allows comparisons between populations with different age distributions by adjusting for age.
5. The number of deaths due to a specific disease per 100,000 population in a given period.
6. A measure comparing observed deaths to expected deaths after adjusting for age.
7. The proportion of individuals in a defined age group who die within a given time period.

Answers

Q1. Correct answer: C. Begin with a risk factor and control and follow participants over time.

Explanation of the other options:

A. Start with the disease and control and look backwards for risk factors → case–control study.
B. Examine risk factors and outcomes at a single point in time → cross-sectional study.
D. Actively manipulate exposure to a risk factor and look for outcomes → experimental study.
E. Use group-level data to assess relationships → ecological study.

Q2. Correct answer: C. Cross-sectional study

Q3. Correct answer: E. Ecological studies

Q4. The two lists should be paired as:

1. G (prevalence)
2. D (crude death rate)
3. E (incidence)
4. H (Standardized (age-adjusted) rate)
5. C (cause-specific death rate)
6. F (standardized mortality ratio)
7. A (age-specific death rate)

Further Reading

Ahmad OB, Boschi-Pinto C, Lopez AD, et al. *Age Standardization of Rates: A New WHO Standard.* Geneva: World Health Organization; 2001.

Celentano DD, Szklo M. *Gordis Epidemiology.* 6th ed. Amsterdam: Elsevier; 2019.

Kirkwood BR, Sterne JAC. *Essential Medical Statistics.* 2nd ed. Oxford: Blackwell Science; 2003.

Lash TL, VanderWeele TJ, Haneuse S, Rothman KJ. *Modern Epidemiology.* 4th ed. Philadelphia: Wolters Kluwer; 2021.

Porta M, ed. *A Dictionary of Epidemiology.* 6th ed. Oxford: Oxford University Press; 2014.

Rothman KJ. *Epidemiology: An Introduction.* 2nd ed. Oxford: Oxford University Press; 2012.

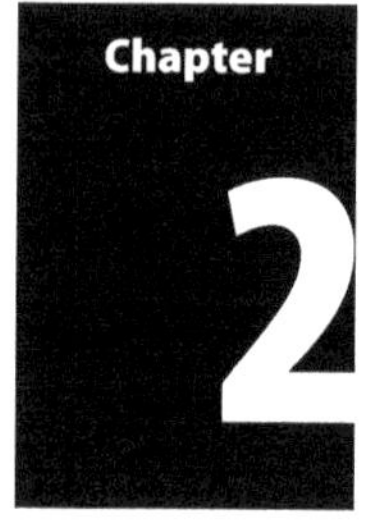

Cross-Sectional and Ecological Studies

Cross-Sectional Studies

Introduction

A cross-sectional study is an observational study that analyses data from a population at *a single point in time.* It is often used to determine the prevalence of a condition, associations between variables, or demographic characteristics within a specific population. Unlike longitudinal studies, which track changes over time, cross-sectional studies provide a snapshot of a particular group at one moment.

Cross-sectional studies can be:

- **descriptive:** focus on describing the prevalence of a particular health outcome, exposure, or characteristic within a population
- **analytical:** assess associations between exposure and outcome at a single point in time
- **exploratory:** used to generate hypotheses when little is known about a topic.

Cross-sectional studies have limitations similar to those discussed in Chapter 3 on case–control studies, as they are prone to biases and **confounding**[1] factors.

Methodology of a Cross-Sectional Study

The methodology of a cross-sectional study typically includes the following steps.

Define the Research Objective

- Identify the hypothesis or research question (e.g. prevalence of depression among university students).

Identify the Population

- Define the target population (e.g. adults aged 18–65 in a specific city).
- Select a sample that represents the population using techniques such as random sampling or stratified sampling.

Data Collection

Data is gathered at a single point in time using methods such as:

- surveys/questionnaires (e.g. self-reported smoking habits)

[1] **Confounding:** Distortion of the exposure–outcome association by a third variable related to both but not on the causal pathway; address via design (randomization, restriction, matching) or analysis (stratification, regression/adjustment).

- interviews (e.g. assessing mental health conditions)
- medical records (e.g. hospital data on depression prevalence)
- laboratory tests (e.g. measuring blood tests in a group).

Measurement of Variables

- Define independent (exposure) and dependent (outcome) variables. For example, studying the association between childhood trauma (independent variable) and major depressive disorder (dependent variable).

Data Analysis

- Use **descriptive statistics**[2] (e.g. mean, percentage, prevalence rates).
- Use **inferential statistics**[3] (e.g. chi-square tests, **logistic regression**)[4] to analyse relationships between variables.

Interpretation and Conclusion

- Summarize findings (e.g. '30% of surveyed individuals reported symptoms of anxiety').
- Identify potential associations but acknowledge that cross-sectional studies cannot establish causation (only correlation).

Strengths and Limitations of Cross-Sectional Studies

Strengths

- Quick and cost-effective
- useful for measuring prevalence of psychiatric conditions
- can assess multiple variables simultaneously
- no risk of loss to follow-up
- good for generating hypotheses for further research
- ethical and feasible without long-term tracking.

Limitations

- Cannot establish causality (only show associations)
- temporal ambiguity – unclear which came first, exposure or outcome
- susceptible to **recall bias**,[5] where participants may inaccurately report past experiences
- **selection bias**[6] – results may not generalize if the sample is not representative

---

[2] **Descriptive statistics:** Methods that summarize data (e.g. mean, median, standard deviation, range, IQR). They provide essential context before inferential analysis.

[3] **Inferential statistics:** Statistical tests to make inferences about a population from a sample.

[4] **Logistic regression:** Regression for binary outcomes modelling the log-odds as a linear function of predictors; yields odds ratios and enables adjustment for confounders (assumes correct model, independence, and linearity in the logit for continuous predictors).

[5] **Recall bias:** Differential accuracy or completeness of remembered exposures between groups (e.g. people with the outcome recall more/less); minimize with objective records, standardized questionnaires, and blinding to study aims.

[6] **Selection bias:** Systematic differences between those included and the target population (or between comparison groups), often from non-response or convenience sampling; can distort prevalence and associations – mitigate via careful sampling, high response, weighting, and sensitivity analyses.

- confounding factors – unmeasured variables may influence the results
- cannot measure incidence – only provides a snapshot, not how conditions develop over time.

Ecological Studies

Introduction

Ecology is the branch of biology that studies the interactions between living organisms and their environment. Ecological studies are a type of epidemiological research that examines how exposures and health outcomes vary across groups or populations, rather than at the individual level. These studies analyse the association between population-level risk factors – such as air pollution, dietary habits, socio-economic status, and income inequality – and health outcomes, including respiratory and cardiovascular diseases or mortality rates. Additionally, ecological studies assess the impact of public health interventions, such as smoking bans or vaccination programmes, on population health.

Key Elements of Ecological Studies

1. Data on risk factors and health outcomes is collected at the group or population level.
2. Ecological studies are observational, meaning researchers do not manipulate exposures or outcomes.
3. These studies do not fit neatly into cohort, case–control, or cross-sectional designs because they focus on groups rather than individuals. However, they can have features of the following:
   - Cohort studies: when exposure data is collected over time to assess associations with outcomes (e.g. tracking smoking rates and lung cancer mortality in different countries).
   - Case–control studies: when populations are classified based on an outcome (e.g. areas with high and low disease rates) to identify potential exposures.
   - Cross-sectional studies: when exposure and outcome data are examined at a single point in time across different populations (e.g. comparing obesity rates and fast food availability across cities in a given year).

Measuring Strength of Association in Ecological Studies

1. Data analysis involves statistical methods tailored for aggregated, group-level data.
2. Descriptive analysis includes measures such as mean, median, and proportion of exposure, and outcome variables, often visualized using scatter plots or time series graphs.
3. Statistical tests such as *t*-tests, ANOVA (analysis of variance), or chi-square can be used to evaluate differences or associations.
4. Correlation analysis measures the strength and direction of the association between two variables, while regression analysis quantifies relationships between exposures and outcomes.

Strengths and Limitations of Ecological Studies

Strengths

- Efficient and inexpensive: uses readily available data, such as census records, hospital statistics, or environmental monitoring.
- Hypothesis generation: useful for identifying potential associations that can be explored further with more rigorous individual-level studies.
- Broad scope: can address large-scale issues involving entire populations.

Limitations

- **Ecological fallacy:**[7] associations observed at the population level may not apply to individuals within that population. For example, a country with high average fat consumption may have high heart disease rates, but not all individuals who consume high-fat diets will develop heart disease.
- Confounding factors: the inability to control for all potential confounders (e.g. genetic factors, lifestyle choices) can affect results.
- Lack of individual data: does not provide information about the specific exposure–disease relationships at the individual level.

Chapter Summary

Cross-Sectional Studies

A cross-sectional study is an observational research method that analyses data from a population at a single point in time. It is commonly used to determine the prevalence of a condition, assess associations between variables, or describe demographic characteristics. These studies can be *descriptive*, *analytical*, or *exploratory*, but share the limitation of being prone to *biases* and *confounding factors* and cannot establish causality.

Methodology of Cross-Sectional Studies

The research process involves:

1. defining the research objective (e.g. prevalence of depression in university students)
2. identifying the population and selecting a representative sample
3. data collection using surveys, interviews, medical records, or laboratory tests
4. measurement of variables, distinguishing between independent (exposure) and dependent (outcome) variables
5. data analysis using descriptive and inferential statistics
6. interpretation, summarizing findings while acknowledging the inability to establish causation.

[7] **Ecological fallacy:** Mistakenly inferring individual-level effects from group-level associations; guard against this with individual-level data or multilevel models.

Strengths and Limitations

Cross-sectional studies are quick, cost-effective, and useful for measuring prevalence, but they suffer from selection bias, recall bias, and temporal ambiguity, making them unsuitable for determining causality.

Ecological Studies

Ecological studies are a type of epidemiological research that examines associations between population-level risk factors (e.g. air pollution, socio-economic status) and health outcomes (e.g. cardiovascular diseases, mortality rates). These studies focus on groups rather than individuals and can be cohort-like, case–control-like, or cross-sectional in design.

Statistical methods such as descriptive analysis, correlation, and regression are used to measure associations. Ecological studies are cost-effective, broad in scope, and useful for hypothesis generation, but they are limited by ecological fallacy, confounding factors, and the lack of individual-level data. Despite these limitations, they provide valuable insights into public health trends and the impact of environmental exposures.

Practice Questions

Q1. In an epidemiological study, the incidence of a disease is higher in younger individuals compared to older individuals, but the prevalence is higher in older individuals. What does this suggest?

A. The disease has a longer duration in older individuals.
B. Case fatality is higher in younger individuals.
C. The disease is more severe in younger individuals.
D. Recovery is quicker in younger individuals.
E. Older individuals are more susceptible to reinfection.

Q2. What is the key characteristic of a cross-sectional study?

A. It follows participants over time.
B. It analyses data at a single point in time.
C. It assigns participants to exposure groups.
D. It is always randomized.
E. It measures only mortality rates.

Q3. Cross-sectional studies are most commonly used to measure:

A. Incidence of disease
B. Prevalence of disease
C. Mortality rates over time
D. Risk factors longitudinally
E. Survival rates in different populations

Q4. A study collects data on the smoking habits and current lung disease status of a population on 1 January 2024. This is an example of which of the following types of study?

A. Cohort study
B. Randomized controlled trial

C. Cross-sectional study
D. Case–control study
E. Longitudinal ecological study

Q5. Which of the following is a major advantage of cross-sectional studies?
A. They can establish causality.
B. They are time-efficient and cost-effective.
C. They eliminate recall bias.
D. They track changes in disease status over time.
E. They are always free from selection bias.

Q6. What is one major limitation of cross-sectional studies?
A. They require a long follow-up period.
B. They are very expensive.
C. They cannot establish temporal relationships between exposure and outcome.
D. They always require biological samples for diagnosis.
E. They are the best method to determine disease incidence.

Q7. Cross-sectional studies may be susceptible to which type of bias?
A. Selection bias
B. Recall bias
C. Confounding bias
D. All of the above
E. None of the above

Q8. A researcher conducts a cross-sectional study and finds that 20% of a population has high blood pressure. What epidemiological measure does this represent?
A. Incidence
B. Case fatality rate
C. Prevalence
D. Mortality rate
E. Risk ratio

Q9. Which of the following scenarios best describes an analytical cross-sectional study?
A. Measuring the percentage of people with diabetes in a city.
B. Studying the association between physical activity levels and obesity in a population at a single time point.
C. Following a group of smokers and non-smokers over 10 years to assess lung cancer development.
D. Assigning participants to two groups to test a new vaccine.
E. Comparing mortality rates between two different countries over 20 years.

Q10. Which of the following is an example of an ecological study?
A. Measuring the BMI of individuals and comparing it with their personal dietary habits.

B. Comparing the obesity rates across different cities based on fast food availability.
C. Randomly assigning individuals to high-sodium and low-sodium diets to observe blood pressure changes.
D. Interviewing patients with diabetes to assess their physical activity levels.
E. Collecting detailed case histories of individual patients with cardiovascular disease.

Q11. Which of the following best describes an ecological fallacy?
A. Misinterpreting individual-level findings as applicable to entire populations.
B. Assuming that associations observed at the population level also apply to individuals within that population.
C. Conducting studies with incorrect sample sizes.
D. Failing to control for genetic variations in an observational study.
E. Using self-reported data instead of objective measurements.

Answers

Q1. Correct answer: A. The disease has a longer duration in older individuals.
This suggests that the disease lasts longer in older individuals. If the disease had a short duration in older people, the prevalence would be lower in that age group, even with a lower incidence.
Why other options are incorrect:

B. Case fatality is higher in younger individuals: higher case fatality would lead to lower prevalence in young people.
C. The disease is more severe in younger individuals: severity doesn't directly impact prevalence unless it significantly affects the duration of the disease or leads to death.
D. Recovery is quicker in younger individuals: this would also lead to lower prevalence in young people.
E. Older individuals are more susceptible to reinfection: reinfection could increase prevalence, but it wouldn't explain the higher prevalence in older individuals if the disease duration wasn't also longer in that group.

Q2. Correct answer: B. It analyses data at a single point in time. Cross-sectional studies provide a snapshot of a population, capturing data at one specific point. Unlike cohort studies, they do not track changes over time.
Why other options are incorrect:

A. It follows participants over time: describes a cohort study.
C. It assigns participants to exposure groups: describes an experimental study.
D. It is always randomized: randomization occurs in clinical trials, not cross-sectional studies.
E. It measures only mortality rates: cross-sectional studies measure prevalence, not just mortality.

Q3. Correct answer: B. Prevalence of disease. Since cross-sectional studies collect data at one time point, they are best for estimating prevalence, which measures the proportion of individuals with a disease at a given time.
Why other options are incorrect:

A. Incidence of disease: incidence requires tracking new cases over time (cohort studies).
C. Mortality rates over time: requires longitudinal studies.
D. Risk factors longitudinally: requires cohort or case–control studies.
E. Survival rates in different populations: requires long-term follow-up studies.

Q4. Correct answer: C. A cross-sectional study. Since the study assesses both exposure (smoking) and outcome (lung disease) at a single time point, it fits the cross-sectional study design.
Why other options are incorrect:

A. A cohort study: would require longitudinal tracking.
B. A randomized controlled trial: no randomization or intervention is used.
D. A case–control study: would involve matching cases and controls based on past exposure.
E. A longitudinal ecological study: would involve multiple time points.

Q5. Correct answer: B. They are time-efficient and cost-effective. Cross-sectional studies are quicker and less expensive than cohort or experimental studies since they do not require follow-up.
Why other options are incorrect:

A. They can establish causality: they only show associations, not causation.
C. They eliminate recall bias: recall bias is a problem in self-reported data.
D. They track changes in disease status over time: they do not track changes.
E. They are always free from selection bias: selection bias can occur.

Q6. Correct answer: C. They cannot establish temporal relationships between exposure and outcome. Since exposure and disease are measured at the same time, it is unclear which occurred first.
Why other options are incorrect:

A. They require a long follow-up period: no follow-up occurs.
B. They are very expensive: they are actually cost-effective.
D. They always require biological samples for diagnosis: not necessarily, they often use surveys.
E. They are the best method to determine disease incidence: incidence requires time tracking.

Q7. Correct answer: D. All of the above. Selection bias: if the sample is not representative. Recall bias: if self-reported data is inaccurate. Confounding bias: if other unmeasured factors influence the outcome.

Q8. Correct answer: C. Prevalence. Prevalence measures the total number of cases (new + old) at a given time.
Why other options are incorrect:

A. Incidence: measures new cases over time.
B. Case fatality rate: measures mortality among diseased individuals.
D. Mortality rate: measures death rates.
E. Risk ratio: compares exposed vs unexposed groups.

Q9. Correct answer: B. Studying the association between physical activity levels and obesity in a population at a single time point. Analytical cross-sectional studies examine associations between variables at one time point.
Why other options are incorrect:

A. Measuring the percentage of people with diabetes in a city: descriptive, not analytical.
C. Following a group of smokers and non-smokers over 10 years to assess lung cancer development: cohort study.
D. Assigning participants to two groups to test a new vaccine: randomized controlled trial.
E. Comparing mortality rates between two different countries over 20 years: longitudinal ecological study.

Q10. Correct answer: B. Comparing the obesity rates across different cities based on fast food availability. This study examines population-level exposure (fast food availability) and health outcomes (obesity rates), which is characteristic of ecological studies.

Q11. Correct answer: B. Assuming that associations observed at the population level also apply to individuals within that population. Ecological fallacy occurs when group-level findings are incorrectly generalized to individuals, which can lead to misleading conclusions.

Further Reading

Altman DG. *Practical Statistics for Medical Research*. London: Chapman & Hall/CRC; 1990. https://doi.org/10.1201/9780429258589.

Hosmer DW Jr, Lemeshow S, Sturdivant RX. *Applied Logistic Regression*. 3rd ed. Hoboken, NJ: Wiley; 2013.

Levin KA. Study design III: cross-sectional studies. *Evid Based Dent*. 2006;**7**(1):24–5. https://doi.org/10.1038/sj.ebd.6400375.

Morgenstern H. Ecologic studies in epidemiology: concepts, principles, and methods. *Annu Rev Public Health*. 1995;**16**:61–81. https://doi.org/10.1146/annurev.pu.16.050195.000425.

Piantadosi S, Byar DP, Green SB. The ecological fallacy. *Am J Epidemiol*. 1988;**127**(5):893–904. https://doi.org/10.1093/oxfordjournals.aje.a114892.

Porta M, ed. *A Dictionary of Epidemiology*. 6th ed. Oxford: Oxford University Press; 2014.

Robinson WS. Ecological correlations and the behavior of individuals. *Am Sociol Rev*. 1950;**15**(3):351–7.

Sedgwick P. Cross sectional studies: advantages and disadvantages. *BMJ*. 2014;**348**:g2276. https://doi.org/10.1136/bmj.g2276.

Setia MS. Methodology series module 3: cross-sectional studies. *Indian J Dermatol*. 2016;**61**(3):261–4. https://doi.org/10.4103/0019-5154.182410.

Szklo M, Nieto FJ. *Epidemiology: Beyond the Basics*. 4th ed. Burlington, MA: Jones & Bartlett Learning; 2019.

Chapter 3

Case–Control Studies

Introduction

A case–control study is a retrospective epidemiological study that investigates the association between an exposure (risk factor) and an outcome (disease). It starts by identifying two groups:

- **Cases:** individuals who have the disease or outcome of interest.
- **Controls:** individuals from the same population who do not have the disease.

Researchers then look back in time to determine if cases were more likely to have been exposed to the risk factor than the controls. If a higher proportion of cases were exposed compared to controls, an *association* is inferred between the risk factor and the disease.

However, for a valid association, researchers must first account for chance, confounding, and bias (see also Box 3.1):

Box 3.1 Possible Explanations for an Observed Association

There are four possible explanations for an observed association:

1. chance
2. bias
3. confounders
4. true association.

The first three must be accounted for before concluding true association.

- **Chance** is the possibility that the observed difference in exposure between cases and controls occurred simply by accident rather than reflecting a true effect. It is addressed through *p*-values and confidence intervals.
- **Confounding** occurs when an extraneous variable affects both the exposure and the outcome.
- **Bias** can distort results and must be minimized.

Case–Control Study Design

Figure 3.1 illustrates the structure of a case–control study.

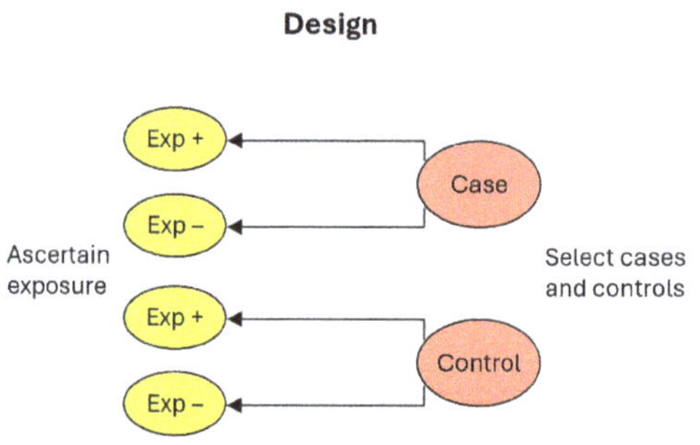

Design

Exp +
Exp –
Case
Ascertain exposure
Select cases and controls
Exp +
Exp –
Control

Figure 3.1 Structure of a case–control study.

Defining Outcomes and Risk Factors

To ensure clarity and reproducibility, researchers must predefine the following:

- **Outcome (disease):** must be clearly defined within the study sample, specifying how the condition is identified or measured (e.g. clinical diagnosis using ICD-10/DSM-5 vs self-reported depression).
- **Exposure (risk factor):** must be precisely defined within the study sample, including how it is measured or categorised (e.g. smoking: ever smoked, current smoker, or smoking ≥10 cigarettes/day?).

Clear definitions enhance the validity and comparability across studies.

Selecting Cases and Controls

Cases and controls must be drawn from the same source population and should be well-matched on all factors other than the exposure under investigation. A useful 'acid test' is to ask whether the controls would have been eligible as cases if they had developed the disease.

When selecting participants, it is essential to ensure that both cases and controls are representative of the source population. At each step, two key questions can be considered (Figure 3.2):

1. Who is missing from the study?
2. Does their exclusion matter?

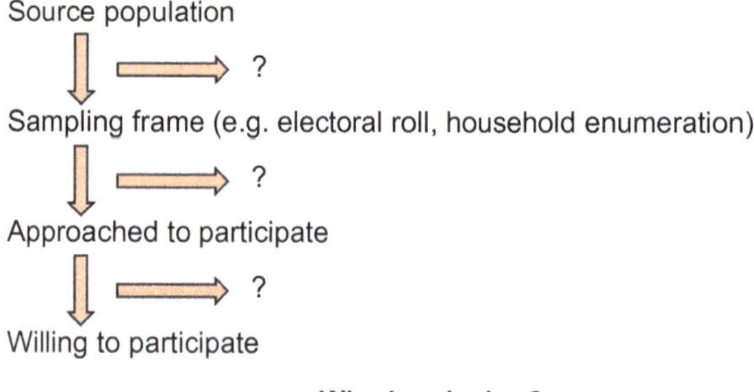

Figure 3.2 Inclusion/exclusion bias (selection bias) in case–control studies: stages where participants may be lost from the source population to study sample.

Data Collection and Minimizing Bias

It is important that data collection methods are decided beforehand and uniformly applied to both the cases and the controls. To reduce **information bias,**[1] researchers should:

- use objective markers (e.g. blood tests) instead of subjective questionnaires
- rely on medical records rather than recall-based data
- apply consistent data collection methods to both cases and controls
- blind interviewers and participants to study hypotheses to prevent bias.

Bias in Case–Control Studies

Bias is a systematic error in the design and execution of a study that distorts findings. Unlike confounding, bias cannot be adjusted for in analysis and must be prevented. Bias is a fundamental issue in both study design and critical appraisal of a case–control study.

There are two main types of bias in case–control studies (i.e. inclusion/exclusion (section) bias and information (measurement) bias), both of which can be introduced either by researchers or participants, leading to four distinct subtypes:

1. selection bias introduced by researchers
2. selection bias introduced by participants
3. information bias introduced by observers
4. information bias introduced by participants.

Inclusion/Exclusion (Selection) Bias

Selection bias occurs when cases and controls are not selected from the same population or are not comparable. It can be introduced by the researchers and/or the participants.

Selection Bias Introduced by Researchers

This occurs when cases and controls are selected differently, leading to non-equivalent groups. For example, a study finds an inverse association between arthritis and Alzheimer's disease. However, the cases (patients with Alzheimer's disease) are recruited from dementia wards while controls are recruited from GP waiting areas. Individuals attending their GP are more likely to have arthritis, as they often seek medical care for chronic conditions. As a result, arthritis becomes artificially more common in the control group. The flawed selection results in inflated arthritis prevalence among controls, distorting findings.

Selection Bias Introduced by Participants

This occurs when cases and controls agree to participate at different rates, leading to non-representative samples. For example, in a study using mailed questionnaires, depressed patients may be less likely to complete and return mailed questionnaires compared to controls, leading to underrepresentation of depressed subjects and biased results.

[1] **Information bias:** Systematic error arising from inaccurate measurement or misclassification of exposure, outcome, or covariates. State expected direction (towards/away from null) and describe design/analysis strategies to mitigate it.

Information Bias in Case–Control Studies

Information bias occurs when errors arise in data collection, measurement, or classification. It can be differential (systematic differences between cases and controls) or non-differential (random error affecting both groups equally).

- **Systematic error:** a consistent, repeatable error affecting all participants, leading to bias.
- **Random error:** no predictable pattern; reduces precision but can be minimized by increasing sample size.

Information bias can be introduced by researchers or participants:

Information Bias Introduced by Observers (Measurement Bias)

This occurs when researchers collect data differently for cases and controls. For example, in a study investigating childhood abuse and emotionally unstable personality disorder (EUPD), researchers probe cases more rigorously, leading to inflated associations.

Information Bias Introduced by Participants (Recall Bias)

Cases and controls may differentially recall or report exposures. For example:

- In a study on EUPD and childhood abuse, cases are more likely to recall past abuse if they know they have the diagnosis.
- In a study on *Salmonella* infection and egg ingestion, cases may be more likely than controls to recall eating eggs, seeking explanations for their illness ('effort after meaning' bias).

Confounding in Case–Control Studies

A confounder is a third variable that is associated with both the exposure and the outcome and it distorts the true relationship between them. It is not on the causal pathway between exposure and outcome.

For example, suppose a study finds an association between grey hair (risk factor) and death (outcome). Age is a confounder, as it is associated with both grey hair (older people more likely to have grey hair) and death (higher mortality in older individuals) (Figure 3.3).

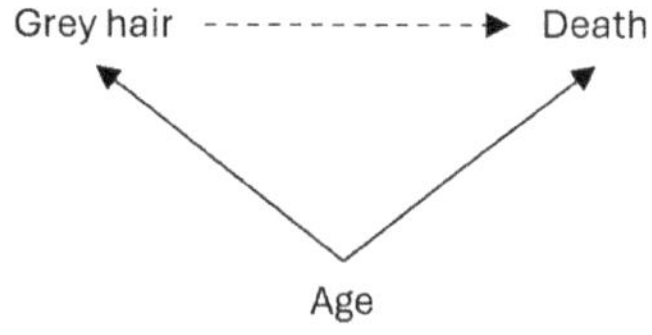

Age (the confounder) is strongly and independently associated both with the outcome (dying) and with the exposure (grey hair).

Figure 3.3 Illustration of confounding in case–control studies.

Identifying Confounders

There is no statistical test to identify confounders; they must be evaluated based on study context. It is usually helpful to start by considering demographic factors such as age, sex, social class, and education as possible confounding factors. Residual confounding occurs when confounders are not measured or are inaccurately measured.

Unlike bias, confounders can be controlled during study design or data analysis.

Controlling for Confounders in Study Design

Methods to control for confounders are:

- **Matching:** for each case with a confounder, a control with the same confounder is selected.

  Advantage: simple and intuitive.

  Drawback: becomes complex when matching multiple confounders (e.g. finding a control for a 90-year-old, university-educated, migrant female would be difficult).

- **Restriction:** a method of controlling for confounding by limiting study participants to a specific category of a variable. This ensures that subjects with the confounding factor are excluded from the study.

  Example: if gender is a confounder in a study on anorexia nervosa, restricting participants to females only eliminates gender as a confounder.

  Drawback: reduces generalizability (e.g. findings are not applicable to males if males are excluded from the anorexia nervosa study in above example).

- **Randomization:** the process of allocating study participants to groups purely by chance. This ensures that confounders are evenly distributed between groups.

  Advantage: controls for both known and unknown confounders.

  Drawback: not feasible for case–control studies (only applicable to randomized trials).

Controlling for Confounders during Data Analysis

Methods to control for confounders during analysis are:

- **Stratified analysis (e.g. Mantel–Haenszel adjustment):** controls confounding by dividing data into strata of the confounder and estimating the exposure–outcome association *within each stratum*. If stratum-specific estimates are similar, *pooled Mantel–Haenszel* estimate can be reported; if they differ, *stratum-specific* estimates should be reported.

  Example: in a 'grey hair → death' study, stratifying by age often removes the crude association, revealing age as the confounder.

  Advantages: transparent; minimal modelling.

  Drawback: awkward for continuous confounders or many strata (sparse cells).

- **Multivariable analysis (regression adjustment):** controls for confounding by fitting a regression model for the outcome that includes the exposure and measured confounders (choose the model to match the outcome: linear for continuous outcomes; logistic for binary outcomes including case–control; log-binomial/Poisson with robust standard errors for risk ratio; Cox regression for time-to-event). Use flexible terms for continuous confounders (e.g. splines) and include interaction terms if effect modification is plausible.

  Advantages: adjusts for multiple confounders simultaneously; generally more precise.

  Drawback: needs adequate sample size/events, correct model specification; only adjusts for *measured* confounders.

Further Considerations in Confounding

It is important to consider other factors that go beyond basic confounding, as illustrated in Figure 3.4.

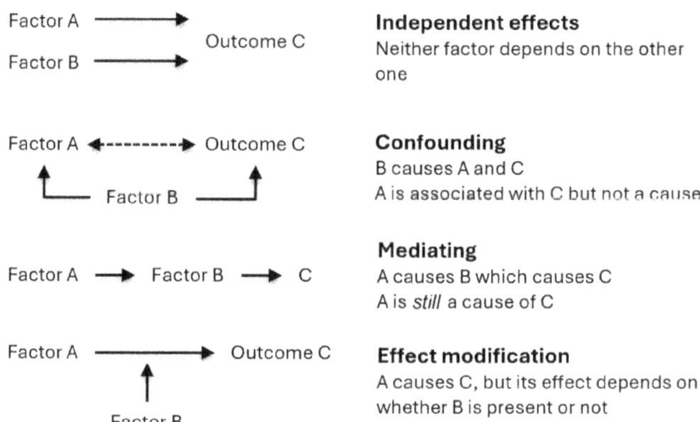

Figure 3.4 Further considerations in confounding: independent effects, mediators, and effect modification.

Independent Effects and Synergism

Two risk factors may independently contribute to an outcome without depending on each other.

When the combined effect of these two risk factors on the outcome is greater than the sum of their individual effects, this phenomenon is known as synergism. The concept of synergism (or interaction) is important in epidemiology and biostatistics. It implies that the presence of one risk factor enhances the effect of the other on the outcome, leading to a more-than-additive effect. If the combined effect is less than additive, this is referred to as antagonism.

Examples of synergism are the effect of:

- obesity and a sedentary lifestyle on risk of cardiovascular disease
- smoking and asbestosis on lung cancer
- alcohol and sedatives on the central nervous system.

Examples of antagonism are:

- Naloxone competitively antagonizing opioid receptors, reversing both analgesic and respiratory depressant effects of opioids.
- Antipsychotics (e.g. haloperidol) blocking dopamine D2 receptors, while dopaminergic agents (e.g. levodopa in Parkinson's disease) increase dopamine signalling. When co-prescribed, their therapeutic effects may be diminished due to opposing pharmacological actions.

Mediating Factor

A mediating factor is a variable that serves as an intermediate step between the risk factor and outcome. An example is obesity → hyperlipidaemia → cardiovascular disease (where hyperlipidaemia is the mediator).

Effect Modification

An effect modifier is a variable that changes the strength or direction of an exposure–outcome relationship. In other words, the association between exposure and outcome varies depending on the level or presence of the effect modifier.

Examples of effect modification are:

- Exercise and heart disease in the elderly: the impact of strenuous exercise on heart disease risk depends on fitness level. In fit elderly individuals, exercise may reduce risk, while in unfit individuals it may trigger ischaemic heart disease (Figure 3.5).

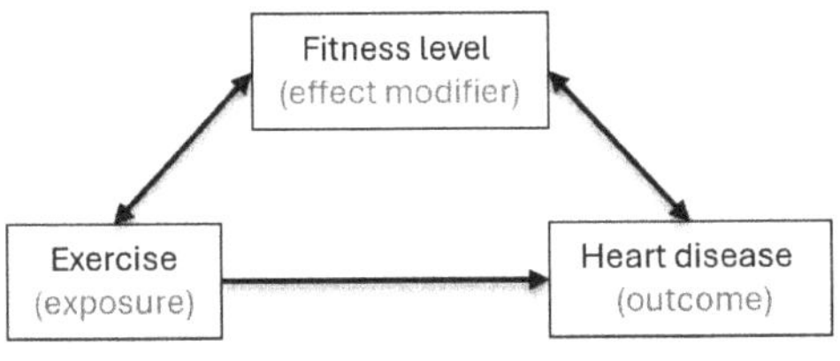

- Exercise is associated with heart disease
- Fitness level modifies the association

Figure 3.5 Effect modification: exercise (exposure) and heart disease (outcome) with fitness level as the effect modifier.

- Alcohol and lung cancer with smoking as an effect modifier: drinking alcohol is associated with lung cancer, but the effect is substantially stronger in individuals who also smoke (Figure 3.6).

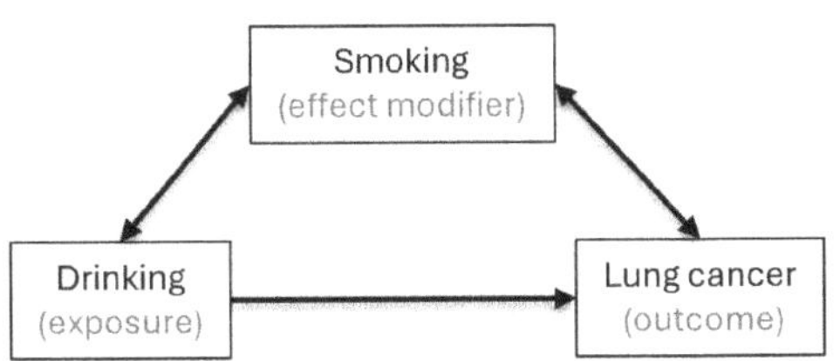

- Drinking is associated with lung cancer
- Smoking is an effect modifier

Figure 3.6 Effect modification: smoking as an effect modifier in the relationship between drinking alcohol and lung cancer.

Confounding by Indication

Confounding by indication occurs when treatment assignment is related to prognosis rather than being randomly assigned.

Examples of confounding by indication are:

- Comparing the efficacy of clozapine versus other atypical antipsychotics, the clozapine group may be worse off to start with because clozapine is prescribed to treatment-resistant cases.
- Comparing depot antipsychotics with oral antipsychotics, the depot antipsychotic group may be worse off to start with because depot antipsychotics are typically prescribed to those with poor compliance.

Reverse Causality in Case–Control Studies

Reverse causality refers to a situation where the direction of cause and effect is unclear, meaning the outcome may influence the exposure rather than the exposure influencing the outcome. A major limitation of case–control studies is the inability to establish causality since both the disease and the risk factor have already occurred at the time of study.

For example, a study finds an association between antidepressant use and obesity. However, does antidepressant use cause obesity, or are obese individuals more likely to be prescribed antidepressants?

Measuring the Strength of Association in Case–Control Studies

In case–control studies, the strength of association between an exposure and an outcome is measured using the **odds ratio (OR)**.[2] Importantly, case–control studies cannot measure incidence or **absolute risk**,[3] as the total population at risk is unknown. Unlike **relative risk (RR)**,[4] which is used in cohort studies, the OR does not provide a direct measure of risk but rather the relative odds of exposure among cases versus controls. When the outcome is rare, the OR approximates RR (rare disease assumption), making it a useful measure. Most diseases studied in epidemiology are rare, and that makes OR a useful measure.

The formula for OR is:

$$\text{Odds ratio} = \frac{\text{Odds of exposure in cases}}{\text{Odds of exposure in controls}}.$$

and a step-by-step calculation is presented in Box 3.2.

Box 3.2 Step-by-Step Calculation of Odds Ratio

1. Construct a 2 × 2 table (Table 3.1), where:

   a is the number of exposed individuals with the outcome
   b is the number of exposed individuals without the outcome
   c is the number of unexposed individuals with the outcome
   d is the number of unexposed individuals without the outcome.

Table 3.1 2 × 2 table for OR

Status	Cases	Controls
Exposed	a	b
Unexposed	c	d
Total	$a + c$	$b + d$

[2] **Odds ratio (OR):** A measure comparing the odds of an outcome between two groups. It approximates the relative risk when outcomes are rare.

[3] **Absolute risk:** The probability that an event (e.g. disease onset) will occur in a defined population over a specified time period. Unlike relative risk, it conveys the actual likelihood of occurrence and is useful for patient-facing communication.

[4] **Relative risk (RR):** The ratio of risk in the exposed group to that in the unexposed group. Values above 1 indicate increased risk; values below 1 indicate protection.

Box 3.2 (cont.)

2. Calculate the odds of exposure in the cases group:

$$\text{Odds of exposure (cases group)} = \frac{a}{c}.$$

Note: Odds of exposure in cases is *a/c* rather than *a/a* + *c* because the numerator is not included in the denominator in odds. For example, when throwing a dice, the *probability* of any number coming up is 1/6, but the *odds* of any number coming up are 1/5 (one success for every five failures).

3. Calculate the odds of exposure in the control group:

$$\text{Odds of exposure (control group)} = \frac{b}{d}.$$

4. Calculate the **odds ratio:**

$$\text{Odds Ratio (OR)} = \text{OR} = \frac{\text{Odds of exposure (cases)}}{\text{Odds of exposure (controls)}} = \frac{a/c}{b/d} = \frac{ad}{bc}.$$

Interpretation of OR

OR = 1: no association between exposure and outcome.

OR > 1: positive association (exposure may increase the risk of the outcome).

OR < 1: negative association (exposure may decrease the risk of the outcome).

Confidence Intervals and Statistical Significance

The OR is often reported with a 95% confidence interval (CI). If the value '1' does not fall within the range of CI, the association is considered statistically significant.

Odds Ratio vs Relative Risk

Relative risk, which is calculated in cohort studies, is often considered a better measure as it compares probabilities, which are directly related to real-world events. It is intuitive and directly answers the question, 'How much more likely is the outcome in the exposed group?' For example, an RR of 2.0 means that the exposed group is twice as likely to develop the outcome as the unexposed group. The OR compares odds, which are less intuitive and can exaggerate the perceived strength of an association when the outcome is common.

Why Can't Relative Risk Be Used in Case–Control Studies?

Incidence (new cases of disease) cannot be calculated in case–control studies because:

1. The study starts with cases and controls (people already have or do not have the disease).
2. The total population at risk is unknown.
3. Relative risk requires incidence rates in both exposed and unexposed groups, which case–control studies cannot provide.

Thus, OR is the best measure of association in case–control studies.

Strengths and Limitations of Case–Control Studies

Strengths

- Good for rare diseases
- useful for diseases with long latency
- no need for follow-up
- requires smaller sample size
- cost-effective and time-efficient
- allows study of multiple exposures.

Limitations

- Not ideal for rare exposures
- prone to selection and information bias
- prone to confounding
- unclear temporal relationships (reverse causality)
- cannot measure incidence or prevalence
- limited to a single outcome.

Comparison with Cohort Studies

Table 3.2 summarizes the key differences between case–control and cohort study designs.

Table 3.2 Comparison of case–control studies with cohort studies

Case–control studies	Cohort studies
Retrospective	Prospective
Rare disease	Rare exposure
Multiple exposures	Multiple outcomes
More bias	Less bias
Loss to follow-up is infrequent	Loss to follow-up is critical
Cheap, quick, easy	Expensive, lengthy, difficult

Critical Appraisal of a Case–Control Study

Since case–control studies are prone to biases and confounding, critical appraisal should focus on:

1. Selection bias:

   Were cases and controls selected from the same population?

   Were eligibility criteria well defined?

2. Information bias

   Were data collection methods the same for cases and controls?

   Was there blinding of participants/interviewers?

3. Confounding

   Were potential confounders identified and controlled for?

   Was matching, restriction, or statistical adjustment used?

4. Reverse causality

   Can the study confirm whether exposure preceded disease?

   Were alternative explanations for the association considered?

5. Statistical validity

   Were ORs and CIs reported?

   Did the CI of OR exclude the value of 1 (statistical significance)?

Chapter Summary

A case–control study begins by identifying cases and controls and then looks back in time to determine exposures to potential risk factors. If more cases are found to be exposed to the risk factor(s) compared to controls, this suggests an association between the risk factor(s) and the development of the outcome (Figure 3.1).

1. Design
2. Pitfalls and critical appraisal points: case–control studies are prone to bias and confounding, making it crucial to carefully assess these factors when critically appraising such studies.
3. Bias: systematic errors in the design or execution of a study can distort findings.
4. Advantages of case–control studies include that they are good for rare diseases, can study multiple exposures, and are quick and easy to do.

Bias and Confounding

1. Inclusion/exclusion (selection) bias occurs when cases and controls are not matched. It can occur due to investigators or participants.
2. Information bias occurs when errors arise in the collection, measurement, or classification of data within a study. It can be due to observers (measurement bias) or participants (recall bias).
3. Confounder: a variable that is associated with both the risk factor and the outcome and creates a spurious association between the two. It is different from an intervening variable (a variable on the causal chain) or effect modifier variable that modifies the strength or direction of the relationship between the exposure and outcome.
4. Confounders can be controlled in the design of the study by restriction, matching, or randomization.
5. Confounders can also be controlled during data analysis either by stratified analysis or by multivariate analysis.
6. Strength of association is calculated by the OR:

$$\text{OR} = \frac{\text{Odds of exposure (cases)}}{\text{Odds of exposure (controls)}} = \frac{a/c}{b/d} = \frac{ad}{bc}.$$

Practice Questions

For Q1–Q5: A study was conducted to investigate the relationship between social media use and the prevalence of anxiety disorders among adolescents aged 13–18 years. Investigators interviewed 200 adolescents diagnosed with generalized anxiety disorder and social anxiety disorder based on DSM-5 criteria. They also interviewed 200 age- and gender-matched adolescents without anxiety disorders, recruited from community schools. Participants were surveyed regarding their average daily social media use in hours and types of platforms used. Overall, 140 adolescents with anxiety disorder reported high social media use (more than 3 hours per day) compared to 80 adolescents without anxiety disorders.

Q1. Which type of study design is used in this study?

A. Retrospective cohort study
B. Case–control study
C. Survey
D. Randomized controlled trial
E. Prospective cohort study

Q2. What measure of association is appropriate for this study?

A. Relative risk
B. Incidence rate ratio
C. Odds ratio
D. Hazard ratio
E. Attributable risk

Q3. What is the absolute risk of anxiety disorder between high vs low social media use?

A. 1.75
B. 3.5
C. 0.5
D. 1.25
E. It cannot be calculated.

Q4. Which of the following is true regarding this study?

A. High social media use causes anxiety disorders.
B. Adolescents with anxiety disorders have 3.5 times higher odds of high social media use than those without anxiety disorders.
C. High social media use reduces the risk of anxiety disorders by 3.5 times.
D. There is no association between social media use and anxiety disorders.
E. The study proves a direct causal link between social media and anxiety.

Q5. Which of the following is a potential limitation of this study design?

A. High cost and long duration
B. Recall bias regarding social media use
C. Inability to calculate an odds ratio

D. Lack of control over exposure status
E. Difficulty in establishing associations between variables

Q6. In a study on smoking and lung cancer, age is found to influence smoking behaviour. Age may be considered as a

A. Confounder
B. Effect modifier
C. Intervening variable
D. Mediator
E. Independent variable

Q7. Which of the following is *not* a method of controlling the confounders in a case–control study:

A. Restriction
B. Stratified analysis
C. Multivariate analysis
D. Matching
E. Blinding

Q 8. Among individuals with a family history of alcohol dependence, exposure to childhood trauma increases the risk of developing alcohol use disorder in adulthood. However, among those without a family history of alcohol dependence, childhood trauma has a much weaker association with alcohol use disorder. Family history of alcohol dependence can be considered:

A. A confounder
B. A necessary cause
C. A risk factor
D. A sufficient cause
E. An effect modifier

Q9. In a study investigating the relationship between a sedentary lifestyle and type 2 diabetes, what would weight gain be considered to be?

A. Confounder
B. Effect modifier
C. Intervening variable
D. Necessary cause
E. Independent variable

For Q10–Q11: A case–control psychological autopsy study was conducted to identify major risk factors associated with suicides. The psychological autopsy method was employed to obtain information. The main sources of information were the close family members of 100 suicide victims, who were matched for age, gender, and area of residence with 100 living controls. The data is given in Table 3.3.

Table 3.3 Table of ICD-10 principle diagnosis.

Diagnosis	Cases (*n* = 100)	Controls (*n* = 100)
Moderate depressive episode (F32.1)	30	1
Severe depressive episode (F32.2)	43	0
Severe depressive episode with psychotic symptoms (F32.3)	6	2
Schizophrenia (F20)	6	2
Adjustment disorders (F43.2)	3	0
Acute stress reaction (F43.0)	5	0
Alcohol use (F10.0)	0	0
Substance abuse (F11.0)	1	0
Mental retardation (F79)	1	0
Personality disorder (F60)	1	1
No psychiatric diagnosis	4	94

Source: Khan MM, Mahmud S, Karim MS, Zaman M, Prince M. Case–control study of suicide in Karachi, Pakistan. *Br J Psychiatry*. 2008;193(5):402–5. doi: https://doi.org/10.1192/bjp.bp.107.042069.

Q10. What are the odds of depression in individuals who committed suicide?

A. 2.50
B. 3.76
C. 4.52
D. 5.25
E. 6.10

Q11. What is the odds ratio of having a psychiatric diagnosis in individuals who committed suicide compared to controls?

A. 150
B. 220
C. 320
D. 376
E. 425

Answers

Q1. Correct answer: B. Case–control study. The study begins with cases and controls and looks back to assess exposure to social media use, a hallmark of case–control studies.

Q2. Correct answer: C. Odds ratio. Odds ratio is the appropriate measure for case–control studies, as it compares the odds of exposure among cases and controls.

Q3. Correct answer: E. It cannot be calculated because this is a case–control study. Absolute risk cannot be determined from a case–control study because the underlying population at risk is not known.

Q4. Correct answer: B. Adolescents with anxiety disorders have 3.5 times higher odds to have high social media use compared to adolescents without anxiety disorders. See Table 3.4.

Table 3.4 2 × 2 contingency table for Q4

Social media use	Anxiety disorder cases	Controls
High	140 (a)	80 (b)
Low	60 (c)	120 (d)
Total	200	200

- Odds of exposure in cases = a/c = 140/60 = 2.33
- Odds of exposure in controls = b/d = 80/120 = 0.66
- Odds ratio = 2.33/0.66 = 3.53.

An OR of 3.5 indicates a strong association but does not establish causation, as case–control studies cannot prove causality.

Q5. Correct answer: B. Recall bias regarding social media use. In case–control studies, participants may not accurately recall past exposure, leading to recall bias, especially when estimating social media usage retrospectively, or they may recall differentially depending on whether they have the social anxiety disorder or not.

Q6. Correct answer: A. Confounder. Age is associated with smoking behaviour, as smoking prevalence often varies by age group. Age is also associated with lung cancer risk, as older age increases cancer risk regardless of smoking status. Age is not directly part of the causal chain linking smoking to lung cancer, but failing to control for age could bias the association between smoking and lung cancer.

Q7. Correct answer: E. Blinding. Blinding is a technique used to prevent bias in clinical trials by masking the treatment assignment from participants and/or researchers. It's not relevant to controlling confounders in a case–control study, which is an observational study design.

Why other options are incorrect:

Restriction: limiting the study to participants who fall within a certain range of the confounder (e.g. only including non-smokers).

Stratified analysis: analysing the data separately for different levels of the confounder (e.g. analysing smokers and non-smokers separately).

Multivariate analysis: using statistical techniques to adjust for multiple confounders simultaneously.

Matching: selecting controls who are similar to cases in terms of the confounder (e.g. matching on age and sex).

Q8. Correct answer: E. An effect modifier. In this scenario, the presence of a family history of alcohol dependence modifies the effect of childhood trauma on the risk of developing alcohol use disorder. This is a classic example of effect modification, where the relationship between an exposure (childhood trauma) and an outcome (alcohol use disorder) differs depending on the presence of a third factor (family history of alcohol dependence).

Q9. Correct answer: C. Intervening variable. A intervening variable (mediator) is a variable that lies on the causal pathway between an exposure and an outcome, explaining part of the causal process.

In this scenario, exposure is sedentary lifestyle. Outcome is type 2 diabetes. The intervening variable is weight gain. A sedentary lifestyle often leads to weight gain, and weight gain then increases the risk of type 2 diabetes. This mediating effect of weight gain clarifies the pathway through which sedentary behaviour contributes to diabetes risk.

Why other options are incorrect:

A. Confounder: a confounder would need to be associated with both the exposure and the outcome, but not part of the causal pathway. Weight gain is part of the causal chain, not an external variable influencing both sedentary lifestyle and diabetes independently.
B. Effect modifier: an effect modifier changes the strength or direction of the association between exposure and outcome, which is not the case here. Instead, weight gain explains how a sedentary lifestyle leads to diabetes, fitting the definition of an intervening variable.
D. Necessary cause: a necessary cause is required for an outcome to occur. Type 2 diabetes can occur through mechanisms other than weight gain, so weight gain is not a necessary cause.

Q10. Correct answer: B (3.76). See Table 3.5 for the 2 × 2 table for depression.

Table 3.5 2 × 2 table for Q10

Depression	Suicide cases	Controls	Total
Present	**79** (30 + 43 + 6)	**3** (1 + 0 + 2)	82
Absent	21	97	118
Total	100	100	200

$$\text{Odds of exposure in the cases} = \frac{a}{c} = \frac{79}{21} = 3.76.$$

Q11. Correct answer: D (376). See Table 3.6 for the 2 × 2 table for ICD-10 psychiatric diagnosis.

Table 3.6 2 × 2 table for Q11

Psychiatric diagnosis	Suicide cases	Controls	Total
Present	96 (*a*)	6 (*b*)	102
Absent	4 (*c*)	94 (*d*)	98
Total	100	100	200

$$\text{Odds of psychiatric diagnosis in suicide cases} = \frac{a}{c} = \frac{96}{4} = 24.$$

$$\text{Odds of psychiatric diagnosis in controls} = \frac{b}{d} = \frac{6}{94} = 0.0638.$$

$$\text{Odds ratio (OR)} = \frac{\text{Odds in cases}}{\text{Odds in controls}} = \frac{a/c}{b/d} = \frac{ad}{bc} = \frac{96 \times 94}{6 \times 4} \approx 376.$$

Further Reading

Breslow NE, Day NE. *Statistical Methods in Cancer Research. Vol. 1: The Analysis of Case-Control Studies*. Lyon: IARC; 1980.

Delgado-Rodríguez M, Llorca J. Bias. *J Epidemiol Community Health*. 2004;**58**(8):635–41. doi: https://doi.org/10.1136/jech.2003.008466.

Greenland S, Robins JM. Identifiability, exchangeability, and epidemiological confounding. *Int J Epidemiol*. 1986;**15**(3):413–19.

Grimes DA, Schulz KF. Bias and causal associations in observational research. *Lancet*. 2002;**359**(9302):248–52. doi: https://doi.org/10.1016/S0140-6736(02)07451-2.

Hosmer DW Jr, Lemeshow S, Sturdivant RX. *Applied Logistic Regression*. 3rd ed. Hoboken, NJ: Wiley; 2013. doi: https://doi.org/10.1002/9781118548387.

Miettinen OS, Cook EF. Confounding: essence and detection. *Am J Epidemiol*. 1981;**114**(4):593–603. doi: https://doi.org/10.1093/oxfordjournals.aje.a113225.

Schlesselman JJ. *Case-Control Studies: Design, Conduct, Analysis*. New York: Oxford University Press; 1982.

Wacholder S, McLaughlin JK, Silverman DT, Mandel JS. Selection of controls in case-control studies: I. Principles. *Am J Epidemiol*. 1992;**135**(9):1019–28.

Wacholder S, Silverman DT, McLaughlin JK, Mandel JS. Selection of controls in case-control studies: II. Types of controls. *Am J Epidemiol*. 1992;**135**(9):1029–41.

Wacholder S, McLaughlin JK, Silverman DT, Mandel JS. Selection of controls in case-control studies: III. Design options. *Am J Epidemiol*. 1992;**135**(9):1042–50.

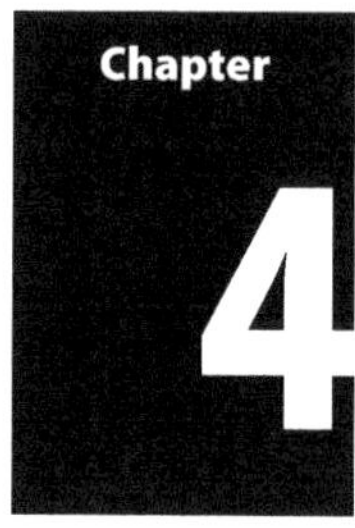

Diagnostic Studies

What Is a Good Test?

Diagnostic tests play a crucial role in the assessment and management of patients. Tests may serve various purposes, including:

- **screening tests** to identify risk factors or detect disease in asymptomatic individuals
- **diagnostic tests** to confirm or rule out a suspected disease in symptomatic individuals
- **prognostic tests** to estimate the likely course or outcome of a disease.

An ideal diagnostic test would always provide the correct result, yielding a positive result in everyone with the disease and a negative result in everyone without the disease. Additionally, it should be quick, safe, simple, painless, reliable, and cost-effective. However, in clinical practice it is rarely possible to have a perfect test. Therefore, it is essential to understand how to assess the usefulness of imperfect tests.

The usefulness of a test may be assessed based on the following criteria:

- **accuracy:** how well the test correctly identifies or excludes a condition
- **reproducibility (precision):** consistency of the test results when repeated under the same conditions
- **feasibility:** practicality of performing the test in a clinical setting
- **effect on clinical decisions:** whether the test influences diagnosis or treatment strategies
- **effect on outcomes:** whether the test improves patient outcomes.

Accuracy of a Test

The accuracy of a test is commonly assessed through its **sensitivity**[1] and **specificity**.[2]

Sensitivity (True Positive Rate)

Sensitivity is the ability of a test to correctly identify individuals with the disease. Statistically, sensitivity is the proportion of people with the disease who have a positive test result.

---

[1] **Sensitivity:** The proportion of true positives correctly identified by a test. High sensitivity is useful for ruling out disease.

[2] **Specificity:** The proportion of true negatives correctly identified. High specificity helps rule in disease.

Specificity (True Negative Rate)

Specificity is the ability of a test to correctly identify individuals without the disease. Statistically, specificity is the proportion of people without the disease who have a negative test result.

Accuracy

Accuracy refers to the proportion of correctly classified subjects (both with and without the condition) among all tested subjects. It can be calculated by drawing a 2 × 2 contingency table, as in Table 4.1.

Table 4.1 2 × 2 contingency table for evaluating diagnostic test accuracy (raw counts)

Test result	Disorder present	Disorder absent	Total
Test positive	a	b	$a+b$
Test negative	c	d	$c+d$
Total	$a+c$	$b+d$	$a+b+c+d$

Using Table 4.1, the sensitivity and specificity of the test can be calculated as follows:

$$\text{Sensitivity} = \frac{a}{a+c},$$

$$\text{Specificity} = \frac{d}{b+d},$$

$$\text{Accuracy} = \frac{a+d}{a+c+b+d}.$$

The 2 × 2 contingency table can also be drawn as in Table 4.2.

Table 4.2 2 × 2 contingency table with true positives, false positives, false negatives, and true negatives labelled

Test result	Disorder present	Disorder absent	Total
Test positive	TP (a)	FP (b)	TP + FP ($a+b$) (total of row)
Test negative	FN (c)	TN (d)	FN + TN ($c+d$) (total of row)
Total	TP + FN ($a+c$) (total of column)	FP + TN ($b+d$) (total of column)	–

TP, true positive; TN, true negative; FP, false positive; FN, false negative.

Using table 4.2, the sensitivity, specificity, and accuracy can be expressed as follows:

$$\text{Sensitivity} = \frac{\text{True positives}}{\text{True positives} + \text{false negatives}} = \frac{\text{True positives}}{\text{All those who have the condition}},$$

$$\text{Specificity} = \frac{\text{True negatives}}{\text{False positives} + \text{true negatives}} = \frac{\text{True negatives}}{\text{All those who do not have the condition}},$$

$$\text{Accuracy} = \frac{\text{True positives} + \text{true negatives}}{\text{True positives} + \text{false negatives} + \text{false positives} + \text{true negatives}}$$

$$= \frac{\text{Correct results with the test}}{\text{All results with the test}}.$$

Predictive Values

While sensitivity and specificity are characteristics of a test and are used to 'test' the test itself, patients are often more concerned about the practical implications of their test i.e., they want to know the likelihood of having the disease if a test result is positive, and the likelihood that a disease has been excluded if a test result is negative. These questions are addressed by the predictive values of a test.

Positive Predictive Value

The **positive predictive value** (PPV)[3] represents the proportion of individuals with a positive test result who actually have the disease. Using the 2 × 2 contingency table, this is calculated as:

$$\text{PPV} = \frac{a}{a+b} = \frac{\text{True positives}}{\text{True positives} + \text{false positives}}.$$

Negative Predictive Value

The **negative predictive value** (NPV)[4] indicates the proportion of individuals with a negative test result who do not have the disease. Using the 2 × 2 contingency table, this is calculated as:

$$\text{NPV} = \frac{d}{c+d} = \frac{\text{True negatives}}{\text{False negatives} + \text{true negatives}}.$$

'Rule In' and 'Rule Out' Concept

When a patient presents with a clinical complaint, the clinician begins by taking a detailed history, performing a physical examination, and conducting a mental state examination to

[3] **Positive predictive value (PPV):** The proportion of positive test results that are true positives. PPV increases with prevalence and test specificity.

[4] **Negative predictive value (NPV):** The probability that individuals with a negative test truly do not have the disease. Predictive values depend on disease prevalence; consider reporting across plausible prevalence ranges.

develop a list of potential differential diagnoses. Tests are then ordered to 'rule out' less likely diagnoses. At this stage, tests with high sensitivity are preferred to minimize the false negative rate and avoid missing true cases of the disease. While this may lead to more false positives, these can be addressed subsequently.

After narrowing down the list of differential diagnoses, the clinician may order a highly specific test to 'rule in' or confirm a diagnosis. An example would be a biopsy for confirming a cancer diagnosis. Therefore, an ideal screening test should have high sensitivity, whereas a confirmatory test should have high specificity.

A mnemonic can be used to aid recall:

- Highly **sp**ecific tests are used to rule **in** a diagnosis: **SPIN**.
- Highly **sen**sitive tests are used to rule **out** a diagnosis: **SNOUT**.

Effect of Disease Prevalence on Predictive Values

The prevalence of a disease in the population where a test is applied does not directly affect the sensitivity or specificity of the test, as these are intrinsic properties of the test itself. However, predictive values (both PPV and NPV) are highly influenced by disease prevalence.

When a test is validated in a population with a high prevalence (e.g. 50%), such as an inpatient ward where every other person may have the disease, the PPV can be high. For example, in Population 1 (Table 4.3), where prevalence is 50%, the PPV is 94%:

Table 4.3 High-prevalence population (50%)

Test result	Disorder present	Disorder absent	Total
Positive	48	3	51
Negative	2	47	49
Total	50	50	100

- Prevalence = 50/100 = 50%
- Sensitivity = 48/50 = 96%
- Specificity = 47/50 = 94%
- PPV = 48/51 = 94%
- NPV = 47/49 = 96%.

However, when the same test is applied to a low-prevalence population (e.g. 2%), the PPV can drop significantly.

In Population 2 (Table 4.4), with a prevalence of 2%, the PPV of the same test decreases to 24%:

Table 4.4 Low-prevalence population (2%)

Test result	Disorder present	Disorder absent	Total
Positive	192	588	780
Negative	8	9,212	9,220
Total	200	9,800	10,000

- Prevalence = 200/10,000 = 2%
- Sensitivity = 192/200 = 96%
- Specificity = 9,212/9,800 = 99.91%
- PPV = 192/780 = 24.6%
- NPV = 9,212/9,220 = 99.9%.

Likelihood Ratios

Likelihood ratios (LRs)[5] are valuable in assessing how much a positive or negative test result changes the probability of having a disease. They combine sensitivity and specificity in a single measure to evaluate the clinical utility of a test:

- **LR+ (likelihood ratio of a positive test)** indicates how much the odds of having the disease increase if the test is positive.
- **LR– (likelihood ratio of a negative test)** indicates how much the odds of having the disease decrease if the test is negative.

Likelihood Ratio of Positive Test (LR+)

The LR+ compares the probability of a positive test result in those without the disease (sensitivity) to the probability of a positive test result when there is no disease (false positive error rate). Essentially, LR+ is the ratio of sensitivity to the false positive error rate:

$$\text{LR+} = \frac{\text{sensitivity}}{1 - \text{specificity}} = \frac{\frac{a}{a+c}}{\frac{b}{b+d}}.$$

The LR+ represents a ratio of what clinicians want (sensitivity) to what they do not want (false positive error rate). The higher the LR+, the better the test. An LR+ of 1 indicates that the test is equally likely to produce a positive result for individuals with and without the disease, offering no diagnostic value. For a test to be clinically useful, the LR+ should be much larger than 1, ideally above 10, indicating a strong likelihood of disease presence when the test is positive.

Likelihood Ratio of Negative Test (LR–)

The LR– compares the probability of a negative test result in someone with the disease (false negative error rate) to the probability of a negative test result in someone without the disease (specificity):

$$\text{LR} - = \frac{1 - \text{sensitivity}}{\text{specificity}} = \frac{\frac{c}{a+c}}{\frac{d}{b+d}}.$$

[5] **Likelihood ratio (LR+, LR–):** Ratios indicating how much a test result changes the probability of disease. Use with pre-test odds to get post-test odds (Fagan nomogram); LR+ > 10 or LR– < 0.1 provide strong shifts in probability.

In other words the LR− is a ratio of what clinicians do not want (false negative error rate) to what they want (specificity). An LR− of 1 would indicate that the test result is equally likely to be negative in individuals without the disease and in those with the disease, offering no diagnostic value. Ideally, LR− should be less than 1 and as closer to 0 as possible i.e. smaller values indicate a better test.

Likelihood Ratios of Commonly Used Tests

The likelihood ratios of commonly used medical tests and psychiatric rating scales are given in Tables 4.5 and 4.6, respectively. The likelihood ratios shown represent approximate values derived from selected studies and may vary depending on population characteristics, disease prevalence and test thresholds.

Table 4.5 Likelihood ratios of commonly used medical diagnostic tests

Disorder	Test/screening tool	LR+	LR−
Acute cholecystitis	Abdominal ultrasound	23.8	0.05
Acute pulmonary embolism	Pulmonary CT angiography	29.1	0.05
Appendicitis	Abdominal CT	18.8	0.06
C. difficile colitis	*C. difficile* toxin-positive	19.6	0.02
Systemic lupus erythematosus (SLE)	Antinuclear antibody	4.5	0.125
Deep vein thrombosis (DVT)	D-dimer test	1.6	0.25
Myocardial infarction (MI)	Troponin I	30.0	0.04
Bacterial meningitis	CSF gram stain	21.0	0.06
Strep. pharyngitis	Rapid *Strep.* test	45.0	0.03
Osteomyelitis	MRI	42.0	0.04

Table 4.6 Likelihood ratios of psychiatric rating scales

Disorder	Test/screening tool	LR+	LR−
Major depressive disorder (MDD)	PHQ-9 (score ≥10)	5.6	0.19
Generalized anxiety disorder (GAD)	GAD-7 (score ≥10)	4.2	0.2
Bipolar disorder	Mood disorder questionnaire (MDQ)	9.6	0.1
Schizophrenia	PANSS positive scale (≥5 on delusions/ hallucinations)	15.0	0.08
ADHD (Adults)	ASRS (score ≥4 in part A)	6.3	0.22
Autism spectrum disorder (ASD)	AQ-10 (score ≥6)	7.5	0.12
PTSD	PCL-5 (score ≥33)	8.0	0.14
Dementia (Alzheimer's disease)	Mini-Mental State Exam (MMSE <24)	10.3	0.1

The examples listed in these two tables illustrate how LRs can vary across different medical and psychiatric conditions. The interpretation of LRs may depend on the specific study, patient population, and testing methods used.

Pre- and Post-Test Probabilities

Understanding pre- and post-test probabilities is essential for interpreting diagnostic tests accurately. This concept is closely linked to Bayes' Theorem, which integrates pre-test probabilities with diagnostic test results to refine the likelihood of a disease.

Bayes' Theorem

Bayes' Theorem is a foundational principle in probability theory that outlines how to update beliefs about an event based on new evidence. In simpler terms, it demonstrates how our perception of probability should change when presented with additional information.

In medical diagnostics, Bayes' Theorem helps refine the estimated probability of disease following a test result. It establishes that the estimated probability of a condition in an individual is influenced by the prior probability (often approximated by population prevalence). Each test result incrementally modifies the probability of disease, because each successive test result effectively reclassifies the population group to which the patient belongs.

Key Concepts in Pre- and Post-Test Probabilities

- **Probability:** the likelihood that an event will occur, expressed as a proportion ranging from 0 to 1 (or 0% to 100%). For example, a probability of 0.7 means the event is expected to occur in 7 out of 10 instances.
- **Odds:** the ratio of the probability that an event occurs to the probability that it does not occur. For example, if the probability of an event is 0.8, the odds are 4 to 1 (0.8/0.2).
- **Pre-test probability (prior probability):** the initial estimation of the likelihood that a patient has a disease before any diagnostic test is performed. This is often based on the prevalence of the disease in the population or the clinician's assessment of risk factors. Denoted as P(A).
- **Pre-test odds:** the odds of disease before the test.
- **Likelihood ratio:** a measure of how much a test result will change the pre-test probability of disease. It reflects the 'power' of a test in modifying the likelihood of disease presence. A positive likelihood ratio indicates how much more likely a positive test result is in diseased individuals compared to non-diseased, while a negative likelihood ratio indicates the reverse.
- **Post-test odds:** the odds of disease after incorporating the test result.
- **Post-test probability (posterior probability):** the revised probability of disease after considering the test result. It is calculated by combining the pre-test probability with the likelihood ratio using Bayes' Theorem. This is our updated belief about the probability of having the disease after considering the test result. It is denoted as P(A|B).

Calculation of Post-Test Probability from Pre-Test Probability

Step 1: Convert Pre-Test Probability to Pre-Test Odds

Example: If the pre-test probability of a condition is 50%, this can be expressed as a 1 in 2 chance. The odds would be even (1:1) because for every person with the condition, there is one person without the condition:

$$\text{Odds} = \frac{\text{Probability}}{1 - \text{Probability}} = \frac{0.5}{1 - 0.5} = 1:1.$$

Conversely, when odds are even, the probability is 1 in 2 ($P = 0.5$):

$$\text{Probability} = \frac{\text{Odds}}{1 + \text{Odds}} = \frac{1}{1+1} = \frac{1}{2} = 0.5.$$

Step 2: Calculate Post-Test Odds

Post-test odds are derived by multiplying the pre-test odds by the LR+:

Post-test odds = LR+ × Pre-test odds.

Step 3: Convert Post-Test Odds to Post-Test Probability

The post-test probability can then be calculated using:

$$\text{Probability (post-test)} = \frac{\text{Odds (post-test)}}{1 + \text{Odds (post-test)}}.$$

The steps are illustrated in Figure 4.1.

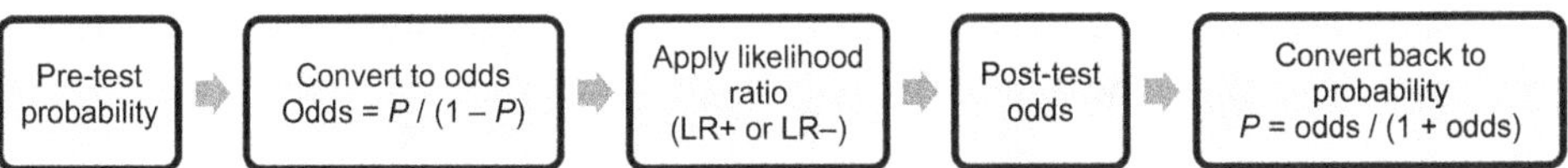

Figure 4.1 Visual flow diagram showing the calculation of post-test probability from a pre-test probability using Bayes' Theorem.

Worked Examples

For a positive test (using probability (prevalance) = 50% and LR+ = 3):

- pre-test probability = 50%
- pre-test odds = $\frac{0.5}{1-0.5}$ = 1.0 (1:1)
- LR+ = 3
- post-test odds = 1 × 3 = 3
- post-test probability = $\frac{3}{1+3}$ = 0.75 (75%).

Interpretation: A positive result increases the probability of disease from 50% to 75%.

For a negative test (using probability (prevalance) = 50% and LR– = 0.25):

- pre-test probability = 50%
- pre-test odds = $\frac{0.5}{1-0.5}$ = 1.0 (1:1)
- LR– = 0.25
- post-test odds = 1 × 0.25 = 0.25
- post-test probability = $\frac{0.25}{1+0.25}$ = 0.20 (20%).

Interpretation: A negative result reduces the probability of disease from 50% to 20%.

Interpretation of 2 × 2 Contingency Table Cells

The 2 × 2 contingency table is a valuable tool in diagnostic test evaluation, allowing clinicians to calculate various test performance metrics including sensitivity, specificity, predictive values, and likelihood ratios. Table 4.7 shows an example 2 × 2 table, which can be interpreted as follows:

Table 4.7 Interpretation of 2 × 2 contingency table cells

Test result	Diseased	Non-diseased	Total
Positive	a	b	$a + b$
Negative	c	d	$c + d$
Total	$a + c$	$b + d$	$a + b + c + d$

- a = number of subjects with the disease × sensitivity (or **prevalence** × **sensitivity** if the population is normalised to 1).
- b is subjects with a **false positive** test result.
- c is subjects with a **false negative** test result.
- d is subjects with a **true negative** test result = **specificity** × **(1 – prevalence)**.
- $a + b$ is all subjects with a **positive** test result.
- $c + d$ is all subjects with a **negative** test result.
- $a + c$ is all subjects with the disease.
- $b + d$ is all subjects without the disease = **1 – prevalence**.
- $a + b + c + d$ is all study subjects (total population).

Key Formulae for Diagnostic Test Evaluation

The 2 × 2 contingency table allows for the calculation of critical metrics used in diagnostic test evaluation, including sensitivity, specificity, predictive values, and likelihood ratios (Table 4.8).

Table 4.8 Key formulae for diagnostic test evaluation

Metric	Formula	Description
Sensitivity	$a / (a + c)$	Proportion of true positives among all diseased subjects
Specificity	$d / (b + d)$	Proportion of true negatives among all non-diseased subjects
False positive error rate[a]	$b / (b + d)$ *or* 1 – specificity	Likelihood of a false positive result among non-diseased subjects
False negative error rate[b]	$c / (a + c)$ *or* 1 – sensitivity	Likelihood of a false negative result among diseased subjects
PPV	$a / (a + b)$	Probability that positive test result indicates presence of disease
NPV	$d / (c + d)$	Probability that negative test result indicates absence of disease

Table 4.8 (cont.)

Metric	Formula	Description
LR+	Sensitivity / (1 – specificity) or $\frac{a/(a+c)}{b/(b+d)}$ or $\frac{a/b}{(a+c)/(b+d)}$	Indicates how much a positive test increases disease odds
LR–	(1 – sensitivity) / specificity or $\frac{c/(a+c)}{d/(b+d)}$ or $\frac{c/d}{(a+c)/(b+d)}$	Indicates how much a negative test decreases disease odds
Prevalence	$(a + c) / (a + b + c + d)$	Proportion of population that actually has the disease

[a] Also called alpha error rate or type I error rate. [b] Also called beta error rate or type II error rate.

Deciding the Appropriate Cut-Off for a Test

When a disease is defined by a threshold on a continuous scale, the test characteristics can be altered by changing the threshold or cut-off point. Lowering the threshold (e.g. Beck's Depression Inventory (BDI) score) improves sensitivity, but often at the cost of lowered specificity (i.e. more false positives). Conversely, raising the threshold improves specificity, but may reduce sensitivity (i.e. more false negatives). This consideration is especially important when the distribution of a characteristic is unimodal, such as blood pressure, cholesterol, weight, etc.

Key Considerations When Selecting a Cut-off

Clinical Consequences of False Positives vs False Negatives

If missing the disease is dangerous (e.g. cancer, sepsis, myocardial infarction), higher sensitivity (lower cut-off) is preferred. If false positives lead to unnecessary interventions (e.g. invasive procedures), higher specificity (higher cut-off) is preferred.

Prevalence of Disease in the Population

In a high-prevalence setting, a higher cut-off may reduce false positives. In a low-prevalence setting, a lower cut-off improves early disease detection.

Receiver Operating Characteristic Curve

The **receiver operating characteristic** (ROC)[6] curve is a widely used tool for evaluating the performance of diagnostic tests. The term 'ROC curve' originated from military radar operators and electrical engineers during World War II, who developed it to distinguish enemy aircraft from background noise. In medical research and clinical practice, the ROC curve serves a similar purpose: separating individuals with disease from those without disease.

[6] **Receiver operating characteristic (ROC) curve:** A plot of sensitivity versus 1 – specificity across thresholds that visualizes discrimination. The AUC summarizes overall test accuracy.

An ROC curve is generated by plotting sensitivity (true positive rate) on the vertical axis against 1 – specificity (false positive rate) on the horizontal axis across all possible cut-off points of the test. This allows one to visualize how test discrimination changes at different thresholds.

Key points to note regarding the ROC are:

- The **area under the curve** (AUC)[7] is a summary measure of the ROC curve representing the overall diagnostic accuracy of a test; values range from 0.5 (no discrimination) to 1.0 (perfect discrimination).
- The ROC curve helps identify the optimal cut-off by examining the trade-off between sensitivity and false positives.
- The most desirable cut-off point is the one closest to the upper-left corner of the graph, representing 100% sensitivity and 0% false positive rate.
- The ideal ROC curve would rise steeply from the lower-left corner and then run horizontally along the top of the graph, indicating excellent diagnostic performance.
- In contrast, if sensitivity equals the false positive rate, the ROC curve will form a diagonal line from the bottom-left to the top-right, indicating a test with no discriminatory value (equivalent to chance).

When ROC curves of different tests are plotted together, they can be compared to evaluate which test performs better in diagnosis, screening, or assessment of a particular disorder. Figure 4.2 illustrates how ROC curves of varying shapes represent different levels of diagnostic accuracy.

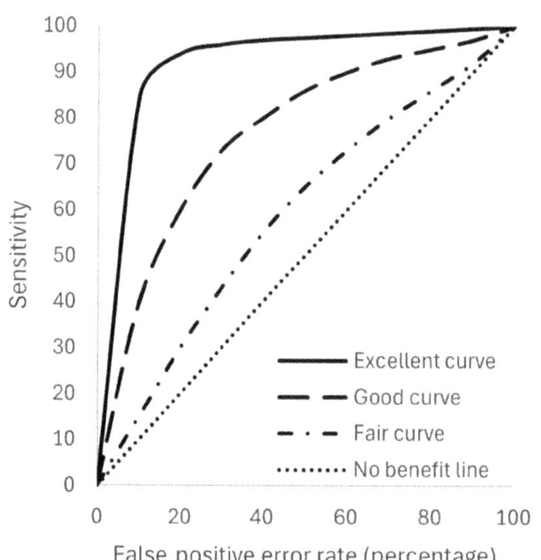

Figure 4.2 Receiver operating characteristic curves illustrating different levels of diagnostic test performance: excellent, good, fair, and no benefit

[7] **Area under the curve (AUC):** A measure summarizing the overall diagnostic accuracy of a test based on the ROC curve. Values range from 0.5 (no discrimination) to 1.0 (perfect discrimination). AUC is threshold-independent but ignores clinical thresholds; pair with sensitivity/specificity at decision-relevant cut-points.

Table 4.9 Sensitivity and specificity at different MMSE cut-off scores

MMSE cut-off	Sensitivity (true positive rate)	Specificity (true negative rate)	Youden Index (J)
24	0.95	0.80	0.75
23	0.90	0.85	0.75
22	0.85	0.90	0.75
21	0.80	0.93	0.73
20	0.75	0.96	0.71

The Youden Index is often used as a summary measure of the ROC curve. It permits the selection of an optimal threshold value or cut-off point:

$$\text{Youden Index } (J) = \text{Sensitivity} + \text{specificity} - 1$$

- The Youden Index ranges from 0 to 1.
- A value of 1 indicates a perfect test with 100% sensitivity and 100% specificity.
- A value of 0 indicates a test that is no better than a random guess.

Table 4.9 presents an example ROC analysis for the Mini-Mental State Examination (MMSE) in diagnosing dementia.

Cut-off scores of 24, 23, and 22 yield the highest Youden Index (0.75). The choice among these depends on whether sensitivity or specificity is prioritized.

The appropriate cut-off is shown for a different variable (cholesterol) is shown in Figure 4.3.

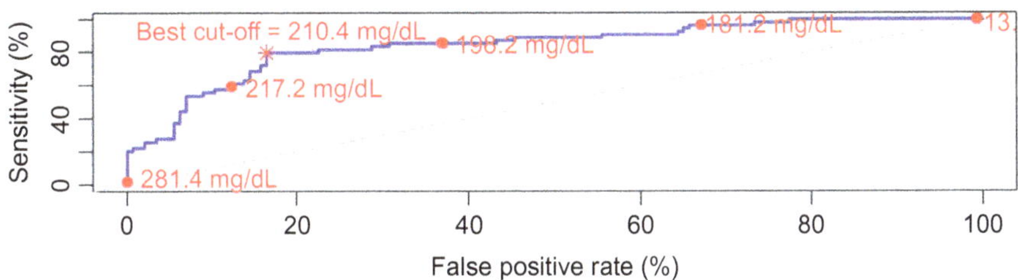

Figure 4.3 Receiver operating characteristic curve for cholesterol: area under the curve (AUC) 0.84; optimal cut-off 210.4 mg/dL.

Biases in Diagnostic Studies

Biases in diagnostic studies can significantly affect the accuracy and generalizability of test results. Understanding common biases is crucial for accurate test interpretation.

Spectrum Bias

Definition: spectrum bias arises when a study population includes only 'clear' or 'definite' cases of the disease and 'clear' healthy controls, thereby not representing the full spectrum of disease presentation.

Impact: this can lead to an overestimation of test accuracy, as the test may perform better in the selected study population than in the broader population.

Example: a study exploring a new screening test for autism spectrum disorder (ASD) in children includes only severe ASD cases and neurotypical controls, excluding mild ASD cases. The test might appear more accurate in this artificially stratified population than in a real-world setting.

Purity Diagnostic Bias

Definition: also known as comorbidity bias, this selection bias occurs when researchers exclude patients with comorbidities from the study population.

Impact: this purity of sample may lead to overestimated diagnostic accuracy, as real-world clinical presentations often involve comorbid conditions.

Example: a study evaluating the accuracy of a new structured clinical interview for diagnosing schizophrenia excludes cases with prodromal symptoms and schizoaffective disorder, resulting in unrealistically high diagnostic specificity for pure schizophrenia cases.

Purity bias and spectrum bias are compared in Table 4.10.

Table 4.10 Comparison of purity bias and spectrum bias

Type of bias	What it affects	Example
Purity bias	Tests only 'pure' cases, excluding borderline conditions	Excluding cases of schizoaffective disorder when testing a schizophrenia diagnosis tool
Spectrum bias	Tests only extreme cases, excluding mild or moderate presentations	Testing ASD screening tool in severe ASD cases and healthy controls

Lead-Time Bias

Definition: lead-time bias occurs when early detection of a disease (through screening) gives the false impression of improved survival, while in reality it only increases the time a patient is aware of their diagnosis without changing the actual disease course.

Mechanism: this bias is common in diseases with poor prognosis and limited treatment options.

Example: a colon cancer screening programme detects cancer at age 50 instead of age 55, when symptoms appear. The patients in both scenarios died at age 60, regardless of detection time.

Without screening: survival time is 5 years (55–60 years old).

With screening: survival time is 10 years (50–60 years old).

The survival time appears doubled (5 vs 10 years), but the actual outcome (death at age 60) remains unchanged.

Length Bias

Definition: length bias occurs when screening is more likely to detect slower-growing, less aggressive diseases, giving the illusion of increased screening effectiveness.

Mechanism: these slower-growing diseases often have a better prognosis, regardless of detection timing. This bias can inflate the perceived benefits of screening programmes.

Example: A disease results in two types of tumours:

- aggressive (fast-growing)
- indolent (slow-growing).

Screening is more likely to detect indolent tumours, as they have a longer pre-clinical phase (time before symptoms appear). Even without screening, individuals with indolent tumours tend to live longer. This scenario can misleadingly suggest that the screening programme improves survival, when it is actually detecting less aggressive cases.

Lead-time bias and length bias are compared in Table 4.11.

Table 4.11 Comparison of lead-time bias and length bias

Feature	Lead-time bias	Length bias
Mechanism	Earlier detection	Preferential detection of less aggressive disease
Impact	Inflates survival time	Overestimates the effectiveness of screening
Focus	Time of diagnosis	Type of disease detected

Validity

Validity refers to the degree to which a test accurately measures what it is intended to measure. There are three main types, each with their own subtypes, as shown in Figure 4.4.

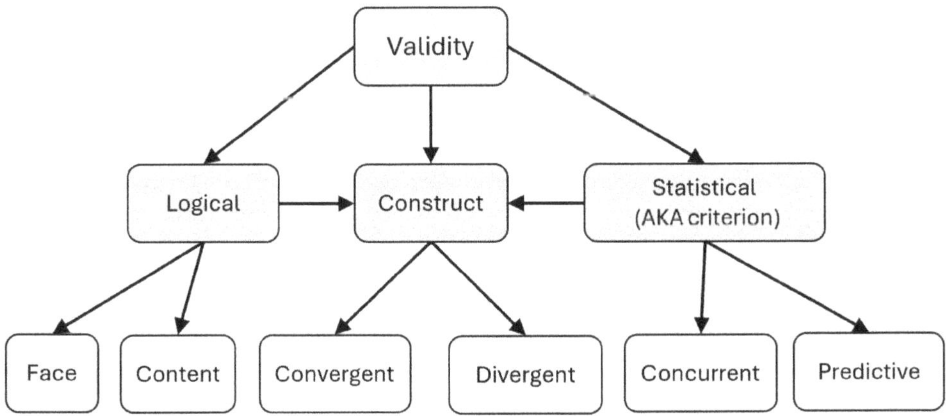

Figure 4.4 Types of validity: logical, construct, and statistical (criterion), with their subtypes.

Logical Validity

Logical validity refers to non-statistical judgements about whether a test appears meaningful and appropriate based on theory and expert opinion. It has two further subtypes, face validity and content validity.

Face Validity

Whether the test looks as if it measures what it claims to measure at face value based on a surface-level or intuitive judgement; for example, a depression questionnaire should ask about mood, sleep, and energy levels.

Content Validity

Whether the test fully covers all aspects of the concept being measured; for example, the screening test for ASD should include three core domains of ASD: social difficulties, communication difficulties, and restricted, repetitive, and stereotyped patterns of behaviour.

Statistical Validity (Criterion Validity)

Statistical validity relies on quantitative or statistical evidence to prove accuracy. It has two subtypes, concurrent and predictive validity.

Concurrent Validity

Whether the test agrees with another established or previously validated test measuring the same concept; for example, does a new anxiety scale correlate with an existing, established anxiety scale?

Predictive Validity

Whether the test accurately predicts future outcomes; for example, does a medical school entrance exam predict future doctor performance?

Construct Validity

Construct validity refers to the extent to which a test accurately measures the theoretical concept (construct) it claims to measure. It is divided into convergent and divergent validity.

Convergent Validity

Measures whether a test correlates well with other tests that measure the same construct. Measures of the same construct (or very similar constructs) should converge or correlate highly with each other. For example, if a test of sleep quality includes two measures – a sleep quality questionnaire and a wrist-worn device – and there is a strong relationship between the two scores, it demonstrates convergent validity.

Divergent Validity (Discriminant Validity)

Measures that theoretically should not be related to each other are observed to not be related to each other in the test – that is, the ability to discriminate between dissimilar constructs. For example, a depression rating scale (e.g. PHQ-9) should not correlate highly with a memory test.

Reliability

Reliability refers to the consistency and stability of a measurement over time, across different raters, and in different conditions. A test is considered reliable if it produces similar results when repeated under the same circumstances. It is important to note that a test can be reliable without being valid, but it cannot be valid without being reliable.

Test–Retest Reliability (Stability Over Time)

This measures whether a test yields similar results when given to the same person at different points in time. For example a depression scale (PHQ-9) should give similar scores when administered two weeks apart, assuming the patient's condition has not changed.

Inter-Rater Reliability (Agreement Between Raters)

This measures the degree of agreement between different observers or clinicians using the same test. For example, two psychiatrists independently diagnosing a patient using the DSM-5 criteria should reach the same diagnosis for high inter-rater reliability.

Parallel-Forms Reliability (Equivalence Between Test Versions)

This measures whether different versions of the same test give similar results. For example, two different versions of an ADHD screening questionnaire should give equivalent scores.

Internal Consistency (Consistency within the Test)

This measures how closely related the items in a test are. Cronbach's alpha (α) measures internal consistency (should be >0.7 for good reliability). Split-half reliability splits a test into two halves to check consistency between them. For example, a GAD-7 test should have high internal consistency, meaning all questions about anxiety should correlate well.

Chapter Summary

Accuracy and Value of Tests

Sensitivity (True Positive Rate)

Sensitivity is the ability of a test to correctly identify individuals with the disease. Statistically, sensitivity is the proportion of people with the disease who have a positive test result. The formula using a 2 × 2 contingency table is: sensitivity = $a/(a + c)$.

Specificity (True Negative Rate)

Specificity is the ability of a test to correctly identify individuals without the disease. Statistically, specificity is the proportion of people without the disease who have a negative test result. The formula using a 2 × 2 contingency table is: specificity = $d / (b + d)$.

Accuracy

Accuracy refers to the proportion of correctly classified subjects (both with and without the condition) among all tested subjects. The formula using a 2 × 2 contingency table is: accuracy = $(a + d) / (a + c + b + d)$.

Positive Predictive Value

The PPV represents the proportion of individuals with a positive test result who actually have the disease. The formula using a 2 × 2 contingency table is: PPV = a / (a + b) = (true positives) / (true positives + false positives).

Negative Predictive Value

The NPV indicates the proportion of individuals with a negative test result who do not have the disease. The formula using a 2 × 2 contingency table is: NPV = d / (c + d) = (true negatives) / (false negatives + true negatives).

The sensitivity and specificity of the test remain constant, but the predictive values vary with changes in the prevalence of the disease in the population.

'Rule In' and 'Rule Out' Concept

Highly **sp**ecific tests are used to rule **in** a diagnosis: **SPIN**.

Highly **sen**sitive tests are used to rule **out** a diagnosis: **SNOUT**.

Likelihood Ratio of Positive Test

The LR+ compares the probability of a positive test result when the disease is present (sensitivity) to the probability of a positive test result in those without the disease (false positive error rate). Essentially, LR+ is the ratio of sensitivity to the false positive error rate. The formula using a 2 × 2 contingency table is: LR+ = sensitivity / (1 − specificity) = (a / (a + c)) / (b / (b + d)).

Likelihood Ratio of Negative Test

The LR− compares the probability of a negative test result in a person with the disease (false negative error rate) to the probability of a negative test result in someone without the disease (specificity). The formula using a 2 × 2 contingency table is: LR− = (1 − sensitivity) / specificity = (c / (a + c)) / (d / (b + d)).

Calculation of Post-Test Probability from Pre-Test Probability

Step 1: Convert Pre-Test Probability to Pre-Test Odds

$$\text{Odds} = \frac{\text{Probability}}{1 - \text{probability}}$$

Step 2: Calculate Post-Test Odds

Post-test odds = LR+ × Pre-test odds

Step 3: Convert Post-Test Odds to Post-Test Probability

$$\text{Probability (post-test)} = \frac{\text{Odds (post-test)}}{1 + \text{Odds (post-test)}}$$

Key Considerations When Selecting a Cut-Off

Clinical Consequences of False Positives vs False Negatives

If missing the disease is dangerous (e.g. cancer, sepsis, myocardial infarction), higher sensitivity (lower cut-off) is preferred. If false positives lead to unnecessary interventions (e.g. invasive procedures), higher specificity (higher cut-off) is preferred.

Prevalence of Disease in the Population

In a high-prevalence setting, a higher cut-off may reduce false positives. In a low-prevalence setting, a lower cut-off improves early disease detection.

Receiver Operating Characteristic Curve

An ROC curve plots sensitivity (vertical axis) versus 1 – specificity (horizontal axis) across all possible cut-off points. The best cut-off point is closest to the upper-left corner, representing a sensitivity of 100% and a false positive error rate of 0%.

Biases in Diagnostic Studies

Spectrum bias arises when a study population includes only 'clear' or 'definite' cases of the disease and 'clear' healthy controls, thereby not representing the full spectrum of disease presentation.

Purity diagnostic bias, also known as comorbidity bias, occurs when researchers exclude patients with comorbidities from the study population.

Lead-time bias occurs when early detection of a disease (through screening) gives the false impression of improved survival, while in reality it only increases the time a patient is aware of their diagnosis without changing the actual disease course.

Length bias occurs when screening is more likely to detect slower-growing, less aggressive diseases, giving the illusion of increased screening effectiveness.

Validity

Validity refers to the degree to which a test accurately measures what it is intended to measure.

Logical validity refers to non-statistical judgements about whether a test appears meaningful and appropriate based on theory and expert opinion. It has two further subtypes:

- Face validity: whether the test looks as if it measures what it claims to measure at face value (superficial judgement).
- Content validity: whether the test fully covers all aspects of the concept being measured.

Statistical validity relies on quantitative or statistical evidence to prove accuracy. It has two subtypes:

- Concurrent validity: whether the test agrees with another established or previously validated test measuring the same concept.
- Predictive validity: whether the test accurately predicts future outcomes.

Construct validity refers to the extent to which a test accurately measures the theoretical concept (construct) it claims to measure. It is divided into two subtypes:

- Convergent validity: measures whether a test correlates well with other tests that measure the same construct. Measures of the same construct (or very similar constructs) should converge or correlate highly with each other.

- Divergent validity (discriminant validity): measures that theoretically should not be related to each other are observed to not be related to each other in the test – that is, ability to discriminate between dissimilar constructs.

Reliability

Reliability refers to the consistency and stability of a measurement over time, across different raters, and in different conditions.

Test–retest reliability measures whether a test yields similar results when given to the same person at different points in time.

Inter-rater reliability measures the degree of agreement between different observers or clinicians using the same test.

Parallel-forms reliability measures whether different versions of the same test give similar results.

Internal consistency measures how closely related the items in a test are. Cronbach's alpha (α) is a statistic used to measure internal consistency; values above 0.7 are generally considered to indicate good reliability. Split-half reliability is another method of testing internal consistency, where a test is divided into two halves and the consistency of results across the two halves is compared.

Practice Questions

For Q1–Q4: A woman is concerned about her risk of diabetes and decides to take a home glucose tolerance test (GTT). The product brochure for the test provides the data shown in Table 4.12.

Table 4.12 2 × 2 contingency table for home GTT in diabetes screening

True disease	Home GTT positive	Home GTT negative	Total
Diabetes present	150	30	180
Diabetes absent	20	200	220
Total	170	230	400

Q1. If the test indicates diabetes, what is the probability that she truly has diabetes?

A. 13%
B. 83%
C. 87%
D. 88%
E. 90%

Q2. If the test indicates no diabetes, what is the probability that she truly does not have diabetes?

A. 13%
B. 83%
C. 87%

D. 88%
E. 90%

Q3. If she truly has diabetes, what is the probability that the test will detect it?
A. 13%
B. 83%
C. 87%
D. 88%
E. 90%

Q4. Why might the test results not be applicable to her specific situation?
A. The false positive error rate of the test is high.
B. The prevalence of diabetes in the population tested is unknown.
C. The prevalence of diabetes in the tested population may not match her prior probability.
D. The test sensitivity is unknown.
E. The test specificity is unknown.

Q5. Pre-test odds of a disease are 1:4. A diagnostic test with a sensitivity of 80% and a specificity of 90% is performed and returns a positive result. What are the post-test odds of the disease?
A. 1:1
B. 2:1
C. 4:1
D. 8:1
E. 1:4

Q6. A patient has a 20% pre-test probability of having a particular infection. The test used has a sensitivity of 95% and a specificity of 85%. If the test is positive, what is the probability that the patient truly has the infection?
A. 51%
B. 61%
C. 71%
D. 81%
E. 91%

For Q7–Q11: A new test for adult ASD screening was developed and applied to 200 subjects. According to the 'gold standard' Autism Diagnostic Interview (ADI-R), 20 of the 200 subjects had ASD. The new test detected 12 cases of ASD, of which 8 were true positives according to the 'gold standard', while 4 were false positives.

Q7. What is the sensitivity of the new test?
A. 40%
B. 60%
C. 67%
D. 94%
E. 98%

Q8. What is the specificity of the new test?

A. 40%
B. 60%
C. 67%
D. 94%
E. 98%

Q9. What is the PPV of the new data?

A. 40%
B. 60%
C. 67%
D. 94%
E. 98%

Q10. What is the NPV of the new test?

A. 40%
B. 60%
C. 67%
D. 94%
E. 98%

Q11. What is the LR+ of the new data?

A. 2
B. 8
C. 18
D. 30
E. 40

For Q12–Q13: Assume that the sensitivity and specificity of the new adult ASD screening test from the previous example remain unchanged. However, this time the test is applied to a different population, in which a diagnostic reference standard (e.g. DISCO) identified 150 out of 200 individuals as having adult ASD.

Q12. What is the PPV of the new adult ASD screening test in this population?

A. 35%
B. 40%
C. 60%
D. 75%
E. 98%

Q13. What is the NPV of the new adult ASD screening test in this population?

A. 35%
B. 40%
C. 60%
D. 75%
E. 98%

For Q14–Q16: A principal of a school with 1,000 students wishes to screen the students for dyslexia. He finds a screening test in the literature that can detect dyslexia with a sensitivity of 94% and a specificity of 90%. The prevalence of dyslexia in the student population is estimated to be 5%.

Q14. What percentage of positive screening test results would be false positives if the test is implemented?

A. 10%
B. 35%
C. 67%
D. 90%
E. 99%

Q15. What would be the PPV of the screening test if it is implemented?

A. 10%
B. 33%
C. 67%
D. 90%
E. 99%

Q16. How many cases of dyslexia would be missed if 1,000 children were screened?

A. 3
B. 47
C. 95
D. 760
E. 855

Q17. The prevalence of a certain disease in the population is 5%. A diagnostic test for this disease has a sensitivity of 90% and a specificity of 95%. If a person tests positive, what is the post-test probability that they actually have the disease?

A. 24%
B. 49%
C. 64%
D. 70%
E. 94%

Q18. The short, dotted curve in Figure 4.5 represents subjects with the disease, while the tall, solid curve represents subjects without the disease. The cut-off point (indicated by the arrow) is used to classify individuals as positive or negative based on test results. If the cut-off is moved to the right, which of the following will decrease?

A. PPV
B. Area under the ROC curve
C. False positive error rate
D. True negative rate
E. False negative error rate

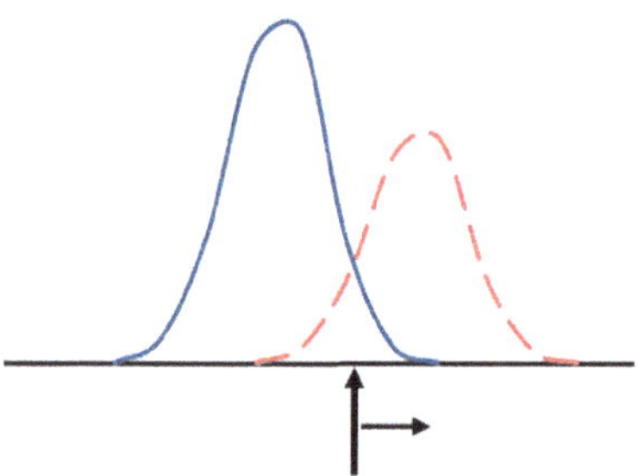

Figure 4.5 Overlapping distributions of test results in two populations, with a cut-off point used for classification.

Q19. The short, dotted curve in Figure 4.6 represents subjects with the disease, while the tall, solid curve represents subjects without the disease. The cut-off point (indicated by the arrow) is used to classify individuals as positive or negative based on test results. If the cut-off is moved to the left, which of the following will decrease?

A. NPV
B. Sensitivity
C. False positive rate
D. PPV
E. True positive rate

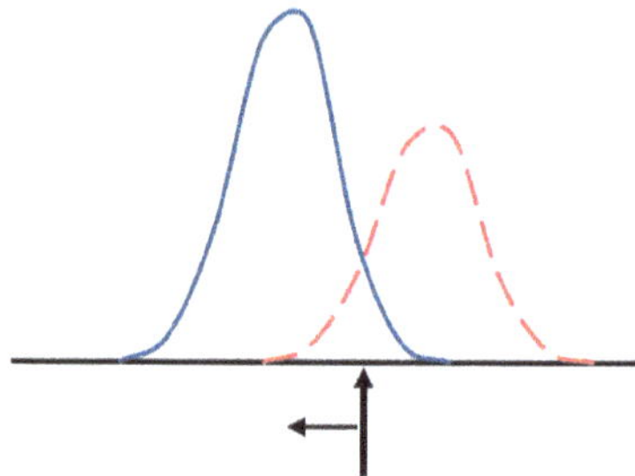

Figure 4.6 Overlapping distributions of test results in two populations, with a cut-off point used for classification.

Q20. A researcher develops a new anxiety questionnaire that only assesses cognitive symptoms of anxiety (e.g. excessive worry, rumination) but does not measure physiological symptoms such as increased heart rate or muscle tension. What type of validity is most likely compromised?

A. Predictive validity
B. Construct validity
C. Content validity
D. Face validity
E. Convergent validity

Q21. A research team develops a new anxiety questionnaire and finds that its scores strongly correlate with scores from an already well-established anxiety scale when administered to the same group at the same time. This demonstrates which type of validity?

A. Face validity
B. Concurrent validity
C. Predictive validity
D. Construct validity
E. Content validity

Answers

Q1. Correct answer: D. 88%. This is the PPV.

- PPV = true positives / total positive results *or* $\frac{a}{a+b}$
- PPV = 150 / 170 = 0.88 = 88%

Q2. Correct answer: C. 87%. This is the NPV.

- NPV = true negatives / total negative results *or* $\frac{d}{c+d}$
- NPV = 200 / 230 = 0.87 = 87%

Q3. Correct answer: B. 83%. This is the sensitivity of the test.

- Sensitivity = true positives / total diabetic *or* $\frac{a}{a+c}$
- Sensitivity = 150 / 180 = 0.83 = 83%

Q4. Correct answer: C. The most relevant reason is that the prevalence in the population tested may not match her prior probability. Predictive values (PPV and NPV) are influenced by the prevalence of the condition in the tested population.

Q5. Correct answer: B. 2:1.

- Pre-test odds = 1:4 = 0.25
- LR+ = Sensitivity / (1 – specificity) = 0.80 / 0.10 = 8
- Post-test odds = Pre-test odds × LR+ = 0.25 × 8 = 2 = 2:1

Q6. Correct answer: B. 61%.

- Pre-test probability = 20% = 0.20
- Pre-test odds = 0.20 / (1 – 0.20) = 0.25
- LR+ = 0.95 / (1 – 0.85) = 6.33
- Post-test odds = 0.25 × 6.33 = 1.58
- Probability = 1.58 / (1 + 1.58) = 0.61 ≈ 61%

Q7. Correct answer: A. 40%. The 2 × 2 contingency table for this would be as shown in Table 4.13.

Table 4.13 2 × 2 contingency table for new adult ASD screening test versus gold standard (ADI-R)

New test	DISCO positive	DISCO negative	Total
New test positive	8	4	12
New test negative	12	176	188
Total	20	180	200

A total of 20 cases tested positive with the gold standard. Of these, 8 tested positive with the new adult ASD screening test.

Sensitivity $= \frac{a}{a+c} = \frac{8}{20} = 40\%$.

Q8. Correct answer: E. 98%. Specificity can be calculated from the table provided in the answer to Q7. Of the 180 individuals who tested negative according to the gold standard, 176 were correctly identified as negative by the new test.

$$\text{Specificity} = \frac{d}{c+d} = \frac{176}{180} = 98\%.$$

Q9. Correct answer: C. 67%. The PPV can be calculated from the table provided in the answer to Q7. Of the 12 cases identified as positive by the new test, 8 were confirmed as positive by the gold standard.

$$\text{PPV} = \frac{a}{a+b} = \frac{8}{12} = 67\%.$$

Q10. Correct answer: D. 94%. The NPV can be calculated from the table provided in the explanation for Q7. Of the 188 individuals who tested negative with the new test, 176 were confirmed as negative by the gold standard.

$$\text{NPV} = \frac{d}{c+d} = \frac{176}{188} = 94\%.$$

Q11. Correct answer: C. 18. The LR+ can be calculated from the table provided in the explanation for Q7 using one of the formulas for LR+. An example calculation is:

$$\text{Sensitivity} = \frac{a}{a+c} = \frac{8}{20} = 0.40,$$

$$\text{Specificity} = \frac{d}{b+d} = \frac{176}{180} = 0.9777,$$

$$\text{LR+} = \frac{\text{Sensitivity}}{1-\text{Specificity}} = \frac{0.40}{1-0.9777} = 18.$$

Q12. Correct answer: E. 98%. The sensitivity and specificity of the test remain constant, but predictive values change with variations in the prevalence of the disease within the population. The new test is now applied to a population with a higher prevalence of adult ASD, as indicated by a diagnostic reference standard (e.g. DISCO). The new diagnostic reference standard identified 150 cases of adult ASD out of 200 tested individuals.

- DISCO positive $(a + c)$: 150
- DISCO negative $(b + d)$: 200 – 150 = 50.

From Table 4.13 we know:

- sensitivity = 40% (0.4)
- specificity = 98% (0.98).

Filling the 2 × 2 contingency table:

1. Calculate cell (a): sensitivity × $(a + c)$ = 0.4 × 150 = 60
2. Calculate cell (c): $(a + c) - a$ = 150 – 60 = 90
3. Calculate cell (d): specificity × $(b + d)$ = 0.98 × 50 = 49
4. Calculate cell (b): $(b + d) - d$ = 50 – 49 = 1

Table 4.14 shows the new 2 × 2 contingency table.

Table 4.14 2 × 2 contingency table for new adult ASD screening test applied in a different population (ASQ as gold standard)

New test	ASQ positive	ASQ negative	Total
New test positive	60 (*a*)	1 (*b*)	61
New test negative	90 (*c*)	49 (*d*)	139
Total	150 (*a* + *c*)	50 (*b* + *d*)	200

From this table, the PPV can be calculated: PPV $= \frac{a}{a+b} = \frac{60}{61} = 98\%$.

Q13. Correct answer: A. 35%. The NPV can be calculated using the constructed table from Q12:

$$\text{NPV} = \frac{d}{c+d} = \frac{49}{139} = 35\%.$$

Q14. Correct answer: C. 67%. We can construct a 2 × 2 contingency table using the given data. The test is applied to 1,000 students with a dyslexia prevalence of 5%, which means:

- Cell $(a + c)$ = 50 (true positive + false negative)
- Cell $(b + d)$ = 1,000 – 50 = 950 (true negative + false positive)

Sensitivity of the screening test: 94%.

- Calculate cell (a): 0.94 × 50 = 47

Specificity of the screening test: 90%

- Calculate cell (d): 0.90 × 950 = 855
- Calculate cell (c): 50–47 = 3
- Calculate cell (b): 950–855 = 95

A 2 ×2 table can be constructed from these values as given in table 4.15.

Table 4.15 2 × 2 contingency table for dyslexia screening in a school population

Screening test	Disease present	Disease absent	Total
Screening test positive	47	95	142
Screening test negative	3	855	858
Total	50	950	1,000

Proportion of positive test results that are false positives $= \frac{b}{a+b} = \frac{95}{47+95} = \frac{95}{142} = 67\%$.

Q15. Correct answer: B. 33%. The PPV can be calculated using the 2 × 2 contingency table constructed for Q14:

$$\text{PPV} = \frac{a}{a+b} = \frac{47}{142} = 33\%.$$

Q16. Correct answer: A. 3. Out of the 50 cases of dyslexia, the test, with a sensitivity of 94%, would detect 47 cases:

47 = 0.94 × 50.

The remaining cases that are not detected by the test are the false negative cases:

False negatives = (1 – sensitivity) × prevalence = (1 – 0.94) × 50 = 0.06 × 50 = 3

The three cases represent the false negatives (cell (c) in the table).

Q17. Correct answer: B. 49%.

1. Convert prevalence to pre-test probability: prevalence = 5% = 0.05.
2. Calculate pre-test odds:
   - Pre-test odds = prevalence / (1 – prevalence)
   - Pre-test odds = 0.05 / 0.95 = 0.053.
3. Calculate LR+:
   - LR+ = sensitivity / (1 – specificity)
   - LR+ = 0.90 / (1 – 0.95) = 18.
4. Calculate post-test odds:
   - Post-test odds = pre-test odds × LR+
   - Post-test odds = 0.053 × 18 = 0.954.
5. Convert post-test odds to probability:
   - Post-test probability = post-test odds / (1 + post-test odds)
   - Post-test probability = 0.954 / (1 + 0.954) = 0.49 = 49%.

Q18. Correct answer: C. False positive error rate decreases. The false positive rate (type I error) is the proportion of healthy individuals wrongly classified as diseased: False positive rate $= \frac{FP}{FP + TN}$.

Since moving the cut-off to the right reduces FP, the false positive error rate decreases. The effect of moving the cut-off to the right in the given distribution is:

- FP decrease: fewer healthy individuals are misclassified as diseased.
- FN increase: more diseased individuals are misclassified as healthy.
- TN increase: more healthy individuals are correctly classified.
- TP decrease: fewer diseased individuals are correctly identified.
- PPV generally increases: the proportion of correctly identified positives among all positives improves because FP decreases at a faster rate than TP.

Explanation of the other answer choices:

A. PPV increases, not decreases. PPV is the proportion of true positives among all positives: PPV $= \frac{TP}{TP + FP}$. Since FP decreases faster than TP, the ratio of TP to (TP + FP) improves, leading to an increase in PPV.

B. AUC does not change. Moving the threshold only affects sensitivity and specificity but does not change the AUC, which is an inherent measure of test performance.

D. True negative rate (specificity) increases, not decreases. Specificity (true negative rate) $= \frac{TN}{TN + FP}$. Since FP decreases, specificity increases, meaning it does not decrease.

E. False negative error rate increases, not decreases. False negative rate is the proportion of diseased individuals wrongly classified as negative. False negative rate $= \frac{FN}{FN + TP}$. Since more diseased individuals are misclassified as negative, false negative rate increases, not decreases.

Q19. Correct answer: D. PPV decreases. PPV decreases because

$$PPV = \frac{TP}{TP + FP}.$$

The effects of moving the cut-off left are:

- More individuals are classified as positive (increasing TP and FP).
- However, FP increase at a higher rate than TP.
- Since FP is in the denominator, this reduces the proportion of TP among all positives.
- As a result, PPV decreases.

Explanation of the other answer choices:

A. NPV is incorrect because NPV increases: NPV $= \frac{TN}{TN + FN}$. The effect of moving the cut-off left is: FN decreases, meaning more diseased individuals are correctly identified; TN stays the same or decrease slightly. The effect on NPV is not fixed and depends on prevalence and how TN and FN change.

B. Sensitivity (true positive rate) is incorrect because sensitivity increases. Sensitivity $= \frac{TP}{TP + FN}$. The effect of moving the cut-off left is: more TP are detected (fewer diseased individuals are misclassified as negative); FN decreases. Since TP is in the numerator, as TP increases, sensitivity increases.
C. False positive rate is incorrect because it increases. False positive rate $= \frac{FP}{FP + TN}$. The effect of moving the cut-off left is: more healthy individuals are misclassified as positive; FP increases. Since FP is in the numerator, as FP increases, the FP rate increases.
E. True positive rate (sensitivity) is incorrect because it is the same option as B.

Q20. Correct answer: C. Content validity. Content validity refers to whether a test covers all relevant aspects of the concept it is measuring. In this case, the anxiety questionnaire fails to include physiological symptoms, making it incomplete and reducing its content validity.

Why other options are incorrect:

A. Predictive validity: incorrect because predictive validity refers to whether the test can accurately predict future outcomes (e.g. whether a high score on the anxiety test predicts future clinical diagnosis of anxiety).
B. Construct validity: incorrect because construct validity refers to whether a test measures the theoretical concept it claims to measure. While related, the issue here is not measuring all relevant components, rather than incorrectly measuring anxiety itself.
D. Face validity: incorrect because face validity is about whether a test appears to measure what it claims to measure at first glance. A test can have high face validity but poor content validity if it looks valid but lacks key aspects.
E. Convergent validity: incorrect because convergent validity assesses whether the test correlates well with other established measures of the same construct. The question does not mention comparisons with other tests.

Q21. Correct answer: B. Concurrent validity. Concurrent validity refers to how well a new test correlates with an established test that measures the same construct when both are administered at the same time. Since the new anxiety questionnaire is being compared to a well-established one, this is an example of concurrent validity.

Why other options are incorrect:

A. Face validity: this refers to whether a test appears to measure what it claims to measure, based on subjective judgement, rather than statistical comparison.
C. Predictive validity: this measures how well a test predicts future outcomes, which is not the case here.
D. Construct validity: while related, construct validity is broader and assesses whether a test truly measures the theoretical concept over time, rather than comparing two tests at the same time.
E. Content validity: this refers to whether a test covers all aspects of a concept, rather than how it correlates with another test.

Further Reading

Altman DG, Bland JM. Diagnostic tests 1: sensitivity and specificity. *BMJ*. 1994; **308**(6943):1552. doi: https://doi.org/10.1136/bmj.308.6943.1552.

Altman DG, Bland JM. Diagnostic tests 3: receiver operating characteristic plots. *BMJ*. 1994; **309**(6948):188. doi: https://doi.org/10.1136/bmj.309.6948.188.

Bossuyt PM, Reitsma JB, Bruns DE, et al. STARD 2015: an updated list of essential items for reporting diagnostic accuracy studies. *BMJ*. 2015; **351**:h5527. doi: https://doi.org/10.1136/bmj.h5527.

Cronbach LJ. Coefficient alpha and the internal structure of tests. *Psychometrika*. 1951; **16**(3):297–334. doi: https://doi.org/10.1007/BF02310555.

Deeks JJ, Altman DG. Diagnostic tests 4: likelihood ratios. *BMJ*. 2004; **329**(7458):168–9. doi: https://doi.org/10.1136/bmj.329.7458.168.

Fagan TJ. Letter: Nomogram for Bayes's theorem. *N Engl J Med*. 1975; **293**(5):257. doi: https://doi.org/10.1056/NEJM197507312930513.

Hanley JA, McNeil BJ. The meaning and use of the area under a ROC curve. *Radiology*. 1982; **143**(1):29–36. doi: https://doi.org/10.1148/radiology.143.1.7063747.

Jaeschke R, Guyatt GH, Sackett DL. Users' guides to the medical literature. III. How to use an article about a diagnostic test. A. Are the results of the study valid? *JAMA*. 1994; **271**(5):389–91. doi: https://doi.org/10.1001/jama.271.5.389.

Jaeschke R, Guyatt GH, Sackett DL. Users' guides to the medical literature. III. How to use an article about a diagnostic test. B. What are the results and will they help me in caring for my patients? *JAMA*. 1994; **271**(9):703–7. doi: https://doi.org/10.1001/jama.271.9.703.

Kuder GF, Richardson MW. The theory of the estimation of test reliability. *Psychometrika*. 1937; **2**(3):151–60. doi: https://doi.org/10.1007/BF02288391.

Pepe MS. *The Statistical Evaluation of Medical Tests for Classification and Prediction*. Oxford: Oxford University Press; 2003.

Ransohoff DF, Feinstein AR. Problems of spectrum and bias in evaluating the efficacy of diagnostic tests. *N Engl J Med*. 1978; **299**(17):926–30. doi: https://doi.org/10.1056/NEJM197810262991705.

Streiner DL, Norman GR, Cairney J. *Health Measurement Scales: A Practical Guide to Their Development and Use*. 5th ed. Oxford: Oxford University Press; 2015.

Youden WJ. Index for rating diagnostic tests. *Cancer*. 1950; **3**(1):32–35. doi: https://doi.org/10.1002/1097-0142(1950)3:1<32::AID-CNCR2820030106>3.0.CO;2-3.

Zweig MH, Campbell G. Receiver-operating characteristic (ROC) plots: a fundamental evaluation tool in clinical medicine. *Clin Chem*. 1993; **39**(4):561–77.

Chapter 5

Cohort Studies

Definition of a Cohort

A cohort is a group of individuals who share a common characteristic or experience and are followed over time. Cohorts are frequently used in research to observe outcomes within specific populations. There are different types of cohorts.

Birth Cohort

A birth cohort consists of individuals born within a specific geographic area during a defined period, typically a year. For example, the 1980 birth cohort includes all individuals born in 1980 within a particular region.

Inception Cohort

An inception cohort is defined based on a specific event, such as employment, geographic relocation, or enrolment in a particular programme. For example, all new employees at a company in 2023 could be considered an inception cohort.

Exposure Cohort

An exposure cohort consists of individuals who share exposure to a specific risk factor or environmental condition. For example, a group of individuals who experienced childhood trauma within a particular timeframe, allowing researchers to study that trauma's long-term effects.

Cohort Studies

Cohort studies involve the observation of a cohort (or cohorts) over time to assess outcomes. These studies, often referred to as longitudinal studies or follow-up studies, start with risk factors (exposures) and track participants forwards to observe outcomes. This contrasts with case–control studies, which begin with outcomes and work backwards to identify exposures. Cohort studies are classified into two main types.

Descriptive Cohort Studies

Descriptive cohort studies track a single group without a comparison group. They focus on incidence rates, disease progression, and natural history. Examples are:

- **The Framingham Heart Study (1948, USA)**, which tracked cardiovascular risk factors over decades.

- **The National Child Development Study (1958, UK)**, which followed individuals born in a single week in 1958 to assess lifelong development.

Analytic Cohort Studies

Analytic cohort studies involve comparisons between two or multiple groups to identify associations between exposure and disease. They can be further categorized based on the type of control group used.

Cohort Study with Internal Control

In this design, the control group is drawn from the same cohort as the exposed group. For example, the 1951 British Doctors Study on Smoking included two groups:

- exposed group: doctors who smoked
- control group: doctors who did not smoke.

The study established a strong link between smoking and mortality, particularly lung cancer.

Cohort Study with External Control

In this design, the control group is from a separate population. For example, the 1976 Mortality in Asbestos Workers Study included:

- exposure group: shipbuilders and insulation workers exposed to asbestos
- control group: textile factory workers not exposed to asbestos.

The study found higher mortality from mesothelioma in the asbestos-exposed cohort.

Types of Cohort Studies Based on Timing

Prospective (Classical) Cohort Studies

Prospective cohort studies select exposed and unexposed groups *before the outcome occurs* and follow them over time. Key characteristics are:

- Outcomes occur after study initiation.
- They are useful for establishing temporal relationships between exposure and disease.

Retrospective Cohort Studies

Retrospective cohort studies analyse past records to compare outcomes between exposed and unexposed individuals. Unlike prospective studies, both exposures and outcomes have already occurred by the time the study begins. Researchers identify exposure and control groups using pre-existing data sources (e.g. medical records, registries, or databases) to examine the relationship between exposures and outcomes. Despite being retrospective, the study remains a cohort study because it starts with exposed and unexposed groups, rather than with cases and controls.

Example Retrospective Cohort Study

A study investigating the association between perinatal complications and schizophrenia:

- Researchers review birth records from decades ago to identify individuals who experienced perinatal events (exposed group) and those who did not (non-exposed group).

- They then assess the current incidence of schizophrenia in both groups.
- This allows them to evaluate whether early-life complications are linked to later psychiatric outcomes.

Advantages of Retrospective over Prospective Cohort Studies

- **Time-efficient:** uses pre-existing data, eliminating the need for long-term follow-ups.
- **Cost-effective:** avoids the costs associated with participant recruitment and continuous monitoring.

Key Difference from Case–Control Studies

- Cohort studies start with exposure groups (exposed vs unexposed).
- Case–control studies start with outcome groups (cases vs controls).

Ambispective Cohort Studies

Ambispective studies combine retrospective and prospective elements:

- **Retrospective arm** uses past records to identify exposures.
- **Prospective arm** follows participants into the future for additional outcomes.

Analytic Cohort Study Design

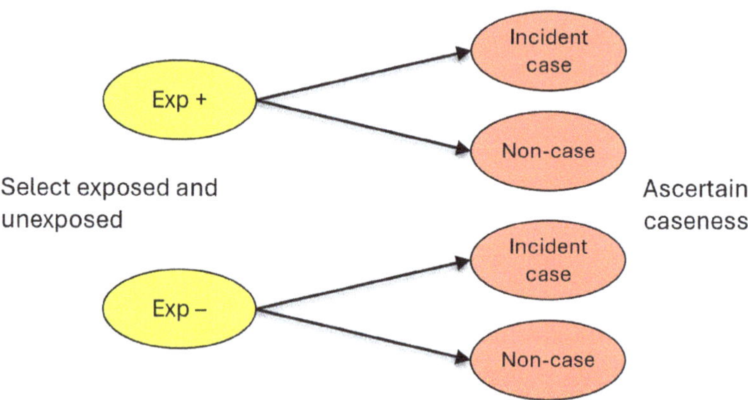

Figure 5.1 Design of an analytic cohort study.

Figure 5.1 illustrates the design of an analytic cohort study.

In this study design, the control group should be as similar as possible to the exposed group in all factors, except for the exposure or risk factor being studied. This ensures comparability and minimizes potential confounding variables.

It is crucial to clearly define both the exposure and the outcome before initiating the study. Specific criteria must be established for what constitutes exposure (e.g. smoking status, occupational exposure) and outcome measures (e.g. clinical diagnosis of depression).

Data collection methods must be decided before the study begins to ensure consistency and reduce bias. Exposure data can be collected through:

- **reviewing records** such as medical records, employment files, or historical data
- **interviewing participants** using structured questionnaires or validated tools
- **clinical examinations** directly assessing exposure status, when appropriate.

Classical cohort studies are often longitudinal, sometimes spanning years or decades. It is important to consider changes in exposure status over time. For example, participants who were smokers at baseline may quit smoking during the study period, potentially altering the exposure classification.

Outcome assessment should be standardized and reliable, using appropriate tools or diagnostic criteria such as rating scales or international diagnostic criteria (e.g. ICD-10, DSM-5).

To preserve data quality, researchers must:

- monitor changes in exposure status regularly
- minimize loss to follow-up, which can bias the results
- ensure consistent data collection methods throughout the study period.

Dropouts in cohort studies occur due to migration, refusal to continue, or death. Researchers should implement strategies to minimize dropouts, such as flagging potential dropouts early and making multiple attempts to maintain contact. At the completion of the study, it is crucial to assess the impact of dropouts on study results, as significant dropout rates may introduce bias and affect the validity of findings.

Measuring the Strength of Association in Cohort Studies

In cohort studies, the strength of association between an exposure and an outcome is typically measured using **relative risk (RR)**[1] and when time-to-event data are analysed, **hazard ratio (HR)**.[2] These measures help quantify how strongly an exposure is associated with development of an outcome.

Relative Risk

Relative risk is a measure used in cohort studies to quantify the strength of association between an exposure and an outcome. It is intuitive and directly answers the research question. For example, RR of 2.0 means that exposure doubles the risk, which is considered as moderate association. The formula for RR is:

$$\text{Relative risk} = \frac{\text{Incidence in the exposed group}}{\text{Incidence in the non-exposed group.}}$$

Step-by-Step Calculation for Relative Risk

1. Construct a 2 × 2 table, as shown in Table 5.1.

---

[1] **Relative risk (RR):** The ratio of risk in the exposed group to that in the unexposed group. Values > 1 indicate increased risk; values < 1 indicate protection.

[2] **Hazard ratio (HR):** Ratio of instantaneous event rates between groups among those still at risk; HR = 1 no difference, >1 higher hazard in the numerator group; typically estimated with a Cox model (assumes proportional hazards).

Table 5.1 Structure of a 2 × 2 table for calculating relative risk in cohort studies

Group	Outcome present	Outcome absent	Total
Exposed	a	b	$a + b$
Not exposed	c	d	$c + d$

a, number of exposed individuals with the outcome; *b*, number of exposed individuals without the outcome; *c*, number of unexposed individuals with the outcome; *d*, number of unexposed individuals without the outcome.

2. Calculate the incidence in exposed group:
   Incidence of outcome in exposed group = $\frac{a}{a+b}$.
3. Calculate the incidence in unexposed group:
   Incidence of outcome in unexposed group = $\frac{c}{c+d}$.
4. Calculate the relative risk:

$$\mathrm{RR} = \frac{\text{Incidence in exposed group}}{\text{Incidence in unexposed group}} = \frac{\frac{a}{a+b}}{\frac{c}{c+d}}.$$

Interpretation

Relative risk can be interpreted as follows:

RR = 1: indicates no association between exposure and outcome.

RR > 1: shows a positive association, meaning the exposure increases the risk of the outcome.

RR < 1: reflects a negative association, where the exposure decreases the risk of the outcome.

Hazard Ratio

Hazard ratio is a measure often used in survival analysis, particularly when the primary interest is in comparing the time to an event (e.g. death, disease onset, recovery) between two or more groups. The HR formula is:

$$\mathrm{HR} = \lambda_1(t)/\lambda_0(t),$$

where:

- $\lambda_1(t)$ is the HR (risk of the event per unit time) for the exposed or treatment group
- $\lambda_0(t)$ is the HR for the unexposed or control group.

Hazard Ratio Example

Suppose a cohort study examines the time to relapse in patients receiving two different treatments:

- Hazard rate for the treatment group: 0.02 per month
- Hazard rate for the control group: 0.04 per month.

The calculation is:

$$HR = \frac{0.02}{0.04} = 0.5.$$

An HR of 0.5 means the treatment group has half the risk of relapse compared to the control group, indicating a protective effect of the treatment.

Strengths and Limitations of Cohort Studies

Strengths

- Good for studying rare exposures.
- Can study multiple disease outcomes.
- Includes prospective elements such as:
  - assessing direction of causality
  - distinguishing incidence from maintenance
  - reducing selection and information bias compared to case–control studies.
- Provides direct estimates of **absolute risk difference** in exposed and unexposed groups.[3]
- Enables calculation of incidence rates and relative risk.
- Can establish a temporal relationship between exposure and outcome, which strengthens causal inference.

Limitations

- Inefficient for rare outcomes, requiring large sample sizes and being relatively expensive to conduct.
- Primarily suited for single exposure studies (classical design).
- Risk of loss to follow-up is a major problem, leading to potential bias.
- Difficult for long-term follow-up when the latency period for the outcome is long.
- Time-consuming and expensive.
- The exposure status of participants may change during the study.

Critical Appraisal of Cohort Studies

Loss to follow-up is a significant challenge in classical cohort studies, as they are often long-term studies, increasing the risk of participant dropout over time.

Key Considerations for Critical Appraisal

- Assess dropout rates: a high dropout rate threatens validity.
- Evaluate bias from attrition: dropouts can introduce selection bias, making results less representative.

[3] **Absolute risk difference (ARD):** Also known as *attributable risk*, this is the numerical difference between the risk of an outcome in an exposed group compared to an unexposed group. It measures the actual change in risk – such as the number of additional cases of a disease – that can be directly attributed to a specific exposure. It is calculated as ARD = risk exposed – risk unexposed.

- Assess methods to manage missing data: did researchers use imputation techniques or make reasonable adjustments for missing data?
- Determine whether follow-up efforts were sufficient: strong cohort studies implement multiple attempts to contact participants and minimize loss.
- A thorough critical appraisal should assess how researchers managed dropouts and whether the study accounted for potential biases introduced by attrition.

Chapter Summary

Cohort

A cohort is a group of individuals who share a common characteristic or trait and move forward together as a unit. Cohorts are widely used in research to observe outcomes over time. Common types of cohorts include:

- Inception cohort: individuals assembled based on a particular factor, such as location or employment.
- Birth cohort: a group born within a specific geographic area during a defined time period, such as all individuals born in 1990.
- Exposure cohort: individuals who share a common exposure, such as a group exposed to a specific environmental factor.

Cohort Studies

Cohort studies involve the systematic observation of a cohort (or cohorts) over time to measure outcomes. The key distinction of cohort studies is that they start with risk factors (exposures) and observe outcomes over time, in contrast to case–control studies, which start with outcomes and look back for risk factors.

Types of Cohort Studies

Descriptive Cohort Studies

- Descriptive cohort studies involve a single group and focus on measuring frequencies and incidence rates of diseases over time or simply describing the natural history of diseases.
- These studies provide baseline data and insights into the progression of health conditions, but do not include comparative groups.

Analytic Cohort Studies

Analytic cohort studies use double-group or multiple-group comparisons to identify differences in outcomes or diseases between exposed and control groups. These studies can be further categorized into various designs.

Prospective (Classical) Cohort Studies

- In prospective cohort studies, exposed and unexposed groups are identified at the study's start and then followed forward over time to observe differences in outcomes.
- These studies are ideal for assessing temporal relationships, as they monitor participants' health status into the future.

Retrospective Cohort Studies

Retrospective cohort studies examine both exposures and outcomes in the past, using existing data sources such as medical records, registries, or historical datasets. Sometimes investigators go back into the past to identify risk groups and a control group and follow the groups up to the present time to assess what outcomes have occurred. This is a retrospective cohort model.

Although data collection is retrospective, the study design remains cohort in nature because it begins by identifying exposed and unexposed groups and then analyses differences in outcomes between these groups. This approach maintains the prospective logic of starting with exposure status and observing outcome variations, even when looking back into historical data, and also retains the ability to calculate absolute risk difference.

Ambispective Cohort Studies

- Ambispective cohort studies combine prospective and retrospective elements, utilizing historical data to identify exposures and then following participants forward in time to observe outcomes.
- This hybrid approach provides comprehensive insights by leveraging past records while incorporating real-time follow-up.

Analytic Cohort Study Design

Ensure fewer dropouts by maintaining contact with participants, as avoiding loss to follow-up is key to the integrity of the cohort study.

Measuring Strength of Association

$$\text{Relative Risk (RR)} = \frac{\text{Incidence in exposed group}}{\text{Incidence in unexposed group}} = \frac{\frac{a}{a+b}}{\frac{c}{c+d}}.$$

Advantages of Cohort Studies

Cohort studies offer numerous advantages in epidemiological research, including:

- Effectiveness for studying rare exposures: ideal for researching rare risk factors, where enough exposed individuals can be followed over time.
- Ability to study multiple outcomes: allows examination of various disease outcomes related to a single exposure.

  Advantages of prospective studies include:

- Assessing direction of causality: helps determine whether exposure precedes the outcome, establishing causal relationships.
- Distinguishing incidence from maintenance: differentiates between new cases (incidence) and ongoing cases (prevalence).
- Reduction of bias: lower risk of selection and information bias compared to case–control studies, as exposure data is collected before outcomes develop.
- Provides direct estimates of absolute risk difference: calculates the risk of an outcome in exposed and unexposed groups, offering clear insights into public health impacts.

- Enables calculation of incidence rates and relative risk: facilitates quantitative analysis of how strongly an exposure influences the risk of developing an outcome.
- Establishes temporal relationships: by tracking participants over time, cohort studies demonstrate the chronological order of exposure and outcome, which strengthens causal inference.

Pitfalls and Critical Appraisal of Cohort Studies

A key pitfall of cohort studies is the attrition rate or loss to follow-up, which can significantly impact the study's validity. When appraising a cohort study, it is crucial to evaluate the extent of attrition, understand the reasons for dropout, and assess how researchers managed missing data.

Practice Questions

For Q1–Q4: A study is conducted to evaluate the impact of physical activity on the development of depression in adults. Researchers enrolled 1,000 adults and classified them into two groups: those who engage in regular physical activity and those who lead a sedentary lifestyle. The participants were followed for five years, and the results are shown in the 2 × 2 contingency table in Table 5.2.

Table 5.2 Example of a 2 × 2 table from a prospective cohort study on physical activity and depression

Lifestyle	Depression present	Depression absent
Physically active	50 (*a*)	450 (*b*)
Sedentary	100 (*c*)	400 (*d*)

Q1. What type of study design is represented in this scenario?
  A. Case–control study
  B. Cross-sectional study
  C. Prospective cohort study
  D. Randomized controlled trial
  E. Retrospective cohort study

Q2. Which of the following measures of association is most appropriate for this study?
  A. Odds ratio
  B. Hazard ratio
  C. Attributable risk
  D. Relative risk
  E. Prevalence ratio

Q3. What is the relative risk of developing depression among sedentary individuals compared to those who are physically active?
  A. 1.0
  B. 1.5

C. 2.0
D. 2.5
E. 3.0

Q4. Which of the following statements best represents the null hypothesis for this cohort study?
A. Physical activity prevents depression.
B. There is no association between physical activity and depression.
C. A sedentary lifestyle causes depression.
D. Physical activity increases the risk of depression.
E. Depression influences physical activity levels.

Q5. Which of the following scenarios best represents a retrospective cohort study?
A. Comparing patients with and without diabetes for the prevalence of chronic kidney disease at the time of the study.
B. Identifying individuals who were exposed to a contaminated water source five years ago and evaluating the incidence of gastrointestinal cancers in this group.
C. Selecting patients currently diagnosed with colorectal cancer and asking about their history of dietary fibre intake.
D. Randomly assigning healthy adults to receive a new influenza vaccine or placebo and monitoring for flu symptoms over the winter season.
E. Following a group of new-borns for the development of asthma based on their parental history of allergies.

Q6. Which of the following is the most important factor to consider when critically appraising a cohort study?
A. Whether participants were randomly assigned to exposure groups
B. The length of follow-up and completeness of outcome data
C. Whether blinding was used for participants and investigators
D. The use of a placebo to prevent measurement bias
E. The statistical significance (p-value) of the study findings

Q7. Which of the following scenarios best represents a retrospective cohort study?
A. Identifying adults with a diagnosis of major depressive disorder and assessing their childhood history of trauma through interviews.
B. Following a cohort of individuals with schizophrenia who are randomly assigned to either cognitive behavioural therapy (CBT) or standard care and monitoring relapse rates.
C. Selecting a group of adolescents who were prescribed antipsychotic medication five years ago and evaluating the incidence of metabolic syndrome using their medical records.
D. Recruiting patients currently hospitalized for bipolar disorder and comparing their family history of mental illness with healthy controls.
E. Conducting a survey to assess the prevalence of anxiety disorders among university students and correlating it with current academic stress levels.

Q8. Which of the following aspects is crucial for assessing the validity when critically appraising a cohort study?

A. Whether the study used randomization to assign exposures
B. The use of double blinding to prevent bias
C. Whether loss to follow-up was adequately reported and addressed
D. The presence of a control group receiving a placebo
E. The use of crossover design to compare outcomes

Answers

Q1. Correct answer: C. Prospective cohort study. This is a prospective cohort study because participants were classified based on their exposure status (physical activity vs sedentary lifestyle) and followed over five years to measure the development of depression, allowing for calculation of incidence and relative risk. This is not a retrospective cohort study as the outcome was looked at in the future, after five years, rather than back in time.

Q2. Correct answer: D. Relative risk. Relative risk is the appropriate measure of association for cohort studies, as it compares the incidence of depression between the exposed (physically active) and unexposed (sedentary) groups.

Q3. Correct answer: C. 2.0.

- Incidence in physically active group = $a / (a + b) = 50/500 = 0.1$
- Incidence in sedentary group = $c / (c + d) = 100/500 = 0.2$

The relative risk is calculated as:

$$RR = \frac{\text{Incidence in sedentary group}}{\text{Incidence in physically active group}} = \frac{0.2}{0.1} = 2.0.$$

Q4. Correct answer: B. There is no association between physical activity and depression. The null hypothesis in a cohort study states that there is no association between exposure (physical activity) and the outcome (depression).

Q5. Correct answer: B. Identifying individuals who were exposed to a contaminated water source five years ago and evaluating the incidence of gastrointestinal cancers in this group. Option B represents a retrospective cohort study because the study starts with identifying individuals based on a past exposure (contaminated water source) and then assesses the development of an outcome (gastrointestinal cancers) using historical data. Why the other options are wrong:

- A is a cross-sectional study (measuring exposure and outcome simultaneously).
- C is a case–control study, starting with the outcome and looking back at exposure.
- D is a randomized controlled trial (prospective and experimental).
- E represents a prospective cohort study, where exposure is assessed at the start, and outcomes are measured in the future.

Q6. Correct answer: B. The length of follow-up and completeness of outcome data. Option B is correct because, in cohort studies, the length of follow-up is crucial to ensure that enough time has passed to observe the outcomes of interest. Additionally, completeness of outcome data is important to minimize attrition bias and maintain the validity of the study.

Why the other options are wrong:

- A is incorrect because random assignment is a characteristic of randomized controlled trials (RCTs), not cohort studies. In cohort studies, participants are categorized based on natural exposure status rather than randomization.
- C is less relevant to cohort studies, as blinding is more commonly associated with experimental studies (e.g. RCTs) to reduce performance and detection bias.
- D is not applicable to cohort studies, as they do not typically involve the use of a placebo. Instead, they observe natural exposures and outcomes.
- E is important for interpreting study findings, but it is not as critical as assessing follow-up duration and data completeness when appraising study quality. A statistically significant *p*-value does not necessarily imply a study is methodologically sound.

Q7. Correct answer: C. Selecting a group of adolescents who were prescribed antipsychotic medication five years ago and evaluating the incidence of metabolic syndrome using their medical records. Option C represents a retrospective cohort study because it involves identifying a cohort based on past exposure (prescription of antipsychotic medication) and then examining an outcome (development of metabolic syndrome) using existing data (medical records).

Why the other options are wrong:

- A is a case–control study, as it starts with an outcome (depression) and looks back at exposure (childhood trauma).
- B is an RCT (prospective and experimental).
- D is also a case–control study, comparing past exposures in those with and without the outcome.
- E represents a cross-sectional study, assessing exposure and outcome simultaneously.

Q8. Correct answer: C. Whether loss to follow-up was adequately reported and addressed. Option C is correct because loss to follow-up can lead to attrition bias, particularly if the dropout rate is high or not similar between the exposed and unexposed groups. Proper reporting and addressing of loss to follow-up helps maintain the study's internal validity.

Why the other options are wrong:

- A is incorrect because randomization is not a feature of cohort studies; it is characteristic of RCTs. Cohort studies involve natural exposure groups rather than assigned exposure groups.
- B is more relevant to RCTs than cohort studies. While blinding can help reduce bias, it is not typically a core component of cohort studies, which are observational by nature.
- D is not applicable, as cohort studies do not involve placebos. Instead, they focus on observing natural exposures and the subsequent development of outcomes.
- E is characteristic of crossover trials, not cohort studies. Crossover designs involve participants serving as their own controls, which is not a typical approach in cohort studies.

Further Reading

Altman DG, Bland JM. Time to event (survival) data. *BMJ.* 1998;**317**(7156):468–9. doi: https://doi.org/10.1136/bmj.317.7156.468.

Cox DR. Regression models and life-tables. *J R Stat Soc B.* 1972;**34**(2):187–220.

Dawber TR, Meadors GF, Moore FE Jr. Epidemiological approaches to heart disease: the Framingham study. *Am J Public Health.* 1951;**41**(3):279–81. doi: https://doi.org/10.2105/ajph.41.3.279.

Grimes DA, Schulz KF. Cohort studies: marching towards outcomes. *Lancet.* 2002;**359**(9303):341–5. doi: https://doi.org/10.1016/S0140-6736(02)07500-1.

Hernán MA, Robins JM. *Causal Inference: What If.* Boca Raton, FL: Chapman & Hall/CRC; 2020.

Lash TL, VanderWeele TJ, Haneuse S, Rothman KJ. *Modern Epidemiology.* 4th ed. Philadelphia: Wolters Kluwer; 2021.

Pedersen AB, Mikkelsen EM, Cronin-Fenton D, et al. Missing data and multiple imputation in clinical epidemiological research. *Clin Epidemiol.* 2017;**9**:157–66. doi: https://doi.org/10.2147/CLEP.S129785.

Spruance SL, Reid JE, Grace M, Samore M. Hazard ratio in clinical trials. *Antimicrob Agents Chemother.* 2004;**48**(8):2787–92. doi: https://doi.org/10.1128/AAC.48.8.2787-2792.2004.

Szklo M, Nieto FJ. *Epidemiology: Beyond the Basics.* 4th ed. Burlington, MA: Jones & Bartlett Learning; 2019.

von Elm E, Altman DG, Egger M, et al. The STROBE statement: guidelines for reporting observational studies. *PLoS Med.* 2007;**4**(10):e296. doi: https://doi.org/10.1371/journal.pmed.0040296.

Chapter 6

Self-Controlled Case Series Studies

Introduction

The Self-Controlled Case Series (SCCS) is an observational study design used to examine the association between transient exposures (e.g. vaccination, medication) and acute outcomes (e.g. adverse reactions, onset of disease). Unlike traditional case–control or cohort studies, the SCCS approach compares different time periods within the same individual, controlling for between-individual confounding due to fixed characteristics.

This design is particularly useful in pharmacoepidemiology and vaccine safety studies due to its efficiency and ability to control for time-invariant (fixed) confounders such as genetics, sex, lifestyle, and long-term comorbidities.

A suitable application is investigating whether exposure to antipsychotic medication increases the risk of stroke in the elderly population. By analysing periods before, during, and after antipsychotic use, researchers can assess whether the incidence of stroke is higher during the exposed period compared to the unexposed period than during the unexposed period.

Key Components of SCCS Design

Figure 6.1 illustrates the general design of a SCCS study. These studies are particularly useful in the following scenarios.

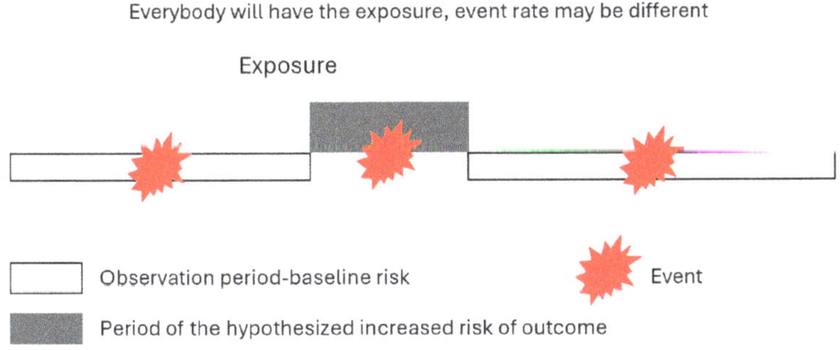

Figure 6.1 Design of a self-controlled case series study.

Sample Selection

- **Inclusion criteria:** only individuals who have experienced the outcome of interest (e.g. stroke, seizure) are included in the study.

- **Exclusion criteria:** individuals who have never experienced the outcome are excluded.
- This makes the SCCS a case-only design, as only individuals who experience the outcome contribute information to the analysis.

Observation Period

The total duration over which individuals are observed for both exposures and outcomes. This period is divided into:

- **Exposed period(s):** time periods when individuals are exposed to the risk factor (e.g. after receiving a vaccine or starting a medication).
- **Unexposed period(s):** time periods when individuals are not exposed to the risk factor.

Exposure

- The exposure must be transient, meaning it occurs for a defined period (e.g. a specific vaccine, medication dose, or short-term infection).
- It should be measurable in time, allowing for precise classification of **exposure windows.**[1]

Outcome

- Typically an acute event (e.g. seizure, allergic reaction, hospitalization).
- The occurrence of the outcome is analysed relative to the timing of exposure.

Analysis

- SCCS models the rate of events during exposed versus unexposed periods within the same individuals.
- **Poisson regression**[2] or other time-dependent statistical models are used to quantify the association.

The primary measure of association is the **incidence rate ratio (IRR).**[3] The IRR is defined as the ratio of the incidence rate of events during exposed periods to the incidence rate during unexposed periods in the same individuals:

$$\text{IRR} = \frac{\text{Event rate during exposed period}}{\text{Event rate during unexposed period}}$$

- **IRR > 1** indicates an *increased risk* during the exposed period.
- **IRR < 1** suggests a *decreased risk* during the exposed period.

---

1 **Exposure window:** A pre-specified period after (or around) exposure when risk may change; define start/length a priori, and consider pre-risk windows to avoid reverse causation.

2 **Poisson regression:** Regression for count data or rates with a log link; in SCCS it is used to estimate the IRR, typically with an offset for time at risk.

3 **Incidence rate ratio (IRR):** The IRR is the event rate during exposed periods divided by the event rate during unexposed periods, within the same individuals; IRR = 1 no difference; >1 higher risk during exposure.

- Key assumptions include that the occurrence of the outcome does not substantially alter the probability of subsequent exposure or censor follow-up time, and that outcome events are independent. The SCCS design may be less suitable for outcomes that are fatal or permanently change exposure status, as this can violate these assumptions.

When Are SCCS Studies Preferable?

Studying Transient Exposures and Acute Events

SCCS is ideal when assessing the association between a short-term exposure and an acute health event. Since individuals serve as their own controls, there is reduced variability caused by individual differences.

Difficulty in Identifying a Suitable Control Group

In certain epidemiological studies, finding an appropriate control group is challenging. For example, in vaccine safety studies it may be difficult to find unvaccinated individuals who are truly comparable to vaccinated individuals in all aspects. SCCS overcomes this challenge by using within-individual comparisons, thus eliminating the need for external controls.

Unclear Population at Risk

In some settings, determining the total population at risk is complex (e.g. tertiary hospitals with poorly defined catchment areas). SCCS allow researchers to bypass this issue by focusing only on individuals who experienced the outcome, rather than estimating incidence rates in a broader population.

Chapter Summary

The SCCS is an observational study design used to assess the association between transient exposures and acute outcomes. Unlike cohort or case–control studies, SCCS compares different time periods within the same individual, eliminating between-individual confounding.

Key Features

- Inclusion: only individuals who have experienced the outcome are included.
- Observation period: divided into exposed (during risk factor exposure) and unexposed periods.
- Analysis: uses the incidence rate ratio to compare event rates in exposed and unexposed periods:
  - IRR > 1: increased risk during exposure.
  - IRR < 1: decreased risk during exposure.

When to Use SCCS

1. To study transient exposures and acute outcomes (e.g. vaccine side effects)
2. when a suitable control group is difficult to find (e.g. vaccine safety studies)
3. when the population at risk is unclear (e.g. hospital-based research).

SCCS is efficient, eliminates fixed confounders, and is widely used in pharmacoepidemiology and vaccine safety studies.

Practice Questions

Q1. Which type of exposure is best suited to an SCCS study?
- A. Chronic exposure lasting several years
- B. Transient exposure occurring at a specific time
- C. Genetic predisposition to a disease
- D. Continuous environmental exposure
- E. Socioeconomic status

Q2. In an SCCS study, what type of event is typically analysed?
- A. Chronic diseases with gradual onset
- B. Acute events with a defined time of occurrence
- C. Long-term behavioural changes
- D. Slowly progressing neurological disorders
- E. Socioeconomic trends over time

Q3. What is the key difference between SCCS and traditional cohort studies?
- A. SCCS uses external control groups, while cohort studies do not.
- B. SCCS compares within-individual changes, while cohort studies compare between individuals.
- C. SCCS requires larger sample sizes than cohort studies.
- D. SCCS cannot be used for vaccine safety research.
- E. SCCS does not account for confounding variables.

Q4. What statistical measure is commonly used in SCCS studies to quantify the association between exposure and outcome?
- A. Relative risk (RR)
- B. Odds ratio (OR)
- C. Incidence rate ratio (IRR)
- D. Hazard ratio (HR)
- E. Standardized mortality ratio (SMR)

Q5. Which of the following is an example of a research question suited for an SCCS study?
- A. Does long-term air pollution exposure increase lung cancer risk?
- B. Does a high-fat diet increase the risk of obesity?
- C. Does vaccination increase the risk of febrile seizures within 14 days post-vaccination?
- D. Does socioeconomic status affect the risk of cardiovascular disease over decades?
- E. Does occupational stress lead to depression in different professions?

Q6. What assumption must hold for SCCS studies to be valid?
- A. The risk of outcome is constant throughout the study.

B. The exposure must be rare in the general population.
C. The occurrence of the outcome does not influence the probability of subsequent exposure.
D. The study must include an equal number of males and females.
E. The study must follow participants for at least 10 years.

Q7. In a self-controlled case series study, which of the following factors typically requires explicit adjustment as a time-varying confounder?
A. Genetic background
B. Sex
C. Socio-economic status
D. Age
E. Ethnicity

Answers

Q1. Correct answer: B. Transient exposure occurring at a specific time. SCCS is best used for short-term (transient) exposures, such as a vaccine dose, medication, or infection, because it allows researchers to examine how the timing of the exposure relates to an acute outcome. Chronic exposures (e.g. long-term pollution) are not ideal for this design as they lack well-defined 'exposed' and 'unexposed' periods.

Q2. Correct answer: B. Acute events with a defined time of occurrence. SCCS is most effective for studying acute events (e.g. seizures, strokes, allergic reactions) that occur shortly after exposure. Chronic conditions (e.g. cancer, diabetes) develop over long periods, making them less suitable for SCCS analysis.

Q3. Correct answer: B. SCCS compares within-individual changes, while cohort studies compare between individuals. In a cohort study, researchers compare exposed and unexposed groups of different people. In contrast, SCCS compares different time periods within the same individuals, which controls for fixed individual confounders.

Q4. Correct answer: C. Incidence rate ratio (IRR). The IRR is the main statistic used in SCCS studies. It compares the rate of events during the exposed period to the rate during the unexposed period. IRR > 1 suggests increased risk, while IRR < 1 suggests reduced risk.

Q5. Correct answer: C. Does vaccination increase the risk of febrile seizures within 14 days post-vaccination? SCCS is best suited for transient exposures (e.g. vaccinations) and acute outcomes (e.g. febrile seizures). The other options involve long-term exposures or chronic diseases, which are not ideal for SCCS.

Q6. Correct answer: C. The occurrence of the outcome does not influence the probability of subsequent exposure. SCCS assumes that the occurrence of the outcome does not influence the probability of subsequent exposure. If experiencing the outcome makes a person more (or less) likely to be exposed again, the SCCS model becomes biased.

Q7. Correct answer: D. Age. In an SCCS study, each individual serves as their own control. This design inherently controls for time-invariant confounders such as genetics, sex, ethnicity, and long-term socioeconomic status.

However, time-varying confounders – factors that change during the observation period and may influence the risk of the outcome – must be explicitly modelled. Age is one of the most important time-varying confounders in SCCS studies because the risk of many outcomes (e.g. seizures, infections, cardiovascular events) changes substantially with age. Therefore, SCCS analyses routinely include age (often in bands or as a time-dependent variable) to avoid biased estimates of the association between exposure and outcome.

Further Reading

Cameron AC, Trivedi PK. *Regression Analysis of Count Data*. 2nd ed. Cambridge: Cambridge University Press; 2013. doi: https://doi.org/10.1017/CBO9781139013567.

Farrington CP. Relative incidence estimation from case series for vaccine safety evaluation. *Biometrics*. 1995;**51**(1):228–35. doi: https://doi.org/10.2307/2533328.

Farrington CP. Control without separate controls: evaluation of vaccine safety using case-only methods. *Vaccine*. 2004;**22**(15–16):2064–70. doi: https://doi.org/10.1016/j.vaccine.2004.01.017.

Farrington CP, Anaya-Izquierdo K, Whitaker HJ, et al. Self-controlled case series analysis with event-dependent observation periods. *J Am Stat Assoc*. 2011;**106**(494):417–26. doi: https://doi.org/10.1198/jasa.2011.ap10108.

McCullagh P, Nelder JA. *Generalized Linear Models*. 2nd ed. London: Chapman & Hall/CRC; 1989.

Musonda P, Farrington CP, Whitaker HJ. Sample sizes for self-controlled case series studies. *Stat Med*. 2006;**25**(15):2618–31. doi: https://doi.org/10.1002/sim.2477.

Petersen I, Douglas I, Whitaker H. Self controlled case series methods: an alternative to standard epidemiological study designs. *BMJ*. 2016;**354**:i4515. doi: https://doi.org/10.1136/bmj.i4515.

Weldeselassie YG, Whitaker HJ, Farrington CP. Use of the self-controlled case-series method in vaccine safety studies: review and recommendations for best practice. *Epidemiol Infect*. 2011;**139**(12):1805–17. doi: https://doi.org/10.1017/S0950268811001531.

Whitaker HJ, Farrington CP, Spiessens B, Musonda P. Tutorial in biostatistics: the self-controlled case series method. *Stat Med*. 2006;**25**(10):1768–97. doi: https://doi.org/10.1002/sim.2302.

Whitaker HJ, Hocine MN, Farrington CP. The methodology of self-controlled case series studies. *Stat Methods Med Res*. 2009;**18**(1):7–26. doi: https://doi.org/10.1177/0962280208092342.

Chapter 7

Causation in Epidemiological Studies

Epidemiological studies (e.g. cross-sectional, case–control, and cohort studies) identify associations between risk factors and outcomes. However, a statistical association does not necessarily imply that the exposure caused the outcome. Distinguishing between mere correlation and true causation is a fundamental challenge in epidemiology and requires a systematic approach. Several frameworks have been developed to assess causation, which offer complementary perspectives for understanding causation in epidemiology.

Bradford Hill Criteria

Proposed by Sir Austin Bradford Hill in 1965, these nine criteria help evaluate whether an observed association is likely to be causal. They are not a definitive checklist, but rather a framework for scientific reasoning.

1. **Strength of association:** stronger associations (e.g. smoking and lung cancer) are more likely to be causal. There is no universal agreement on what constitutes a strong association. However, an odds ratio (OR) or relative risk (RR) of 2 is often considered a moderate association in practice, while a value of 5 or above is considered strong, although interpretation depends on context. The relationship between smoking and lung cancer is an example of strong association, as ORs and RRs in different studies range from 4 to 20.
2. **Consistency:** findings should be replicated in different studies and populations. Consistency is demonstrated if an association is found in repeated studies conducted on different populations, under different circumstances, and with different study designs. For example, the association between cigarette smoking and lung cancer has been consistently demonstrated in a number of different types of epidemiological studies.
3. **Specificity:** a single exposure should be linked to a specific outcome (e.g. tuberculosis and *Mycobacterium tuberculosis*). This is often considered the weakest criterion, as many exposures (like smoking) cause multiple diseases.
4. **Temporality:** the exposure must occur **before** the outcome (best demonstrated in cohort studies). This is the only criterion that is regarded as essential for causation.
5. **Biological gradient:** a dose–response relationship supports causation. When changes in the intensity, frequency, or duration of an exposure correspond to a predictable change in the occurrence of the outcome, this strengthens causal inference. For example, higher levels of cigarette smoking lead to a higher risk of developing lung cancer, or increased alcohol consumption leads to a greater risk of liver cirrhosis.
6. **Plausibility:** the association should be biologically or scientifically explainable. It adds weight to the evidence for causation, guides research, and enhances public acceptance.

For example, it is known that elevated cholesterol contributes to plaque formation in arteries (atherosclerosis), which increases the risk of heart attacks and strokes.

7. **Coherence:** the association should align with existing knowledge and findings. It focuses on whether the cause–effect relationship aligns with the broader body of biological, clinical, and epidemiological evidence. It means that the association 'fits' with what is already known. It is broader than the plausibility criterion because it focuses on the consistency of the association with all available evidence, including biological, clinical, and epidemiological data. For example, the link between high cholesterol and heart disease is coherent because it aligns with epidemiological evidence, clinical findings (e.g. atherosclerosis), and experimental studies.
8. **Experiment:** reducing exposure should reduce the outcome (e.g. smoking bans resulting in lower respiratory illness rates).
9. **Analogy:** similar exposures causing similar effects strengthen causal reasoning. It involves reasoning by comparison. For example, well-established knowledge of asbestos exposure and mesothelioma prompted the analogy that other fibres or particulates might also cause similar respiratory diseases, which in turn prompted studies into silica exposure and lung disease.

Koch's Postulates

In the late nineteenth century, Robert Koch developed a framework for establishing a causal relationship between a microorganism and a disease. These four postulates remain foundational in microbiology and epidemiology:

1. **Presence of the organism:** the microorganism must be found in all individuals suffering from the disease but not in healthy individuals.
2. **Isolation and growth in pure culture:** the microorganism must be isolated from the diseased host and grown in a pure culture.
3. **Reproduction of disease:** when introduced into a healthy individual, the microorganism must cause the same disease.
4. **Re-isolation of the microorganism:** the microorganism must be re-isolated from the experimentally infected host and confirmed as identical to the original pathogen.

Limitations of Koch's Postulates

While revolutionary, Koch's postulates have several limitations in modern epidemiology and microbiology:

- **Asymptomatic carriers:** many microorganisms (e.g. *H. pylori*) exist in healthy individuals without causing disease.
- **Non-culturable microorganisms:** certain pathogens (e.g. *Treponema pallidum*, the cause of syphilis) cannot currently be grown in vitro.
- **Multifactorial diseases:** some diseases (e.g. cancer, autoimmune disorders) arise from a combination of genetic and environmental factors, rather than a single infectious agent.
- **Host susceptibility:** disease manifestation can vary between individuals due to genetic, immune, or environmental factors; the same pathogen does not affect every host identically.

Rothman's Causal Pies Model

Kenneth Rothman introduced the **causal pies model**, shifting away from single-factor explanations of disease and embracing multifactorial causation. His model complements the Bradford Hill criteria by recognizing that diseases often result from multiple interacting factors rather than a single cause.

Key Components of Rothman's Causal Pies Model

1. **Sufficient cause:** a complete set of component causes that, together, inevitably lead to the outcome (disease). For example, homozygosity for sickle cell anaemia is a sufficient cause for sickle cell disease. Multiple sufficient causes may exist for the same outcome (e.g. radon exposure + genetic susceptibility for lung cancer).
2. **Component causes:** individual risk factors or exposures (the 'slices' of the pie) that contribute to a sufficient cause. For example, smoking, genetic susceptibility, exposure to carcinogens, and chronic inflammation all contribute to lung cancer.
3. **Necessary cause:** a component cause that is present in all sufficient causes of the outcome but is not enough on its own to cause disease. For example, the HIV virus is a necessary cause of AIDS, but not all individuals infected with HIV will develop AIDS as it is not a sufficient cause on its own, and other factors influence the progression of the disease.

Susser's Criteria for Cause-and-Effect Relationships

Mervyn Susser proposed a holistic approach to causation, emphasizing that most health outcomes result from the interplay of multiple factors rather than a single cause. These factors include biological agents, behaviours, environmental exposures, and societal conditions.

Key Contributions of Susser's Model

1. **The causal web:** a conceptual framework illustrating how multiple factors interconnect to produce an outcome. It emphasizes the interdependencies between causes rather than a linear relationship.
2. **Adaptability and context:** Susser endorsed the Bradford Hill criteria, but argued they should not be applied rigidly. The weight given to any single criterion should depend on the specific scientific and social context.
3. **Key causal considerations:**
   - Temporal order: the cause must precede the effect.
   - Ruling out **confounding:**[1] rigorous efforts should be made to ensure the association is not due to confounding of 'hidden' third variables.
   - Multifactorial approach: a comprehensive evaluation of all interacting influences is required to truly understand disease distribution.

[1] **Confounding:** Distortion of the exposure–outcome association by a third variable related to both but not on the causal pathway; address via design (randomization, restriction, matching) or analysis (stratification, regression/adjustment).

Susser's integrative approach highlights the systemic and dynamic nature of causation, reinforcing the importance of considering multiple influences when evaluating epidemiological evidence.

Comparison of Approaches to Causation

Table 7.1 presents a comparison of the Bradford Hill criteria, Koch's postulates, Rothman's causal pies model, and Susser's causal web.

Chapter Summary

Epidemiological studies identify associations between risk factors and outcomes, but determining causality requires a systematic approach. Several frameworks help evaluate whether an observed association is truly causal.

Bradford Hill Criteria (1965)

A set of nine criteria used to assess causation:

- strength of association
- consistency
- specificity
- temporality
- biological gradient (dose–response relationship)
- plausibility
- coherence
- experiment
- analogy.

These criteria are widely applied in chronic disease research (e.g. smoking and lung cancer).

Koch's Postulates

A four-step framework used to establish causation between microorganisms and infectious diseases:

- presence of the organism in all cases of the disease but not in healthy individuals
- isolation and growth in pure culture from a diseased individual
- reproduction of disease in a healthy host upon introduction of the microorganism
- re-isolation of the microorganism from the experimentally infected host.

While foundational for microbiology, Koch's postulates have limitations due to asymptomatic carriers, non-culturable pathogens, and multifactorial diseases.

Rothman's Causal Pies Model

A multifactorial causation model recognizing that diseases often result from multiple interacting factors:

- sufficient cause: a complete set of component causes that lead to disease
- component causes: individual factors contributing to disease (e.g. smoking, genetic predisposition)

Table 7.1 Comparison of approaches to causation in epidemiology

Aspect	Bradford Hill (1965)	Koch's postulates	Rothman's causal pie model	Susser's causal web
Primary focus	Criteria for assessing causation in epidemiology	Establishing causation in infectious diseases	Multifactorial causation using component causes	Interconnected causes in a web of relationships
Causation type	Primarily **probabilistic causal reasoning**[2]	**Deterministic**[3]	Probabilistic and multifactorial	Contextual and systemic
Key concepts	Nine criteria, including temporality, strength, consistency, and biological plausibility	A pathogen must meet specific criteria to cause disease	Sufficient cause (a complete set of factors leading to an outcome) vs necessary cause (a factor present in all sufficient causes)	Causal web: interconnected causes at multiple levels Multilevel causation (biological, behavioural, societal)
Flexibility	Moderate: criteria are flexible but not all are essential	Low: rigid, focused on single-agent causation	High: accounts for complex, multifactorial causation	Very high: incorporates broader social and environmental factors
Key strengths	Widely applicable across disciplines Useful for chronic and infectious diseases Combines biological and epidemiological evidence	Clear and definitive for single-agent infectious diseases Strong experimental foundation	Explains multifactorial causation Addresses both necessary and sufficient causes Highlights probabilistic nature of causation	Contextual and adaptable Recognizes interplay of factors Useful for chronic and complex diseases
Key limitations	Not all criteria are essential or equally applicable Limited for complex, multifactorial diseases	Not applicable to non-infectious diseases Cannot address multifactorial or chronic conditions	Does not always specify mechanisms of interaction Complex to apply without detailed data	Requires extensive contextual knowledge Difficult to operationalize quantitatively

[2] **Probabilistic causation:** A cause changes the probability of an outcome rather than guaranteeing it; typical for multifactorial, population-level health outcomes.

[3] **Deterministic causation:** A cause that, if present, is sufficient to produce the effect in a given context (no randomness once conditions are fixed).

Table 7.1 (cont.)

Aspect	Bradford Hill (1965)	Koch's postulates	Rothman's causal pie model	Susser's causal web
Application	Chronic diseases Environmental and occupational health Public health policy	Infectious disease research Pathogen identification	Chronic and multifactorial diseases Public health and epidemiological studies	Chronic diseases Social determinants of health Environmental health
Example	Smoking and lung cancer: assessed using strength, temporality, and dose–response relationship	*Mycobacterium tuberculosis* and tuberculosis	Lung cancer: sufficient cause may include smoking + asbestos exposure + genetic susceptibility	Heart disease: web includes diet, exercise, stress, and healthcare access
Temporal component	Essential: cause must precede effect	Essential: cause must precede disease	Essential: temporal relationship assumed in sufficient cause	Essential: contextual understanding of time emphasized
Complexity of causation	Moderate: can handle some multifactorial causes	Low: single-agent causation	High: emphasizes interplay of multiple component causes	Very high: focuses on dynamic, multilevel causes

- necessary cause: a factor present in all sufficient causes but not sufficient on its own (e.g. HIV for AIDS).

This model highlights the complexity of disease causation beyond single-factor explanations.

Susser's Causal Web Model

A holistic approach emphasizing the interconnected nature of causation, integrating biological, behavioural, environmental, and societal factors:

- the causal web: a network of interdependent causes influencing disease
- adaptability and context: the need for flexible application of causal reasoning
- key causal considerations:
  - temporal order (cause must precede effect).
  - ruling out confounding (ensuring the association is not due to external factors).
  - multifactorial approach (health outcomes arise from multiple interacting factors).

Susser's approach is particularly useful for complex diseases influenced by social and environmental determinants.

Comparison

Each framework has strengths and limitations, with Bradford Hill providing structured guidelines, Koch's postulates being foundational for infectious disease research, Rothman's model addressing multifactorial causation, and Susser's approach incorporating broader societal and environmental influences. Together, these frameworks provide complementary perspectives on causation in epidemiology.

Practice Questions

Q1. Which of the following is *not* one of Bradford Hill's criteria for causation?

A. Strength of association
B. Temporality
C. Necessary cause
D. Biological gradient
E. Coherence

Q2. What is the primary limitation of Koch's postulates in modern epidemiology?

A. It only applies to chronic diseases.
B. It fails to consider multifactorial disease causation.
C. It does not require laboratory evidence.
D. It does not establish causation in infectious diseases.
E. It does not apply to bacterial infections.

Q3. Which model of causation describes a disease as resulting from multiple interacting component causes?

A. Bradford Hill criteria
B. Koch's postulates
C. Rothman's causal pies model

D. Susser's causal web model
E. Henle–Koch model

Q4. In Rothman's causal pies model, what is a 'necessary cause'?
A. A cause that always leads to disease.
B. A cause present in all sufficient causes but not enough on its own.
C. A risk factor that only occurs randomly.
D. A cause that must be eliminated to prevent disease.
E. A cause that is unique to genetic disorders.

Q5. Which of the following best describes Susser's causal web model?
A. It focuses solely on biological determinants of disease.
B. It considers interconnected biological, behavioural, and environmental factors.
C. It applies only to infectious diseases.
D. It follows rigid criteria for causation.
E. It is only relevant to genetic disorders.

Q6. Why does Rothman's causal pies model move away from the specificity criterion of Bradford Hill?
A. It focuses only on infectious diseases.
B. It acknowledges that diseases often have multiple contributing factors.
C. It is based on experimental models only.
D. It rejects the need for component causes.
E. It assumes that every disease has a single cause.

Q7. What does the causal web concept in Susser's model emphasize?
A. Diseases arise from multiple interconnected causes.
B. A single cause is necessary for every disease.
C. Random chance is the primary determinant of disease.
D. Each disease has only one necessary cause.
E. Every exposure leads to a disease outcome.

Q8. Which causation model is most applicable to diseases influenced by social and environmental factors?
A. Koch's postulates
B. Susser's causal web model
C. Bradford Hill criteria
D. Rothman's causal pies model
E. Monocausal disease model

Answers

Q1. Correct answer: C. Necessary cause. The Bradford Hill criteria include strength of association, temporality, and biological gradient, but the concept of a necessary cause is part of Rothman's causal pies model.

Q2. Correct answer: B. It fails to consider multifactorial disease causation. Koch's postulates were designed for infectious diseases, but many modern diseases (e.g. cancer, autoimmune disorders) involve multiple genetic and environmental factors.
Q3. Correct answer: C. Rothman's causal pies model. Rothman's model describes disease causation as a combination of component causes, where a sufficient cause leads to disease only when all required component causes are present.
Q4. Correct answer: B. A cause present in all sufficient causes but not enough on its own. A necessary cause is a component cause that appears in every sufficient cause but does not cause disease by itself (e.g. HIV is necessary for AIDS but does not always lead to AIDS).
Q5. Correct answer: B. It considers interconnected biological, behavioural, and environmental factors. Susser's model recognizes that disease causation is complex, involving multiple interacting factors rather than a single cause.
Q6. Correct answer: B. It acknowledges that diseases often have multiple contributing factors. Unlike Bradford Hill's specificity criterion, Rothman's model recognizes that many diseases have multiple sufficient causes rather than a single cause–outcome relationship.
Q7. Correct answer: A. Diseases arise from multiple interconnected causes. Susser's causal web model illustrates that disease causation involves multiple, interdependent factors, including social and environmental influences.
Q8. Correct answer: B. Susser's causal web model. Explanation: Susser's model incorporates biological, behavioural, and societal factors, making it useful for chronic diseases with social determinants.

Further Reading

Fredricks DN, Relman DA. Sequence-based identification of microbial pathogens: a reconsideration of Koch's postulates. *Clin Microbiol Rev.* 1996;**9**(1):18–33. doi: https://doi.org/10.1128/CMR.9.1.18.

Greenland S, Pearl J, Robins JM. Causal diagrams for epidemiologic research. *Epidemiology.* 1999;**10**(1):37–48.

Hernán MA, Robins JM. *Causal Inference: What If.* Boca Raton, FL: Chapman & Hall/CRC; 2020.

Hill AB. The environment and disease: association or causation? *Proc R Soc Med.* 1965;**58**:295–300.

Krause RM. Koch's postulates and the search for the AIDS agent. *ASM News.* 1984;**50**(8):429–35.

Rothman KJ. Causes. *Am J Epidemiol.* 1976;**104**(6):587–92. doi: https://doi.org/10.1093/oxfordjournals.aje.a112335.

Susser M. *Causal Thinking in the Health Sciences: Concepts and Strategies of Epidemiology.* New York: Oxford University Press; 1973.

Susser M. What is a cause and how do we know one? A grammar for pragmatic epidemiology. *Am J Epidemiol.* 1991;**133**(7):635–48. doi: https://doi.org/10.1093/oxfordjournals.aje.a115939.

Clinical Trials

Randomized Controlled Trials

Randomized controlled trials (RCTs) are experimental studies used to evaluate the effectiveness of an intervention by randomly assigning participants into an intervention group or a control group, and then comparing outcomes between the groups.

Key Features of a Randomized Controlled Trial

Randomization

Participants are randomly assigned to different groups (e.g. treatment vs control), eliminating selection bias and ensuring baseline comparability. There are several types of randomization.

Simple Randomization

Each participant has an equal chance of being assigned to any group, akin to flipping a coin. It is unbiased but may result in unequal group sizes in small trials.

Block Randomization

Block randomization ensures that there are approximately equal numbers of participants in each group throughout the trial. It is commonly used in small trials to prevent major imbalances between groups. Participants are randomized into blocks (e.g. four, six, or eight), with equal allocation to each group within a block. The allocation is determined by randomly selecting one of the predefined sequences.

- **Example:** In a trial with two groups – A (drug) and B (placebo) – the block size must be a multiple of two. Suppose researchers use a block size of four and randomize 20 subjects. The possible sequences could be ABBA, BABA, BAAB, AABB, ABAB, BBAA, ensuring equal distribution across groups. However, if the block size is known, the last one or two assignments may become predictable. To mitigate this issue, **permuted block randomization** is used, where the block sizes are varied randomly (e.g. four, six, or eight), making it harder to predict group assignments.

Stratified Randomization

Stratified randomization ensures the equal distribution of important prognostic characteristics (covariates) across treatment groups, such as age, gender, or disease severity. This reduces confounding and improves comparability. Participants are first categorized into **strata** (subgroups) according to a key prognostic factor, and then randomized within each stratum.

- **Example:** In a depression treatment study, participants may be stratified by depression severity (mild, moderate, severe) before randomization within each severity category to ensure balanced distribution.

Adaptive Randomization

Adaptive randomization adjusts the allocation probability dynamically as the trial progresses, based on accumulated outcomes. This method ensures that groups remain balanced on important characteristics, even if participants are recruited unevenly.

Response-Adaptive Randomization

This is a specific type of randomization where participants are more likely assigned to the treatment that appears more effective based on interim results. For example, if early data indicate that a new antipsychotic is yielding better outcomes, more participants may be assigned to that treatment arm to maximize potential benefits while maintaining scientific rigour.

Minimization

Minimization[1] is a covariate-adaptive method that ensures balance in treatment assignment by considering multiple factors (e.g. age, disease stage, gender) simultaneously. It is not purely random, but uses a probability-based allocation to minimize differences between groups. Minimization works by calculating a measure of imbalance for each possible assignment of a participant to a group. The participant is then assigned to the group that would result in the lowest imbalance in important variables. Unlike pure randomization, this method actively corrects imbalances as the trial progresses. It is particularly useful in studies with small sample sizes, where achieving balance using other methods can be challenging.

Cluster Randomization

Cluster randomization is used in studies where entire groups or 'clusters' of participants are randomly assigned to different treatment conditions rather than individual participants. These clusters can be naturally occurring groups, such as hospitals, wards, or GP surgeries. Cluster randomization is particularly useful for studying interventions that cannot be applied to individuals, such as health education programmes or infection control measures, where cross-contamination between individuals is a concern.

- **Example:** A trial evaluating a mental health intervention in schools might randomize entire schools rather than individual students.
- **Challenges of Cluster Randomization:** It requires a larger sample size to achieve the same statistical power as individually randomized trials because individuals within a cluster tend to be more similar to each other than individuals across different clusters.
- Data analysis is more complex, requiring statistical techniques such as hierarchical modelling (mixed-effects models) or generalized estimating equations (GEE) to account for intra-cluster correlation.

---

[1] **Minimization:** An adaptive allocation method balancing groups on prognostic factors. It improves comparability in small samples but requires allocation concealment.

Comparison of Stratified Randomization, Adaptive Randomization, and Minimization

Table 8.1 presents a comparison of three approaches to randomization.

Table 8.1 Comparison of stratified randomization, adaptive randomization, and minimization

Feature	Stratified randomization	Adaptive randomization	Minimization
Definition	Ensures balance across predefined subgroups (strata) before randomization	Adjusts the allocation probability dynamically based on accumulating trial data	Allocates participants based on the need to minimize imbalance across multiple factors
Purpose	Controls for known confounding factors by ensuring equal distribution within strata (e.g. age, gender)	Modifies treatment assignment probabilities to improve efficiency or ethical considerations	Ensures balanced allocation by considering multiple factors simultaneously
When used	When important baseline characteristics must be balanced between groups before randomization	When ongoing trial data can help optimize group allocation (e.g. in response to early results)	When a study has multiple confounders and a small sample size where randomization may not ensure balance
Methodology	Participants are grouped into strata first, then randomized separately within each stratum	Randomization is adjusted dynamically based on interim trial results	New participants are assigned to the group that minimizes imbalance across all factors
Flexibility	Fixed method: stratification must be determined before randomization begins	Dynamic method: allocation can change as more participants are enrolled	Dynamic method: assignment changes based on previous allocations
Common uses	Clinical trials where factors like age, disease severity, or gender could influence results	Drug trials, personalized medicine, and adaptive clinical trial designs	Small trials where strict balance between groups is needed across many variables
Randomness	Randomly assigns participants within each stratum	Randomization probabilities change based on interim results	Not purely random: a probability-based approach is used to minimize imbalances
Example	In a clinical trial for diabetes treatment, patients are stratified by age before randomization	In a clinical trial for a new drug, more patients may be assigned to the better-performing treatment as data accumulates	In a small cancer trial, new patients are assigned to the group that maintains balance in terms of age, gender, and tumour stage

Control Group

Randomized controlled trials often include a control group, which may be a placebo group or a standard treatment group, to isolate the effect of the experimental intervention.

A placebo is a substance or treatment that has no active therapeutic ingredient but is designed to resemble the intervention being tested. Placebo controls are particularly challenging in psychotherapy trials as it is not always possible to create an 'inactive' version of therapy. Some studies use sham therapy or attention control, where therapists engage with patients but do not provide structured therapy.

The placebo effect refers to a perceived or actual improvement in symptoms after receiving a placebo. This phenomenon is driven by several psychological and biological mechanisms:

- **Expectation:** if a person believes a treatment will work, they may experience a positive outcome even if the treatment is inactive.
- **Conditioning:** past positive experiences with medical treatments may reinforce the belief that receiving treatment leads to improvement.
- **Neurobiological mechanisms:** studies show that the placebo effect can activate brain regions associated with pain relief and mood regulation.

Blinding

Blinding, also known as masking, is used to prevent bias by keeping one or more parties unaware of treatment assignments. It helps reduce bias, enable objective evaluation, and control for the placebo effect.

- **Single-blind:** only participants are unaware of their treatment assignment.
- **Double-blind:** both participants and researchers are unaware of the treatment assignment.
- **Triple-blind:** participants, researchers, and data analysts are all unaware of the treatment assignments.

Blinding is particularly challenging in psychotherapy trials since both therapists and patients are actively involved. Researchers employ a variety of strategies to address these challenges, as shown in Table 8.2.

Table 8.2 Challenges and solutions for blinding in psychotherapy trials

Challenge	Solution
Patients can tell if they are receiving therapy.	Use active control therapies to maintain credibility.
Therapists may unconsciously bias results.	Use scripted protocols and therapist training.
Outcome assessors may know group assignments.	Use independent, blinded raters to assess symptom changes.
Placebo therapy may still have therapeutic effects.	Design 'sham therapy' carefully to avoid active treatment elements.

Types of Analyses

Per-Protocol Analysis

Per-protocol (PP) analysis includes only participants who adhered strictly to the study protocol, meaning they received the intended treatment and completed all follow-up assessments as planned. Participants who deviate from the protocol are excluded. This method does not preserve randomization and provides the **best-case scenario** estimate of treatment effect.

Intention-to-Treat Analysis

Intention-to-treat (ITT) analysis includes all participants as originally assigned, regardless of discontinuation, treatment switching, or non-adherence ('once randomized, always analysed'). Intention-to-treat preserves the benefits of randomization and provides a more realistic estimate of treatment effectiveness. Several methods are used to handle missing data in ITT:

- **Last observation carried forward (LOCF):** the last recorded measurement is carried forward for missing values. However, this method can introduce bias if dropouts are related to treatment failure. For example, in trials of anticholinesterase medications, which aim to slow cognitive decline, using the last recorded measurement may favour the medication group, as these observations are likely to be better than the end-of-trial measurements. This approach implicitly assumes no change after dropout, which is rarely valid and may bias results.

- **Multiple imputation (MI):**[2] a statistical approach that generates multiple plausible datasets to estimate missing values, accounting for uncertainty and reducing bias. It creates several different versions of the dataset with imputed values, analyses each dataset separately, and then combines the results to produce more reliable estimates. Multiple imputation is generally preferred over simpler methods like LOCF, as it provides a more accurate reflection of variability and uncertainty in missing data handling.

- **Mixed models/repeated measures analysis:** a statistical approach used for analysing data where individuals are measured multiple times. It is particularly useful for longitudinal studies that track changes over time. Mixed models account for within-subject correlations, ensuring that repeated measures for an individual are appropriately handled. This method provides flexibility in handling missing data and can adjust for time-dependent covariates.

- **Treatment policy estimator (TPE):**[3] a statistical approach that evaluates a treatment's effect based on its initial assignment, regardless of whether patients continue or switch

---

[2] **Multiple imputation (MI):** Handles missing data by creating several (m) complete datasets using an imputation model that reflects uncertainty, analysing each, then pooling estimates and standard errors using Rubin's rules. Typically assumes data are missing at random, given variables in the imputation model; include predictors of missingness and the outcome, respect variable types (e.g. logistic for binary), and align imputation with the analysis model.

[3] **Treatment policy estimator (TPE):** Targets the effect of initial treatment assignment regardless of post-randomization events (e.g. non-adherence, discontinuation, switching, rescue therapy). Typically operationalized with ITT analyses that include all randomized participants as allocated and use observed outcomes irrespective of adherence.

treatments. It tries to answer the question, 'what is the effect of assigning the treatment regardless of adherence/discontinuation/switching?' Treatment policy estimator reflects real-world scenarios and preserves randomization by analysing outcomes based on initial treatment assignment.

Handling Missing Data

Missing data is a common problem in RCTs, and it can lead to biased results if not handled appropriately. Several techniques can be used to address missing data.

Complete Case Analysis

Under complete case analysis (CCA), only participants with complete data for all variables are included in the analysis. If a participant has a missing value for any variable, they are excluded. This method is appropriate when missing data occurs completely at random. It differs from PP analysis, which excludes participants based on protocol deviations, whereas CCA excludes them due to missing data.

Inverse Probability Weighting

Inverse probability weighting (IPW) assigns weights to participants based on the probability of having complete observed outcomes. Participants who are less likely to be observed receive higher weights, so that the analysis better represents the full study population. Inverse probability weighting can reduce bias due to incomplete follow-up, particularly when missingness is missing at random (MAR) and the model for missingness is appropriately specified.

Example

In a trial comparing an antidepressant to a placebo for major depressive disorder, 30% of participants dropped out before completion, with dropouts more likely in those with severe depression. A logistic regression model predicts dropout likelihood based on baseline depression severity, age, and treatment history. Participants who remain in the trial (low dropout risk) receive lower weights, while those who drop out (high dropout risk) receive higher weights to compensate for missing data.

Mean or Median Imputation

Missing values are replaced with the mean or median of observed values for that variable. This approach is typically only recommended when the amount of missing data is small. Although simple, this approach can distort associations and underestimate variability, and is therefore generally not recommended for primary analyses in RCTs.

Worst-Case Scenario Analysis

This method assumes that all missing participants in the treatment group experienced treatment failure, while missing participants in the control group had the best possible outcome. It is primarily used for binary outcomes and in cases where the experimental group is expected to show substantial superiority, allowing a conservative estimate of treatment efficacy.

Calculating Difference between Groups

A 2 × 2 table is a useful tool for analysing data from RCTs with binary outcomes (see Table 8.3). It helps to visualize and calculate the difference between treatment and control groups.

Table 8.3 A 2 × 2 table for analysing outcomes in RCTs

Group	Improved	Not improved	Total
Treatment	a	b	$a + b$
Control	c	d	$c + d$
Total	$a + c$	$b + d$	–

- **Experimental event rate (EER):** the proportion of experimental subjects experiencing an event:

  $$\text{EER} = \frac{a}{a+b}.$$

- **Control event rate (CER):** the proportion of control subjects experiencing an event:

  $$\text{CER} = \frac{c}{c+d}.$$

- **Absolute benefit increase (ABI):** the difference between the experimental and control event rates:

  $$\text{ABI} = \text{EER} - \text{CER}.$$

Note: Absolute benefit increase (ABI) is equivalent to absolute risk reduction (ARR) when the outcome is beneficial (e.g. symptom improvement)

- **Number needed to treat (NNT):** the number of people who need to be treated with the active intervention to achieve one additional beneficial outcome compared to placebo:

  $$\text{NNT} = 1 / \text{ABI}.$$

- **Relative risk (RR):** the risk of an event in the experimental group compared to the control group:

  $$\text{RR} = \frac{\text{EER}}{\text{CER}}.$$

- **Relative benefit increase (RBI):** the proportional increase in benefit in the experimental group compared to the control group:

  $$\text{RBI} = \frac{\text{EER-CER}}{\text{CER}}.$$

Ethical Considerations

Ethical considerations in RCTs include ensuring the following:

- Informed consent is obtained from all participants.
- Ethical approval is granted by the relevant regulatory bodies.
- Participant safety is prioritized, and withdrawal from the study is allowed at any time without consequences.

Other Types of Trials

Pragmatic Clinical Trials

A pragmatic clinical trial (PCT) evaluates an intervention in 'real-world' clinical practice rather than a tightly controlled research setting.

A common criticism of RCTs is that participating subjects are highly selected and therefore unrepresentative of a typical population – that is, they have good internal validity but poor external validity. The sort of patients who are willing to participate in an RCT are motivated and may not be representative of patients that we often manage in day-to-day practice, especially in psychiatry, where real-life patients are often disengaged and have more comorbidities than the RCT patients. Therefore, a treatment that shows great promise in an RCT might not be effective or feasible in real-world settings due to factors such as non-compliance, comorbidities, or variations in how the treatment is delivered. Pragmatic clinical trials help bridge this gap by providing valuable information on the real-world impact of interventions, aiding clinicians and policymakers in making informed decisions. For example, comparing the effectiveness of two antidepressants in a primary care setting without strict inclusion and exclusion criteria. These trials address the gap between research and clinical practice. A key limitation of traditional RCTs is that participants tend to be highly selected, making the findings less generalizable to broader patient populations.

Purpose

A PCT assesses the effectiveness of an intervention in routine clinical settings.

Design

The study population is often broader and more representative of everyday clinical practice. Pragmatic clinical trials often include all patients with a particular disorder in a location. The key component is that the patients, services, and treatments are representative of what is routinely available. The intervention is applied under usual conditions with minimal restrictions. Treatment protocols are therefore less rigid, allowing adjustments as they would occur in normal clinical settings.

Outcome Measures

The focus is patient-centred outcomes, such as quality of life and functionality. Given their real-world nature, PCTs often include missing data, requiring advanced statistical techniques such as MI.

Generalizability

These studies have high external validity, making the results more applicable to everyday clinical practice.

Crossover Trial

A crossover trial is a type of clinical trial in which participants receive multiple interventions sequentially, with each participant serving as their own control. This design is commonly used to compare the effects of two or more treatments, allowing each participant to experience all treatment conditions in a controlled manner. By switching ('crossing over') between treatments, researchers can directly measure the differences in response within the same individual, reducing variability and increasing statistical power.

Design

- **Randomization:** participants are randomly assigned to different treatment sequences (e.g. A then B or B then A).
- **Treatment periods:** each participant receives both treatments for a specified time. The treatment periods are of equal length and are separated by a washout period to prevent carryover effects.
- **Washout period:** a critical phase where no treatment is given, allowing the effects of the first treatment to dissipate before the next treatment begins. The length of the washout period depends on the half-life of the treatment and the duration of its effects.
- **Outcome assessment:** the same outcome measures are assessed at the end of each treatment period. This allows a direct within-subject comparison of the treatments. Paired *t*-tests, repeated measures ANOVA (analysis of variance) and linear mixed-effects models are used to analyse the data, with mixed-effects models generally preferred in modern analyses due to their flexibility in handling missing data and within-subject correlations.

When to Use Crossover Trials

- Suitable when treatment effects are temporary and reversible.
- Best for conditions that remain stable over time.
- Avoided when interventions have long-lasting or have irreversible effects (e.g. surgery).

Advantages of Crossover Trials

- **Within-subject comparison:** each participant serves as their own control, reducing variability.
- **Smaller sample size:** increased statistical power due to reduced variability.
- **Efficient use of participants:** particularly beneficial when recruitment is challenging.
- **Direct comparison of treatments:** ideal for comparing treatments' effects in the same individual.

Limitations of Crossover Trials

- **Carryover effects:** when the effect of the first treatment carries over into the second treatment period. It is mitigated by an appropriate washout period.

- **Order effects:** order effects occur when the sequence in which treatments are administered influences the outcome. This can introduce bias because the treatment effect may not solely reflect the intervention but rather the position of the treatment in the sequence.
- **Not suitable for all conditions:** it is inapplicable if the condition changes over time (e.g. progressive diseases). It is inappropriate for treatments with permanent effects (e.g. surgery).
- **Participant burden:** participants must undergo multiple treatment phases, which can increase dropout rates. This may lead to the 'fatigue effect' in which participants become tired or disengaged as the study progresses, potentially diminishing the effect of later treatments.
- **Complex statistical analysis:** requires analysis techniques that account for the crossover design, such as paired *t*-tests, repeated measures ANOVA, and mixed-effects models.

N-of-1 Trials

Definition

N-of-1 trials, also known as single-patient trials or individualized clinical trials, are a type of research design in which a single patient receives multiple courses of different treatments (including placebo or standard treatment if applicable) in a randomized or blinded fashion. The goal is to determine the most effective treatment for that individual patient rather than making broad population-level inferences.

How *N*-of-1 Trials Are Conducted

- **Patient identification:** *N*-of-1 trials are most appropriate for patients with chronic conditions where:
  - symptoms fluctuate or are difficult to manage
  - there are several treatment options available
  - the patient and clinician are uncertain about which treatment is best
  - the patient is motivated to participate in the trial.
- **Treatment selection:** the patient and clinician collaboratively decide on the treatments to be compared. This usually includes the current standard treatment and one or more alternative treatments. A placebo arm may also be included.

Trial Design

- **Randomization:** the order in which the patient receives the treatments is randomized. This helps to minimize bias and ensure that any observed differences in outcomes are due to the treatment and not other factors.
- **Blinding:** ideally, the patient and the clinician assessing the outcomes should be blinded to the treatment being administered. This can be challenging in some cases, but every effort should be made to maintain blinding where possible.
- **Treatment cycles:** the patient receives each treatment for a predefined period (treatment cycle). The length of the cycle depends on the condition and the treatments being

studied. It needs to be long enough to allow the treatment to have its full effect, but short enough to be practical.

- **Washout periods (if needed):** between treatment cycles, there should be a washout period during which the patient receives no treatment or a placebo to minimize carryover effects from one treatment to the next. The length of the washout depends on the pharmacokinetics of the medications.
- **Outcome measurement:** during each treatment cycle, the patient's symptoms or other relevant outcomes are measured regularly.
- **Data analysis:** the data from the *N*-of-1 trial are analysed to determine which treatment was most effective for that individual patient. This might involve visual inspection of the data, statistical analysis (e.g. comparing mean symptom scores across treatment periods), or a combination of both.
- **Clinical decision:** based on the results of the *N*-of-1 trial, the patient and clinician make a shared decision about the most appropriate long-term treatment plan.

When Are *N*-of-1 Trials Useful?

N-of-1 trials are particularly useful in the following cases:

- chronic conditions with fluctuating symptoms (e.g. chronic pain, irritable bowel syndrome, asthma, migraines)
- conditions where there are several treatment options with similar efficacy
- situations where the patient and clinician are uncertain about which treatment is best
- patients who are motivated to participate in a trial and are able to reliably assess their symptoms.

Advantages of *N*-of-1 Trials

- **Personalized medicine:** *N*-of-1 trials provide individualized evidence to guide treatment decisions, leading to more personalized and effective care.
- **Improved outcomes:** by identifying the most effective treatment for a specific patient, *N*-of-1 trials can lead to better symptom control, improved quality of life, and reduced healthcare costs.
- **Patient empowerment:** *N*-of-1 trials empower patients to actively participate in their own care and make informed decisions about their treatment.

Disadvantages of *N*-of-1 Trials

- Time-consuming and resource-intensive: conducting multiple treatment cycles can be time-consuming and resource-intensive.
- Carryover effects: carryover effects from one treatment to the next can confound the results.
- Order effect: order effect occurs when the sequence in which treatments are administered influences the outcome.
- Generalizability: the results of an *N*-of-1 trial apply only to the individual patient who participated in the trial. They cannot be generalized to other patients.
- Blinding challenges: blinding can be difficult, especially if treatments have different routes of administration or noticeable side effects.

Field Trials

Definition

Field trials are primarily considered epidemiological studies or community-based trials, although they share some characteristics with clinical trials. They are conducted in real-world settings, such as communities, schools, or workplaces, to evaluate the effectiveness of interventions aimed at improving health outcomes. They differ from traditional clinical trials, which often take place in controlled research environments.

Purpose

These trials are often aimed at preventing diseases or promoting health, such as vaccination programmes or public health campaigns. The focus is on incidence of disease, behavioural changes, or public health impact rather than clinical outcomes alone.

Participants

- Often involve healthy or at-risk individuals rather than patients with specific conditions.
- Participants are randomly assigned to intervention and control groups.

Comparison of Study Types

Table 8.4 presents a comparison of RCTs, pragmatic trials, crossover trials, *N*-of-1 trials, and field trials.

Clinical Trials

Clinical trials are conducted in phases to systematically evaluate the safety, efficacy, and approval of new drugs or treatments before they become widely available. Each phase serves a distinct purpose in the drug development process, ensuring that only safe and effective treatments reach the public.

Preclinical Research

Before human testing, new treatments undergo laboratory and animal studies to:

- assess initial safety, toxicity, and potential efficacy.
- determine whether the treatment is safe enough to proceed to clinical trials.

Phase 0 (Microdosing Studies)

- Involves very small doses administered to a small group (10–15 participants).
- Examines how the drug is processed in the human body, including metabolism and pharmacokinetics.
- Helps determine if the drug has potential for further development.

Phase 1 (Safety and Dosage Trials)

- Conducted on 20–80 healthy volunteers (or patients in specific cases).
- Focuses on safety, establishing a dosage range, and identifying potential side effects.
- Determines the maximum tolerated dose for further testing.

Table 8.4 Comparison of RCTs, pragmatic trials, crossover trials, *N*-of-1 trials, and field trials

Aspect	RCTs	Pragmatic trials	Crossover trials	N-of-1 trials	Field trials
Primary purpose	Evaluate efficacy of an intervention under controlled conditions	Assess effectiveness of an intervention in real-world settings	Compare two or more treatments within the same participants	Determine optimal treatment for individual patients	Evaluate preventive interventions in community settings
Study setting	Controlled clinical settings (e.g. hospitals, research centres)	Routine clinical practice (e.g. primary care, hospitals)	Clinical setting, often outpatient or specialized clinics	Real-world clinical settings, personalized	Community-based, such as schools, neighbourhoods, workplaces
Population	Patients meeting strict inclusion criteria	Broad population, reflecting typical clinical practice	Same patients receive all interventions	Focuses on a single patient, highly individualized	Generally healthy individuals or at-risk groups, not patients
Intervention type	Therapeutic, diagnostic, or preventive	Therapeutic or management strategies	Primarily therapeutic, comparing multiple treatments	Therapeutic, personalized treatment decisions	Preventive measures, public health interventions (e.g. vaccinations)
Design	Randomized, controlled, often double-blind	Randomized, flexible protocols, real-world practice	Randomized, crossover design, with washout periods	Randomized, multiple treatment periods, often blinded	Randomized or quasi-experimental, often group-based
Randomization	Yes, participants are randomly assigned to groups	Yes, with flexibility in treatment application	Yes, but within individuals, not between groups	Yes, randomizes treatment order for individuals	Yes, but often at the community or group level
Control group	Placebo, standard treatment, or no intervention	Typically standard care or usual practice	Each participant serves as their own control	The patient serves as their own control	Placebo, standard practice, or no intervention
Blinding	Usually double-blind	May or may not be blinded, often open-label	Can be blinded, but not always	Ideally blinded, but not always feasible	Rarely blinded, especially in public health interventions

Outcome measures	Clinical endpoints, biomarkers, safety data	Patient-centred outcomes, real-world effectiveness	Compares outcomes across treatment periods	Measures individual treatment response, personalized outcomes	Incidence rates, public health impact, behavioural changes
Analysis method	ITT, per-protocol, statistical testing	Effectiveness measures, practical outcomes, real-world data	Paired *t*-tests, ANOVA, mixed-effects models	Time-series analysis, visual analysis, Bayesian methods	Epidemiological analysis, relative risk, odds ratios
Generalizability	High internal validity, lower external validity	High external validity, applicable to real-world practice	Limited to specific conditions where crossover is suitable	Not directly generalizable, but useful for individualized care	High external validity, generalizable to populations
Duration	Variable, often months to years	Variable, depending on clinical practice needs	Shorter periods, with repeated treatment cycles	Short to medium term, depending on treatment cycles	Often long term, to assess prevention and impact
Examples	Drug trials, surgical interventions, new therapies	Comparing two treatment approaches in routine care	Testing effectiveness of two medications for chronic conditions	Evaluating medication response for treatment-resistant depression	Vaccine trials, community health programmes, public health campaigns
Advantages	Rigorous control, minimizes bias, clear efficacy data	Reflects real-world practice, high external validity	Efficient use of participants, within-subject comparison	Personalized treatment decisions, high internal validity	High external validity, real-world impact, large-scale applicability
Limitations	Expensive, time-consuming, may lack real-world applicability	Less control over variables, heterogeneous populations	Not suitable for all conditions, carryover effects	Not generalizable, time- and resource-intensive	Difficult to control variables, risk of bias, ethical challenges

Phase 2 (Efficacy and Safety Trials)

- Involves 100–300 patients with the target condition.
- Assesses efficacy and continues safety evaluation.
- Helps determine the optimal dose and short-term risks.

Phase 3 (Confirmatory Trials and Regulatory Approval)

- Large-scale trials (300–3,000+ patients) conducted across multiple sites.
- Compares the new treatment with existing standard treatments or a placebo.
- Confirms effectiveness and safety profile for regulatory approval.
- Data from this phase is submitted to regulatory agencies (e.g. MHRA, EMA, FDA) for approval.

Phase 4 (Post-Marketing Surveillance)

- Conducted after regulatory approval and public availability.
- Monitors long-term safety, effectiveness, and rare side effects in real-world settings.
- Identifies any unexpected adverse reactions or drug interactions.

Chapter Summary

Randomized Controlled Trials

Randomized controlled trials are the gold standard for assessing the effectiveness of interventions by minimizing bias and ensuring comparability between treatment groups.

Key Components of RCTs

- Random selection: ensures participants are chosen from a larger population in an unbiased manner.
- Randomization: allocates participants randomly to treatment and control groups, reducing selection bias.
- Blinding: prevents bias by keeping participants, researchers, or data analysts unaware of treatment assignments.
- Control groups: enable comparison between the experimental treatment and standard care, placebo, or no intervention.
- Outcome measures: evaluate treatment effectiveness based on predefined endpoints, such as symptom reduction or disease progression.

Types of Randomization

- Simple randomization: assigns participants randomly to groups, similar to flipping a coin. Effective for large trials but may cause imbalance in small samples.
- Block randomization: ensures equal participant distribution across groups by randomizing within small blocks (e.g. four, six, or eight participants per block).

- Stratified randomization: ensures key prognostic factors (e.g. age, gender, disease severity) are balanced across treatment arms by grouping participants into strata before randomization.
- Adaptive randomization: adjusts group allocation probabilities dynamically based on accumulating trial data, favouring better-performing treatments.
- Minimization: reduces imbalance by considering multiple factors when assigning participants, making it useful for small sample sizes.
- Cluster randomization: assigns entire groups (e.g. hospitals, schools) to treatment conditions instead of individuals, often used for public health interventions.

Analytical Approaches in RCTs

- Per-protocol analysis: includes only participants who adhered to the trial protocol, providing an estimate of the treatment's efficacy under ideal conditions.
- Intention-to-treat analysis: includes all randomized participants, regardless of adherence, preserving the benefits of randomization and reflecting real-world effectiveness.

Methods for Handling Missing Data

- Last observation carried forward: uses the last available measurement for missing data, though it may introduce bias.
- Multiple imputation: creates multiple datasets with plausible values for missing data, improving statistical robustness.
- Mixed models/repeated measures analysis: accounts for within-subject correlations over time, making it useful for longitudinal studies.
- Treatment policy estimator: evaluates treatment effects based on initial assignment, ensuring real-world applicability.

Measuring Strength of Association Using a 2×2 Table

A 2×2 contingency table is commonly used to quantify treatment effects by comparing outcomes in treatment and control groups (see Table 8.3).

From this structure, the following measures can be calculated:

- Experimental event rate: proportion of experimental group experiencing the event: $\text{EER} = a / (a + b)$.
- Control event rate: proportion of control group experiencing the event: $\text{CER} = c / (c + d)$.
- Absolute benefit increase: difference between EER and CER: $\text{ABI} = \text{EER} - \text{CER}$.
- Number needed to treat: number of patients who need to be treated for one additional benefit: $\text{NNT} = 1 / \text{ABI}$.
- Relative risk: likelihood of the event occurring in the treatment group compared to the control group: $\text{RR} = \text{EER} / \text{CER}$.
- Relative benefit increase: proportional increase in benefit in the experimental group: $\text{RBI} = (\text{EER} - \text{CER}) / \text{CER}$.

Alternative Trial Designs

- Pragmatic clinical trials: assess real-world effectiveness by including broader patient populations and flexible treatment protocols.
- Crossover trials: participants receive multiple treatments in sequence, serving as their own control to reduce variability.
- *N*-of-1 trials: individualized trials in which a single patient undergoes multiple treatment cycles to determine the best therapeutic approach.
- Field trials: large-scale epidemiological studies that assess public health interventions in real-world settings, such as vaccination programmes.

Stages of Clinical Trials

- Preclinical research: laboratory and animal studies to assess safety and biological effects.
- Phase 0 (first-in-human trials): small human trials (10–15 participants) to evaluate drug metabolism and pharmacokinetics.
- Phase 1: small group trials (20–80 participants) to assess safety, dosage, and side effects.
- Phase 2: larger group trials (100–300 participants) to test efficacy and monitor short-term side effects.
- Phase 3: large trials (300–3,000 participants) to confirm effectiveness, compare treatments, and assess risks.
- Phase 4: post-marketing surveillance to monitor long-term safety and rare side effects.

Practice Questions

For Q1–Q4: In an open-label, multicentre RCT, 1,015 people with heroin dependence received a variable dose of injectable heroin (n = 515) or oral methadone (n = 500) as control for 12 months. Two response criteria, improvement of physical and/or mental health, and decrease in illicit drug use, were evaluated in an intention-to-treat analysis (Table 8.5).

Table 8.5 Intention-to-treat analysis of heroin versus methadone treatment for opioid dependence

	Heroin *n*	Heroin %	Methadone *n*	Methadone %
Improvement in 'health'	412	80.0	370	74.0
Reduction in illegal drug use	356	69.1	276	55.2

Source: Haasen C, Verthein U, Degkwitz P, et al. Heroin-assisted treatment for opioid dependence: randomised controlled trial. *Br J Psychiatry*. 2007;191:55–62. doi: https://doi.org/10.1192/bjp.bp.106.026112.

Q1. What is the ABI in improvement of 'health' with heroin treatment?

A. 2%
B. 4%
C. 6%
D. 8%
E. 10%

Q2. What is the odds ratio for reduction in illegal drug use with heroin treatment compared to methadone treatment?

A. 1.23
B. 1.52
C. 1.82
D. 2.23
E. 2.52

Q3. What is the relative benefit increase (RBI) in reduction in illegal drug use with heroin treatment compared to methadone?

A. 0.10
B. 0.15
C. 0.25
D. 0.30
E. 0.35

Q4. What is the NTT to bring about one additional case of health improvement with heroin treatment?

A. 10
B. 12
C. 14
D. 17
E. 20

Q5. What is the primary purpose of using randomization in an RCT?

A. To ensure equal sample sizes in each group
B. To eliminate all confounding factors
C. To reduce selection bias and ensure baseline comparability
D. To ensure blinding of participants and researchers
E. To increase the generalizability of study findings

Q6. What is the primary purpose of randomization in an RCT?

A. Ensure that the study sample is representative of the general population.
B. Prevent selection bias by ensuring treatment allocation is determined by chance.
C. Minimize the placebo effect in the study.
D. Guarantee that the treatment and control groups are perfectly matched.
E. Reduce the need for statistical adjustments in data analysis.

Q7. Researchers are investigating the effects of a new migraine medication. They use a computer-generated list to randomly select participants from a registry of migraine sufferers before obtaining consent for the study. What is this method called?

A. Random selection
B. Randomization
C. Stratification

D. Blinding
E. Matching

For Q8–Q12: An RCT was conducted to evaluate the effect of streptomycin plus bed rest versus placebo plus bed rest in patients with acute bilateral pulmonary tuberculosis. The study included 107 participants, with 55 in the streptomycin group and 52 in the placebo group. The six-month mortality was 4 out of 55 in the streptomycin group and 14 out of 52 in the placebo group.

Q8. What is the absolute risk reduction of death with streptomycin treatment compared to placebo?

A. 3.68%
B. 7.3%
C. 19.6%
D. 26.9%
E. 73%

Q9. What is the odds ratio for death with streptomycin compared to placebo?

A. 0.21
B. 0.70
C. 1.30
D. 1.35
E. 4.70

Q10. How many patients need to be treated with streptomycin to prevent one additional death?

A. 3
B. 6
C. 10
D. 9
E. 2

Q11. What does this relative risk reduction indicate?

A. Streptomycin reduces the risk of death by 27% compared to placebo.
B. Streptomycin reduces the risk of death by 73% compared to placebo.
C. Streptomycin increases the survival rate by 26.9%.
D. Streptomycin increases the chance of survival by 19.6%.
E. Streptomycin reduces the risk of TB transmission by 50%.

Q12. If the study population was doubled while event rates remained the same, which of the following would change?

A. Absolute risk reduction
B. Relative risk
C. Relative risk reduction
D. *p*-Value
E. Risk difference

Q13. Which phase of clinical trials primarily focuses on determining the safest dose range of a drug?
A. Phase 0
B. Phase 1
C. Phase 2
D. Phase 3
E. Phase 4

Q14. In which phase of clinical trials is the drug tested for the first time on patients with the target condition?
A. Phase 0
B. Phase 1
C. Phase 2
D. Phase 3
E. Phase 4

Q15. What is the primary goal of preclinical research in the drug development process?
A. To test the drug on a large patient population.
B. To monitor the drug's long-term effects after approval.
C. To determine the optimal dosage for human patients.
D. To assess the drug's safety and potential efficacy in laboratory and animal studies.
E. To explore how the drug is processed in the human body.

Answers

Q1. Correct answer: C (6%). Table 8.6 shows the 2 × 2 table for health improvement.

Table 8.6 The 2 × 2 table for health improvement in heroin (experimental) versus methadone (control) treatment groups

Treatment	Improvement	Non-improvement	Total
Heroin (experimental)	412 (*a*)	103 (*b*)	515
Methadone (control)	370 (*c*)	130 (*d*)	500
Total	782	233	1,015

$$\mathrm{CER} = \frac{c}{c+d} = \frac{370}{500} = 0.74,$$

$$\mathrm{EER} = \frac{a}{a+b} = \frac{412}{515} = 0.8,$$

$$\mathrm{ABI} = \mathrm{EER} - \mathrm{CER} = 0.8 - 0.74 = 0.06 = 6\%$$

Q2. Correct answer: C (1.82). Table 8.7 shows the odds ratio for reduction in illegal drug use.

Table 8.7 The 2×2 table for calculating the odds ratio of reduction in illicit drug use in heroin (experimental) versus methadone (control) groups

Treatment	Reduction in illegal drug use	No reduction in illegal drug use	Total
Heroin (experimental)	356 (*a*)	159 (*b*)	515
Methadone (control)	276 (*c*)	224 (*d*)	500
Total	632	383	1,015

$$\text{OR} = \frac{\text{Odds of reduction in illegal drug use with experimental treatment}}{\text{Odds of reduction in illegal drug use with control treatment}},$$

odds of improvement on experimental treatment $= \frac{a}{b}$ *or* $\frac{\text{EER}}{1-\text{EER}} = \frac{356}{159},$

odds of improvement on control treatment $= \frac{c}{d}$ *or* $\frac{\text{CER}}{1-\text{CER}} = \frac{276}{224},$

$\text{OR} = \frac{356\times224}{159\times276} = \frac{79{,}744}{43{,}884} = 1.82.$

Can also use cross-multiplication: $\text{OR} = \frac{ad}{bc}$.

Q3. Correct answer: C (0.25). Using Table 8.7 from Q2:

$\text{EER} = \frac{356}{515} = 0.69,$

$\text{CER} = \frac{276}{500} = 0.55,$

$\text{RR} = \frac{\text{EER}}{\text{CER}} = \frac{0.69}{0.55},$

Relative risk reduction = RR – 1 *or* $\frac{\text{EER}-\text{CER}}{\text{CER}} = \left(\frac{0.69}{0.55}\right) - 1 = 0.25.$

Q4. Correct answer: D. 17:

$\text{ABI} = \text{EER} - \text{CER} = 0.80 - 0.74 = 0.06,$

$\text{NNT} = \frac{1}{\text{ABI}} - \frac{1}{0.06} = 16.6 = 17$ (rounded up).

Q5. Correct answer: C. To reduce selection bias and ensure baseline comparability.

Randomization means that participants are assigned to either the treatment or control group purely by chance. This is like flipping a coin to decide. The primary goal of this is to create groups that are as similar as possible at the start of the trial in all aspects except for the treatment being studied.

Why the other options are incorrect:

A. To ensure equal sample sizes in each group: while randomization often leads to similar group sizes, it's not the main goal. Sometimes, researchers might even use specific randomization techniques to ensure a certain ratio of participants in each group.

B. To eliminate all confounding factors: randomization helps to reduce the influence of confounding factors (things that might affect the outcome other than the treatment), but it cannot eliminate them entirely.

D. To ensure blinding of participants and researchers: blinding is a separate technique used in RCTs and, while important, it's not the primary purpose of randomization.

E. To increase the generalizability of study findings: generalizability relates to how well the study findings apply to a larger population. Randomization helps with internal validity (accuracy of the study itself), but doesn't guarantee generalizability.

Q6. Correct answer: B. Prevent selection bias by ensuring treatment allocation is determined by chance. Selection bias occurs when the groups being compared in a study are different from the start. This can happen if participants are allowed to choose their treatment, or if researchers assign participants based on their characteristics. Randomization removes this bias by using a chance process (such as flipping a coin) to assign participants to either the treatment or control group. This helps create groups that are similar in all aspects except for the treatment being studied.

Why the other options are incorrect:

A. Ensure that the study sample is representative of the general population: while important, this relates to the study's external validity (how well it applies to a larger population). Randomization focuses on internal validity (accuracy within the study itself).

C. Minimize the placebo effect in the study: blinding helps control for the placebo effect, not randomization.

D. Guarantee that the treatment and control groups are perfectly matched: randomization aims for similarity, but it doesn't guarantee perfect matching. There might still be some differences due to chance.

E. Reduce the need for statistical adjustments in data analysis: randomization can reduce the need for some adjustments, but it's not the main reason for its use.

Q7. Correct answer. A. Random selection. Random selection refers to choosing study participants from a larger population before obtaining consent and assigning them to different groups. This ensures a representative sample and improves external validity (generalizability of results).

Randomization happens after consent is obtained and is used to allocate participants to treatment or control groups in a study.

Why the other options are incorrect:

B. Randomization: randomization occurs after consent, ensuring fair assignment to groups. The question focuses on the selection process before randomization.

C. Stratification: stratification is a technique used after selection to ensure key characteristics (e.g. age, disease severity) are balanced across groups.

D. Blinding: blinding prevents participants or researchers from knowing the treatment allocation to reduce bias, which is unrelated to participant selection.
E. Matching: matching is a method used to ensure groups are comparable based on key variables (e.g. age, gender) but does not involve random selection.

Q8. Correct answer: C. 19.6%. Absolute risk reduction (ARR) is calculated as: ARR = CER − EER:

EER = death rate in streptomycin group = 4/55 = 7.3%,

CER = death rate in placebo group = 14/52 = 26.9%,

ARR = 26.9% − 7.3% = 19.6%.

Q9. Correct answer: A. 0.21. Odds ratio is calculated using a 2 × 2 contingency table (Table 8.8).

Table 8.8 The 2 × 2 contingency table for calculating the OR of mortality in streptomycin versus placebo groups

Outcome	Died	Survived	Total
Streptomycin	4 (*a*)	51 (*b*)	55
Placebo	14 (*c*)	38 (*d*)	52

$OR = \frac{ad}{bc} = \frac{4\times 38}{51\times 14} = \frac{152}{714} = 0.21.$

Since OR < 1, this indicates a protective effect of streptomycin against TB-related mortality.

Q10. Correct answer: B. 6. NNT is calculated as:

EER = death rate in streptomycin group = 4/55 = 7.3%,

CER = death rate in placebo group = 14/52 = 26.9%,

ABI = 0.269 − 0.073 = 0.196,

$NNT = \frac{1}{ABI} = \frac{1}{0.196} = 5.1 = 6$ (because NNT should be rounded up).

Q11. Correct answer: B. Streptomycin reduces the risk of death by 73% compared to placebo. Relative risk reduction (RRR) is calculated as:

$RRR = 1 - RR = \frac{ARR}{CER} = \frac{19.6\%}{26.9\%} = 73\%.$

This means treatment with streptomycin reduces the risk of death by 73% compared to placebo.

Q12. Correct answer: D. *p*-Value. ARR, RR, RRR, and risk difference remain the same if the event rates remain unchanged. *p*-Value will decrease (i.e. become more significant) because larger sample sizes reduce variability and increase statistical power.

Q13. Correct answer: B. Phase 1. Phase 1 trials are first-in-human studies, usually conducted on 20–80 healthy volunteers, with a primary focus on safety and determining the optimal dosage range. Researchers identify the maximum tolerated dose and potential side effects before moving to larger patient studies.

Q14. Correct answer: C. Phase 2. Phase 2 trials involve a larger group of 100–300 patients who actually have the disease or condition being studied. The goal is to evaluate efficacy (how well the drug works) while continuing to monitor safety and optimal dosing.

Q15. Correct answer: D. To assess the drug's safety and potential efficacy in laboratory and animal studies. Preclinical research is the initial stage of drug development. It occurs before any testing is done on human subjects. The primary goal is to gather foundational data on the drug's behaviour in biological systems. This involves:

- Safety assessment: determining potential toxicities and side effects through in vitro (laboratory) and in vivo (animal) studies.
- Efficacy assessment: evaluating whether the drug shows promise in treating the targeted condition in animal models. This stage provides crucial information about the drug's pharmacokinetics (how the body processes the drug) and pharmacodynamics (how the drug affects the body). The results of preclinical research determine whether a drug is considered safe and promising enough to proceed to human clinical trials.

Further Reading

Altman DG. Confidence intervals for the number needed to treat. *BMJ.* 1998;**317**(7168):1309–12.

Altman DG, Andersen PK. Calculating the number needed to treat for trials where the outcome is time to an event. *BMJ.* 1999;319 (7223):1492–5.

Altman DG, Schulz KF. Statistics notes: concealing treatment allocation in randomised trials. *BMJ.* 2001;**323**(7310):446–7.

Campbell MK, Piaggio G, Elbourne DR, Altman DG ; CONSORT Group. CONSORT 2010 statement: extension to cluster randomised trials. *BMJ.* 2012;**345**:e5661.

Cook RJ, Sackett DL. The number needed to treat: a clinically useful measure of treatment effect. *BMJ.* 1995;**310**(6977):452–4.

Dimairo M, Pallmann P, Wason J, et al. The Adaptive designs CONSORT Extension (ACE) statement. *BMJ.* 2020;**369**:m115.

Donner A, Klar N. *Design and Analysis of Cluster Randomization Trials in Health Research.* London: Arnold; 2000.

Dwan K, Li T, Altman DG, et al. CONSORT extension for randomised crossover trials. *BMJ.* 2019;**366**:l4378.

Gupta SK. Intention-to-treat concept: a review. *Perspect Clin Res.* 2011;**2**(3):109–12.

Hopewell S, Chan A-W, Collins GS, et al. CONSORT 2025 statement: updated guideline for reporting randomised trials. *BMJ.* 2025;**389**: e081123.

Hróbjartsson A, Gøtzsche PC. Is the placebo powerless? An analysis of clinical trials comparing placebo with no treatment. *N Engl J Med.* 2001;**344**(21):1594–602.

International Council for Harmonisation. E9: Statistical principles for clinical trials. 1998. Available at: www.ema.europa.eu/en/ich-e9-statistical-principles-clinical-trials-scientific-guideline

International Council for Harmonisation. ICH E9 (R1): Addendum on estimands and sensitivity analysis in clinical trials. 2019. Available at: www.ema.europa.eu/en/documents/scientific-guideline/ich-e9-r1-addendum-estimands-and-sensitivity-analysis-clinical-trials-guideline-statistical-principles-clinical-trials-step-5_en.pdf

Laird NM, Ware JH. Random-effects models for longitudinal data. *Biometrics.* 1982;**38**(4):963–74.

Loudon K, Treweek S, Sullivan F, et al. The PRECIS-2 tool: designing trials that are fit for purpose. *BMJ.* 2015;**350**:h2147.

Mallinckrodt CH, Lane PW, Schnell D, Peng Y, Mancuso JP. Recommendations for the primary analysis of continuous endpoints in longitudinal clinical trials. *Ther Innov Regul Sci (Drug Inf J)*. 2008;**42**:303–19.

Pocock SJ, Simon R. Sequential treatment assignment with balancing for prognostic factors in the controlled clinical trial. *Biometrics*. 1975;**31**(1):103–15.

Robins JM, Hernán MA, Brumback B. Marginal structural models and causal inference in epidemiology. *Epidemiology*. 2000;**11**(5):550–60.

Rubin DB. *Multiple Imputation for Nonresponse in Surveys*. New York: Wiley; 1987.

Schulz KF, Grimes DA. Allocation concealment in randomised trials: defending against deciphering. *Lancet*. 2002;**359**(9306):614–18.

Schulz KF, Altman DG, Moher D; CONSORT Group. CONSORT 2010 statement: updated guidelines for reporting parallel group randomised trials. *BMJ*. 2010;**340**:c332.

Smith PG, Morrow RH, Ross DA (eds). *Field Trials of Health Interventions: A Toolbox*. 3rd ed. Oxford: Oxford University Press; 2015.

Taves DR. Minimization: a new method of assigning patients to treatment and control groups. *Clin Pharmacol Ther*. 1974;**15**(5):443–53.

Thorpe KE, Zwarenstein M, Oxman AD, et al. A pragmatic–explanatory continuum indicator summary (PRECIS). *J Clin Epidemiol*. 2009;**62**:464–75.

Vohra S, Shamseer L, Sampson M, et al. CONSORT extension for N-of-1 trials (CENT) 2015. *BMJ*. 2015;**350**:h1738.

White IR, Royston P, Wood AM. Multiple imputation using chained equations: issues and guidance for practice. *Stat Med*. 2011;**30**(4):377–99.

Zwarenstein M, Treweek S, Gagnier JJ, et al. Improving the reporting of pragmatic trials: an extension of the CONSORT statement. *BMJ*. 2008;**337**:a2390.

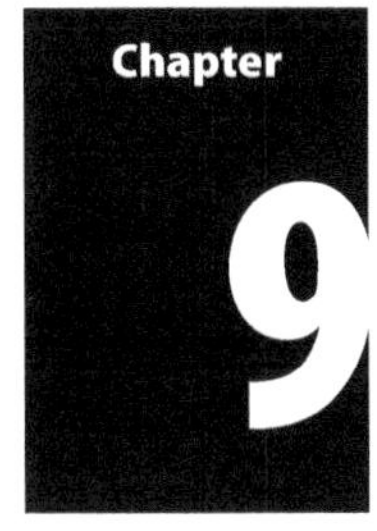

Systematic Review

Introduction

A systematic review in medicine is a structured, comprehensive summary of all available research evidence on a specific clinical question. It follows a rigorous, predefined methodology to identify, evaluate, and synthesize relevant studies, minimizing bias and ensuring reliability.

A meta-analysis is a statistical technique used to combine the results of multiple independent studies on a specific topic. It provides a more comprehensive and precise estimate of the effect of an intervention or exposure than any single study can offer.

Steps in Conducting a Systematic Review

Formulate the Research Question

Clearly define the research question using the **PICO framework** (population, intervention, comparison, and outcome).[1] This guides the entire review process.

Develop a Protocol

Create a detailed plan outlining the review's objectives, inclusion/exclusion criteria, search strategy, data extraction process, and planned analyses. Registering the protocol with a review registry (e.g. PROSPERO) ensures transparency and prevents duplication.

Search for Studies

A comprehensive search is crucial to include all eligible studies. Strategies include:

- **Database search:** searching multiple databases, such as **PubMed,**[2] **Cochrane Library**[3] (for randomized controlled trials (RCTs) and systematic reviews), **Embase**[4] (pharmacological studies), PsycINFO (mental health studies), **CINAHL**[5] (nursing or

---

[1] **PICO framework:** Structure questions and eligibility: population/problem, intervention/exposure, comparator, outcome; often extended to PICOS (adds study design) or PICOT (adds time).

[2] **PubMed:** NLM database with MEDLINE indexing and MeSH terms; use MeSH explosion and field tags to balance sensitivity/specificity.

[3] **Cochrane Library:** Includes CDSR (systematic reviews) and CENTRAL (trial registry of registries); core sources for trial identification. It is a key source for high-quality syntheses.

[4] **Embase:** Emtree-indexed biomedical/pharma database with strong conference abstract coverage – use alongside MEDLINE to reduce retrieval bias; de-duplicate carefully.

[5] **CINAHL:** Nursing and allied-health literature – broadens beyond core biomedical databases.

allied health studies), and **Web of Science/Scopus** (multidisciplinary studies). **Boolean operators**[6] (AND, OR, NOT), parentheses, quotation marks, and truncation enhance search precision.

- **Other sources:** searching grey literature (**HMIC,**[7] **OpenGrey,**[8] NICE evidence), conference proceedings, unpublished studies (**ClinicalTrials.gov,**[9] UK Clinical Trials Gateway, **ICTRP**),[10] hand-searching journals, and checking references of relevant studies.

Screen Studies

Screen titles and abstracts to exclude irrelevant studies. Retrieve full-text articles of potentially eligible studies and assess them against the inclusion/exclusion criteria. This is often done independently by two reviewers to minimize bias. The **PRISMA** (Preferred Reporting Items for Systematic Reviews and Meta-Analyses) flow diagram helps document the study selection process.

Extract Data

Data should be extracted using a standardized form to ensure consistency across studies. Key elements typically include study design, participants, interventions, outcomes, and assessment of risk of bias. An example is provided in Table 9.1.

Table 9.1 Example of a data extraction table

Study	Sample size	Intervention	Comparison	Outcome	Risk of bias
Smith et al. (2022)	200 patients	CBT	Medication	Anxiety score reduction	Low risk
Jones and Williams (2017)	152 patients	CBT	Usual care	Anxiety score reduction	Some concerns
Reed (2016)	37 patients	CBT	Medication	Anxiety score reduction	High risk

[6] **Boolean operators:** Use **AND/OR/NOT**, quotation marks (' ') for phrases, truncation (e.g. therap*), and database-specific proximity operators to tune sensitivity/specificity.

[7] **HMIC:** Health Management Information Consortium – good for health policy, management, and service-delivery evidence.

[8] **OpenGrey:** Database of grey literature (e.g. reports, theses, conference proceedings) not published in traditional journals.

[9] **ClinicalTrials.gov:** Trial registry/results database – helps find ongoing/unpublished studies and assess selective reporting.

[10] **ICTRP (WHO):** Aggregator of national/regional trial registries – improves global ascertainment beyond US/EU databases.

Assess Risk of Bias

Assess the quality of included studies using validated tools. The risk of bias should be evaluated using established tools, such as:

- the Cochrane Risk of Bias Tool for RCTs
- the **Newcastle–Ottawa Scale**[11] for observational studies.

An example is shown in Table 9.2.

Table 9.2 Example of a bias assessment table

Bias type	Risk level
Random sequence generation	Low
Blinding issues	High
Attrition bias	Moderate

Assess for Publication Bias

Publication bias occurs when studies with significant results are more likely to be published. Techniques for assessment of publication bias include:

- **Funnel plot (visual assessment):** a visual method in which asymmetry suggests bias (requires ≥10 studies). Funnel plots provide a visual method for assessing publication bias by plotting study effect sizes against their precision (e.g. standard error). In the absence of publication bias, the plot should resemble a symmetrical inverted funnel, with smaller studies scattered more widely at the bottom and larger studies clustered more tightly at the top. Asymmetry in the funnel plot can suggest publication bias, as it may indicate that smaller studies with non-significant or negative results are missing. Funnel plots are recommended only when there are at least 10 studies, as they are unreliable with fewer studies. Figures 9.1–9.3 illustrate how a funnel plot appears when no publication bias is present versus when publication bias is present.

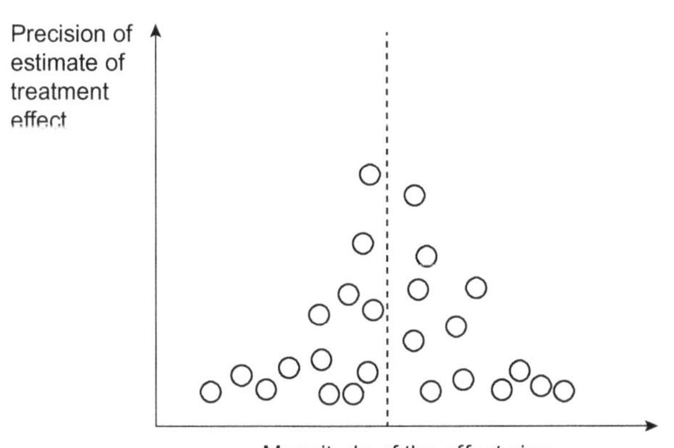

Figure 9.1 Funnel plot showing a symmetrical distribution of studies, indicating no evidence of publication bias (Source: Montori V, Smieja M, Guyatt G. Publication bias: a brief review for clinicians. *Mayo Clinic*. 2001;75:1284–8. doi: https://doi.org/10.4065/75.12.1284).

[11] **Newcastle–Ottawa Scale:** Quality appraisal for non-randomized studies using stars across selection, comparability, and outcome/exposure; provides a quick risk-of-bias signal, not a meta-analytic weight.

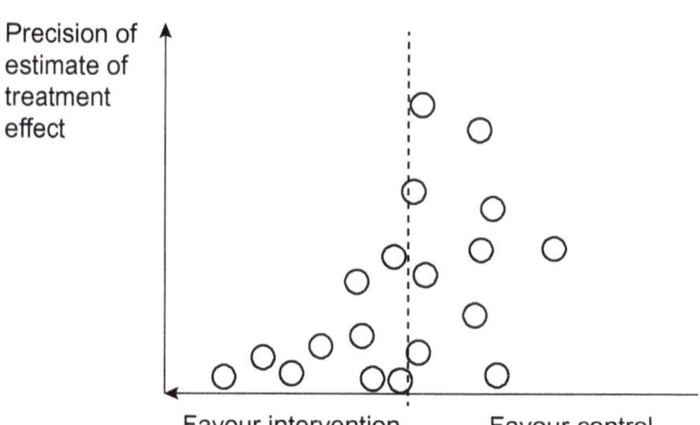

Figure 9.2 Funnel plot showing asymmetrical distribution of studies, indicating the presence of publication bias (Source: Sutton AJ, Duval SJ, Tweedie RL, et al. Empirical assessment of effect of publication bias on meta-analyses. *BMJ* 2000;320:1574. doi: https://doi.org/10.1136/bmj.320.7249.1574

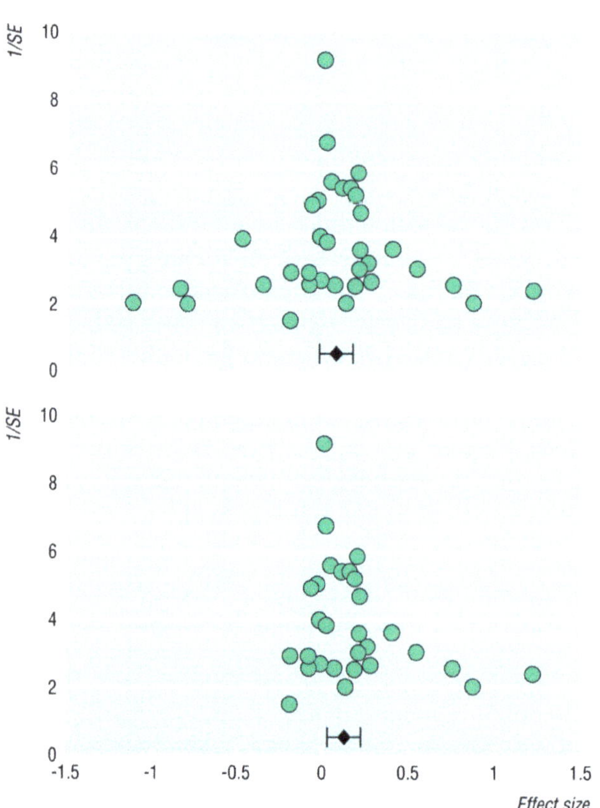

Figure 9.3 Funnel plots illustrating publication bias. The top plot shows results from 35 simulated studies with symmetrical distribution (no bias), while the bottom plot shows the same data with five missing studies, resulting in asymmetry indicative of publication bias (Source: adapted from Sutton AJ, Duval SJ, Tweedie RL, et al. Empirical assessment of effect of publication bias on meta-analyses. *BMJ* 2000;320:1574. doi: https://doi.org/10.1136/bmj.320.7249.1574).

- **Statistical tests:**
  - **Egger's test:** detects small-study effects by analysing funnel plot asymmetry using regression analysis. A significant result ($p < 0.05$) suggests potential publication bias.
  - **Begg's test:** uses rank correlation to assess the relationship between effect size and its variance.

- **Other methods:**
  - **Trim-and-fill method:** imputes missing studies based on observed funnel plot asymmetry and re-estimates the overall effect.
  - **Fail-safe *N*:** calculates the number of unpublished null-result studies required to overturn the conclusions of a meta-analysis.
  - ***p*-curve analysis:** examines the distribution of significant *p*-values in published studies to detect selective reporting (*p*-hacking).
  - **Checking trial registries and grey literature:** involves searching for unpublished studies (e.g. conference abstracts, dissertations) to identify missing data to reduce publication bias.

The different methods available to evaluate the presence of publication bias in systematic reviews and meta-analyses are summarized in Table 9.3.

Table 9.3 Summary of methods for assessing publication bias

Method	Purpose	Best for
Funnel plot	Visual check for missing studies	Meta-analyses with ≥10 studies
Egger's test	Statistical test for small-study effects	Continuous outcomes
Begg's test	Alternative statistical test	Small sample sizes
Trim-and-fill method	Adjusts for missing studies	Meta-analyses showing funnel plot asymmetry
p-curve analysis	Detects selective reporting of significant results	Checking for *p*-hacking
Trial registry comparison	Finds unpublished studies	Identifying missing trials

Assess Heterogeneity

Heterogeneity refers to the variation or inconsistency in the findings of the individual studies included in the review. It is important to look for heterogeneity as it can affect the interpretation and generalizability of the review's results.

Heterogeneity can be classified into three main types, as given in Table 9.4:

Table 9.4 Types of heterogeneity in systematic reviews

Type	Definition	Example
Clinical heterogeneity	Differences in study populations, interventions, and outcomes	One study uses CBT for 4 weeks, another for 12 weeks
Methodological heterogeneity	Differences in study design, risk of bias, or execution	One study is double-blind, another is open-label
Statistical heterogeneity	Differences in effect sizes across studies	Some studies show a large treatment effect, others show no effect

Methods to Assess Heterogeneity

The following methods can be used to assess heterogeneity.

Visual Inspection of Forest Plots

A forest plot provides a graphical way to assess effect sizes and their confidence intervals (CIs) across studies. Confidence intervals indicate the range within which the true effect size is likely to lie. When the confidence intervals of studies do not overlap or only minimally overlap, this suggests high heterogeneity and inconsistent results. However, overlap of confidence intervals is only a rough guide; statistical measures such as I^2 and τ^2 should be used to quantify heterogeneity.

Figure 9.4 shows a forest plot with significant heterogeneity. The wide variation in effect sizes and the lack of overlapping CIs across studies demonstrate substantial variability.

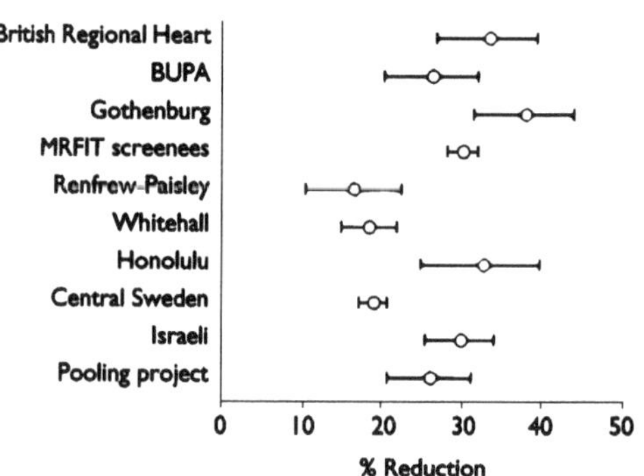

Figure 9.4 Forest plot showing percentage reduction in risk of ischaemic heart disease (with 95% CIs) associated with a 0.6 mmol/L reduction in serum cholesterol across 10 prospective studies of men (Source: Thompson SG. Systematic review: why sources of heterogeneity in meta-analysis should be investigated. *BMJ* 1994;309:1351. doi: https://doi.org/10.1136/bmj.309.6965.1351).

Galbraith Plot (Radial Plot)

A Galbraith plot is another graphical method used to assess heterogeneity. It plots standardized effect sizes against their precision (inverse standard error). The Galbraith plot helps visually detect heterogeneity, outliers, and potential sources of inconsistency.

- Each study's standardized effect size is plotted on the *y*-axis.
- Each study's precision (1/standard error) is plotted on the *x*-axis.
- A central regression line is drawn through the data points, representing the overall pooled estimate.
- Additional lines (typically at ±2 standard deviations) help identify studies that deviate significantly from the pooled effect.

If points scatter widely or diverge from the central line, heterogeneity is high (Figure 9.5).

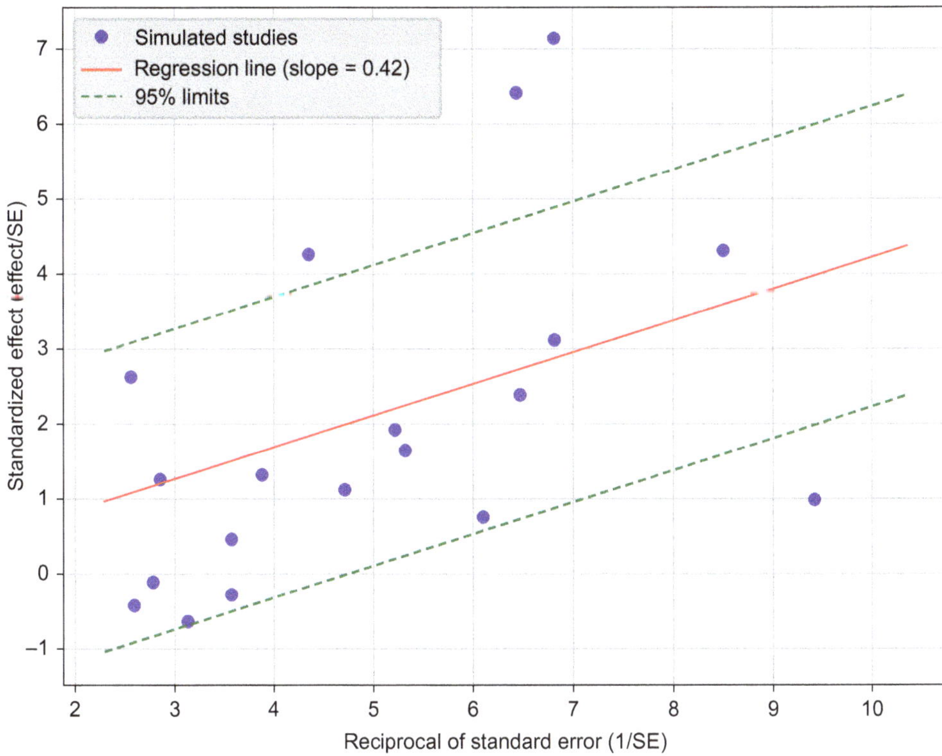

Figure 9.5 Galbraith plot of simulated studies with heterogeneity.

If most points cluster closely around the central line, heterogeneity is low (Figure 9.6). Outliers (points far from the main cluster) indicate studies that might contribute significantly to heterogeneity.

Statistical Tests to Quantify Heterogeneity

Several statistical tests are available to measure the degree of heterogeneity in meta-analyses:

- **Cochran's Q test:** tests whether effect sizes differ more than expected by chance. A significant result ($p < 0.05$) suggests significant heterogeneity.
- **I^2 statistic:** quantifies the percentage of total variation across studies that is due to heterogeneity rather than chance. Higher I^2 values indicate greater heterogeneity:

  0–40%: might not be important

  30–60%: may represent moderate heterogeneity

  50–90%: may represent substantial heterogeneity

  75–100%: considerable heterogeneity.

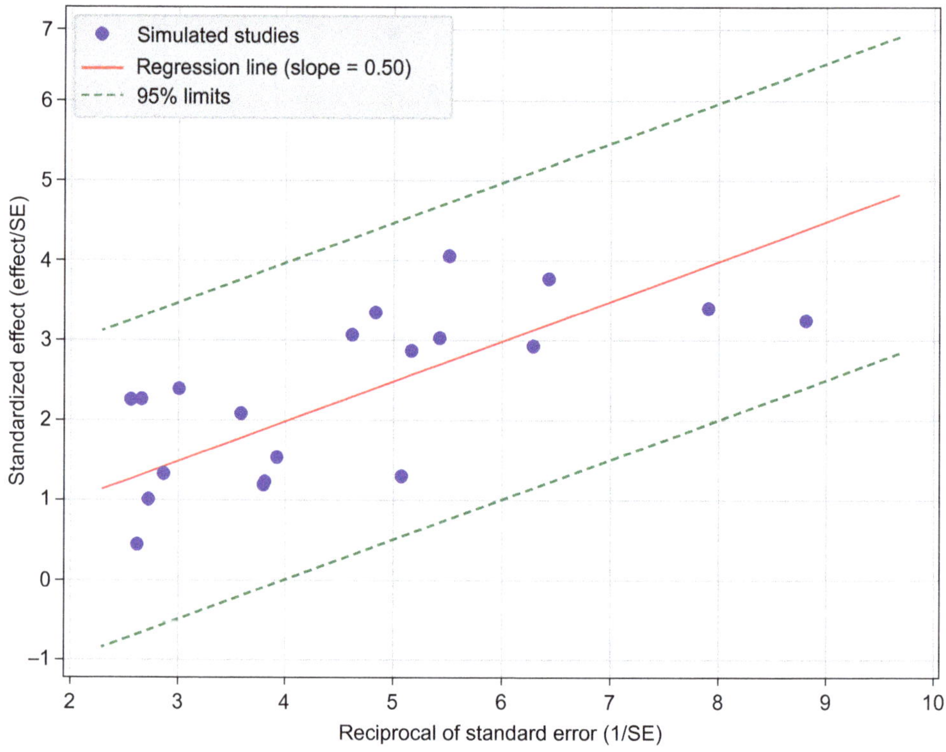

Figure 9.6 Galbraith plot of simulated studies with no heterogeneity.

- **Tau² (τ^2):** measures variance between studies in a random-effects model. Larger values indicate more variability in treatment effects.
- When substantial heterogeneity is present, investigators should explore clinical or methodological differences between studies before interpreting pooled estimates. Moreover if substantial heterogeneity is detected, investigators may then address it using random-effects models, subgroup analyses, or meta-regression.

Table 9.5 summarizes methods to assess heterogeneity in systematic reviews.

Table 9.5 Summary of methods to assess heterogeneity in systematic reviews

Step	Action
Eyeballing forest plot (visual inspection)	Check forest plots for overlapping confidence intervals
Galbraith (radial) plot	Identify outliers and studies contributing to heterogeneity
Cochran's Q test	$p < 0.05$ suggests significant heterogeneity
I^2 statistic	Measures the percentage of variability due to heterogeneity
Tau² (τ^2) test	Measures variance across studies in a random-effects model

Synthesize Findings

Combine study findings via:

- narrative synthesis[12] if data is too heterogeneous for pooling
- **meta-analysis** when data is sufficiently similar.

Meta-analysis

Effect Size Metric

The effect size quantifies the impact of an intervention or association across studies. The choice of effect size depends on the type of data:

- **Binary outcomes: odds ratio** (OR),[13] relative risk (RR), and **risk difference** (RD).[14]
- **Continuous outcomes: mean difference (MD)**[15] for studies using the same scale, and standardized mean difference (SMD) when studies use different measurement scales.

Statistical Models

When performing a meta-analysis, statistical models are used to combine the results of multiple studies and calculate a pooled effect size. The two primary models used are:

- **Fixed-effects model:** this is used when heterogeneity is low. It assumes that all included studies estimate the same true effect size and the confidence interval describes how uncertain we are about the estimate. Weights are given to studies based on their precision (**inverse variance weighting**).[16] It gives greater weight to larger studies and is appropriate when heterogeneity is low.
- **Random-effects model:** this is used when heterogeneity is greater between studies. It assumes that the true treatment effects in the individual studies may be different from each other and these different true effects are normally distributed. The meta-analysis therefore estimates the mean effect while accounting for between-study variance (τ^2).

Assigning Weights

Studies are weighted based on precision and sample size because studies vary in quality, precision, and size. Larger studies and those with small variance receive higher weights, commonly using inverse variance weighting. Meta-analysis software automatically calculates weights based on the chosen method and study data. Figure 9.7 shows a forest plot of simulated studies and Figure 9.8 shows how a forest plot should be read.

---

[12] **Narrative synthesis:** Structured, textual integration when pooling isn't appropriate: group studies, summarize effect directions and certainty, and explain heterogeneity (consider logic models/harvest plots).

[13] **Odds ratio (OR):** A measure comparing the odds of an outcome between two groups. It approximates the relative risk when outcomes are rare.

[14] **Risk difference (RD):** Absolute risk in exposed – risk in comparator (EER – CER). Same as absolute risk reduction/increase.

[15] **Mean difference (MD):** Difference between group means on the same scale (e.g. mmHg, points); typically pooled with inverse-variance methods and shown with a 95% CI. Use SMD instead if studies use different scales.

[16] **Inverse variance weighting:** Study weight $w_i = 1/\mathrm{Var}(\theta^i)$; more precise studies contribute more. Consider REML/DL estimators and Hartung–Knapp CIs when heterogeneity is substantial.

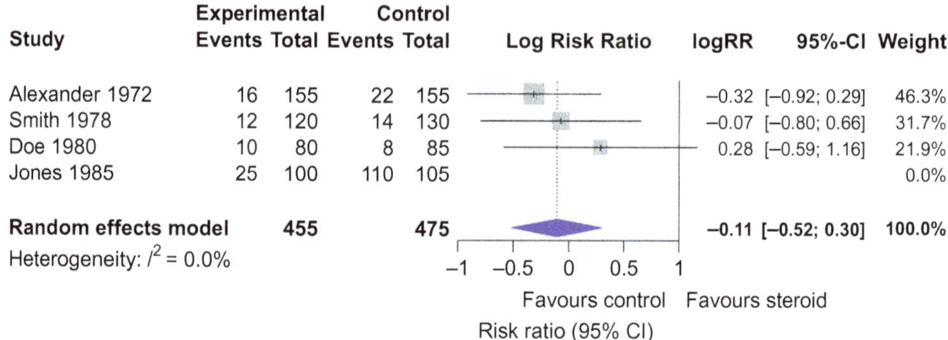

Figure 9.7 Forest plot of four RCTs comparing steroid treatment with control. The pooled effect estimate (diamond) shows no significant difference between groups (log risk ratio = −0.11, 95% CI −0.52 to 0.30).

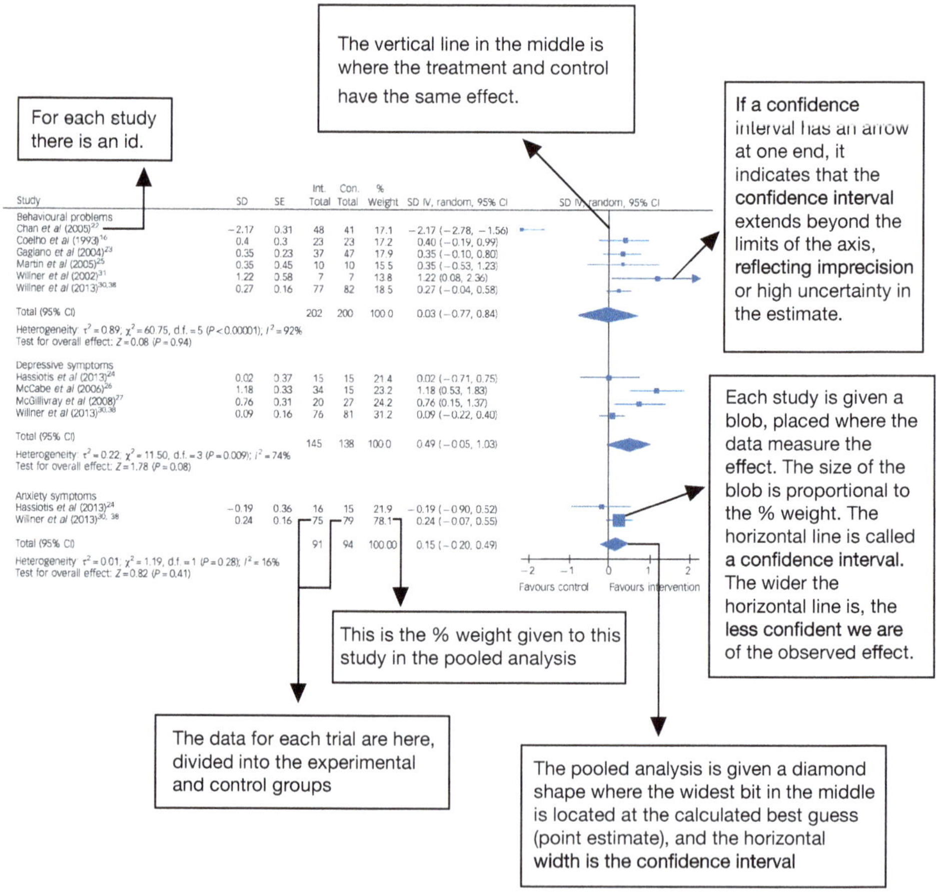

The vertical line in the middle is where the treatment and control have the same effect.

For each study there is an id.

If a confidence interval has an arrow at one end, it indicates that the confidence interval extends beyond the limits of the axis, reflecting imprecision or high uncertainty in the estimate.

Study	SD	SE	Int. Total	Con. Total	% Weight	SD IV, random, 95% CI
Behavioural problems						
Chan *et al* (2005)[22]	−2.17	0.31	48	41	17.1	−2.17 (−2.78, −1.56)
Coelho *et al* (1993)[16]	0.4	0.3	23	23	17.2	0.40 (−0.19, 0.99)
Gaglano *et al* (2004)[23]	0.35	0.23	37	47	17.9	0.35 (−0.10, 0.80)
Martin *et al* (2005)[25]	0.35	0.45	10	10	15.5	0.35 (−0.53, 1.23)
Willner *et al* (2002)[31]	1.22	0.58	7	7	13.8	1.22 (0.08, 2.36)
Willner *et al* (2013)[30,38]	0.27	0.16	77	82	18.5	0.27 (−0.04, 0.58)
Total (95% CI)			202	200	100.0	0.03 (−0.77, 0.84)
Heterogeneity: $\tau^2 = 0.89$; $\chi^2 = 60.75$, d.f. = 5 ($P < 0.00001$); $I^2 = 92\%$						
Test for overall effect: $Z = 0.08$ ($P = 0.94$)						
Depressive symptoms						
Hassiotis *et al* (2013)[24]	0.02	0.37	15	15	21.4	0.02 (−0.71, 0.75)
McCabe *et al* (2006)[26]	1.18	0.33	34	15	23.2	1.18 (0.53, 1.83)
McGillivray *et al* (2008)[27]	0.76	0.31	20	27	24.2	0.76 (0.15, 1.37)
Willner *et al* (2013)[30,38]	0.09	0.16	76	81	31.2	0.09 (−0.22, 0.40)
Total (95% CI)			145	138	100.0	0.49 (−0.05, 1.03)
Heterogeneity: $\tau^2 = 0.22$; $\chi^2 = 11.50$, d.f. = 3 ($P = 0.009$); $I^2 = 74\%$						
Test for overall effect: $Z = 1.78$ ($P = 0.08$)						
Anxiety symptoms						
Hassiotis *et al* (2013)[24]	−0.19	0.36	16	15	21.9	−0.19 (−0.90, 0.52)
Willner *et al* (2013)[30,38]	0.24	0.16	75	79	78.1	0.24 (−0.07, 0.55)
Total (95% CI)			91	94	100.00	0.15 (−0.20, 0.49)
Heterogeneity: $\tau^2 = 0.01$; $\chi^2 = 1.19$, d.f. = 1 ($P = 0.28$); $I^2 = 16\%$						
Test for overall effect: $Z = 0.82$ ($P = 0.41$)						

SD IV, random, 95% CI

−2 −1 0 1 2

Favours control Favours intervention

Each study is given a blob, placed where the data measure the effect. The size of the blob is proportional to the % weight. The horizontal line is called a confidence interval. The wider the horizontal line is, the less confident we are of the observed effect.

This is the % weight given to this study in the pooled analysis

The data for each trial are here, divided into the experimental and control groups

The pooled analysis is given a diamond shape where the widest bit in the middle is located at the calculated best guess (point estimate), and the horizontal width is the confidence interval

Figure 9.8 How to read a forest plot (Source: adapted from Koslowski N, Klein K, Arnold K, et al. Effectiveness of interventions for adults with mild to moderate intellectual disabilities and mental health problems: systematic review and meta-analysis. *Br J Psychiatry*. 2016;209(6):469–74. doi: https://doi.org/10.1192/bjp.bp.114.162313).

Interpret Results

Summarize the main findings of the review. This involves summarizing the main results, assessing the strength and quality of the evidence, and considering their implications for clinical practice, policy, and future research. The **GRADE framework** (Grading of Recommendations, Assessment, Development, and Evaluations)[17] is often used to rank the quality (certainty) of evidence across outcomes as high, moderate, low, or very low, based on factors such as risk of bias, inconsistency, indirectness, imprecision, and publication bias. The implications of the findings for clinical practice, policy, and future research should then be discussed.

Conduct Subgroup, Meta-Regression, and Sensitivity Analyses

Subgroup Analysis

Subgroup analysis involves dividing studies into categories (subgroups) based on study-level characteristics (e.g. age, intervention type) and analysing effect sizes separately within each subgroup. It is done by performing meta-analyses separately for different subgroups (e.g. based on age, disease severity, or intervention type). The aim is to determine whether treatment effects differ systematically between groups.

The purposes of subgroup analysis are to

- explore possible sources of heterogeneity
- generate or test hypotheses about effect modifiers
- improve interpretation of pooled results.

Examples of subgroup analysis include the following:

- **Antidepressant efficacy in depression:** studies can be subgrouped by severity of depression (mild, moderate, severe). Meta-analyses often find that antidepressants show larger effect sizes in severe depression, whereas placebo effects dominate in mild depression.
- **Antipsychotic trials in schizophrenia:** studies can be subgrouped by illness duration (first-episode vs chronic). Evidence suggests early-phase patients respond more robustly to antipsychotics than those with long-term, treatment-resistant illness.

Limitations of subgroup analysis are:

- increased risk of spurious findings due to multiple subgroup comparisons
- often underpowered, as few studies fall into each subgroup
- should ideally be prespecified in the review protocol rather than conducted post hoc.
- subgroup findings should be interpreted cautiously unless supported by strong prior hypotheses.

Meta-regression Analysis

Meta-regression is an extension of subgroup analysis. Instead of dividing studies into categories, it uses regression modelling to examine the relationship between study-level characteristics (predictors) and effect sizes (outcomes).

[17] **GRADE framework:** Rates certainty of evidence (high → very low) across risk of bias, inconsistency, indirectness, imprecision, and publication bias; keeps certainty distinct from recommendation strength.

The purposes of meta-regression are to:

- identify whether variation in effect size can be explained by study characteristics
- formally test for linear or non-linear trends.

Examples of meta-regression analysis include:

- **Psychotherapy for depression:** meta-regression can test whether the number of therapy sessions predicts effect size. Longer therapy (≥12 sessions) may be associated with larger effects compared with brief interventions.
- **Antipsychotic efficacy in schizophrenia:** meta-regression can examine whether chlorpromazine-equivalent dose predicts treatment response. Some meta-analyses find a plateau effect at standard therapeutic doses, with minimal additional benefit from higher doses but increased side-effect burden.

Limitations of meta-regression analysis are:

- Ecological fallacy: associations at the study level may not reflect individual-level effects.
- Requires a relatively large number of studies (ideally ≥10–15 per covariate) to provide robust results.
- Risk of false-positive findings when many covariates are tested.

Sensitivity Analysis

Sensitivity analysis is a method used in systematic reviews and meta-analyses to test how robust (reliable) the overall findings are to changes in the assumptions, decisions, or methods used during the review. In simple terms, it asks: 'If we change certain criteria, do our results stay the same or do they change dramatically?' It involves repeating the meta-analysis with slight variations in the inclusion criteria, data extraction methods, or statistical models.

The purposes of sensitivity analysis are to:

- ensure that conclusions are not driven by a few influential studies or methodological choices
- assess the stability and credibility of findings
- increase confidence in conclusions if results remain consistent.

Examples of sensitivity analysis include:

- **Excluding high-risk-of-bias studies:** in psychotherapy trials for depression, removing studies with poor blinding or high dropout rates.
- **Varying inclusion criteria:** excluding unpublished or non-English language studies.
- **Changing statistical models:** comparing fixed-effect versus random-effects models.
- **Removing outliers:** testing whether excluding a large antipsychotic trial alters pooled results.
- **Testing outcome definitions:** comparing definitions such as ≥50% reduction in depression scores versus remission.

Table 9.6 summarizes the comparison between regression analysis, sensitivity analysis, and subgroup analysis in systematic reviews.

Table 9.6 Comparison of regression analysis, sensitivity analysis, and subgroup analysis in systematic reviews

Feature	Meta-regression analysis	Sensitivity analysis	Subgroup analysis
Primary goal	Explore relationships between study characteristics and results	Assess robustness of meta-analysis results to variations	Examine treatment effect variations across subgroups
Data used	Study-level data (e.g. sample size, year of publication) and effect sizes	Meta-analysis results (overall effect size)	Study-level data (subgroup classifications) and effect sizes
Method	Statistical modelling (e.g. meta-regression)	Rerunning meta-analysis with different parameters	Separate meta-analyses for each subgroup
What it reveals	How study characteristics influence reported effects	How robust the overall effect size is to changes in methods or assumptions	Whether treatment effects differ across specific groups
Example	Does publication year influence reported effect size?	Does excluding high-risk-of-bias studies change the overall conclusion?	Is the treatment more effective in younger vs older patients?
Interpretation	Identifies potential sources of heterogeneity or bias	Provides confidence in the reliability of the findings	Highlights potential variations in treatment effectiveness
Limitations	Can be complex; potential for ecological fallacy	Can be subjective; choice of variations can influence results	Can be underpowered; risk of spurious findings due to multiple comparisons

Report Findings and Publish

Once the systematic review is complete, findings should be written up and disseminated in a transparent and structured way. Reporting should follow internationally recognized standards such as the PRISMA guidelines. The PRISMA checklist ensures that reviews are reported clearly, enabling readers to assess the validity and reliability of the findings. It includes 27 essential items covering all sections of the report. A typical structure is as follows (briefly summarized in Box 9.1):

Box 9.1 Key Sections of a Systematic Review Report Following PRISMA Guidelines

1. **Abstract:** summary of key findings
2. **Introduction:** research question and background
3. **Methods:** search strategy, inclusion criteria, risk of bias
4. **Results:** study selection (PRISMA flow diagram), key findings
5. **Discussion:** interpretation of findings, strengths, limitations
6. **Conclusion:** clinical implications and future research

1. **Abstract:** provides a concise summary of the review, including background, objectives, methods, main results, and conclusions. Structured abstracts are recommended.
2. **Introduction:** states the research question, rationale for the review, and its clinical or scientific importance. Should clearly specify objectives (e.g. using the PICO framework).
3. **Methods:** describes the review protocol, eligibility criteria, search strategy (databases, grey literature, trial registries), study selection process, data extraction, risk of bias assessment, and statistical analyses (e.g. meta-analysis methods, heterogeneity tests). Reference to PROSPERO registration strengthens transparency.
4. **Results:** presents the number of studies identified, screened, included, and excluded, typically displayed in a PRISMA flow diagram. Summarizes characteristics of included studies and provides quantitative results (e.g. pooled effect sizes, forest plots, heterogeneity estimates).
5. **Discussion:** interprets findings in the context of existing evidence. Discusses strengths and limitations of the review, potential biases, and implications for clinical practice, policy, and research.
6. **Conclusion:** summarizes the main take-home messages. Highlights clinical relevance, gaps in knowledge, and directions for future research.

By adhering to PRISMA, authors ensure that their review is comprehensive, transparent, and reproducible. This increases its likelihood of being published in high-impact journals such as the *Cochrane Database of Systematic Reviews* and ensures transparency through advance protocol registration (e.g. in PROSPERO).

In summary, a systematic review follows a structured process designed to minimize bias and maximize transparency. Each stage involves defined steps, tools, and outputs to ensure reproducibility. Table 9.7 provides a summary of the main stages in conducting a systematic review.

Table 9.7 Summary of the systematic review workflow

Stage	Description	Key actions taken
Define the research question	Use PICO to frame the review	Specify population, intervention, comparison, and outcome
Develop a protocol and register	Ensure transparency and avoid duplication	Register in PROSPERO, Cochrane, etc.
Conduct a comprehensive literature search	Identify all relevant studies	Search PubMed, Cochrane, Embase, PsycINFO
Select and screen studies	Apply inclusion/exclusion criteria	Use PRISMA flow diagram for tracking
Extract data from included studies	Extract key study characteristics and outcomes	Use a data extraction table
Assess risk of bias (study-level biases)	Evaluate internal validity of individual studies	Use Cochrane RoB tool, ROBINS-I, Newcastle–Ottawa Scale
Assess publication bias	Check for missing studies that may distort findings	Use funnel plot, Egger's test, trim-and-fill method

Table 9.7 (cont.)

Stage	Description	Key actions taken
Assess heterogeneity	Determine variability in study results before meta-analysis	Use Cochran's Q test, I^2 statistic, τ^2, subgroup analysis
Synthesize findings (narrative or meta-analysis)	Summarize results qualitatively or quantitatively	Conduct meta-analysis if appropriate
Interpret results and assess certainty of evidence	Evaluate the strength of findings	Use GRADE framework
Report findings and publish	Present review transparently	Follow PRISMA guidelines

Network Meta-analysis

Network meta-analysis (NMA) is an advanced statistical method that allows for the comparison of multiple treatments in a single analysis. The hallmark of NMA is its ability to facilitate indirect comparisons of treatments that have never been compared head-to-head in clinical trials. For instance, if Treatment A is four times more effective than placebo and Treatment B is twice as effective as placebo, NMA allows us to infer that Treatment A is likely twice as effective as Treatment B, even without a direct comparison.

The validity of an indirect comparison relies on the assumption of transitivity, meaning that the included randomized trials are similar in all crucial aspects except for the interventions being compared. The combination of direct and indirect evidence is called *mixed evidence*.

Network Diagram

A network diagram (Figure 9.9) provides a visual overview of the treatment comparisons included in an NMA. It illustrates both the structure and strength of the available evidence.

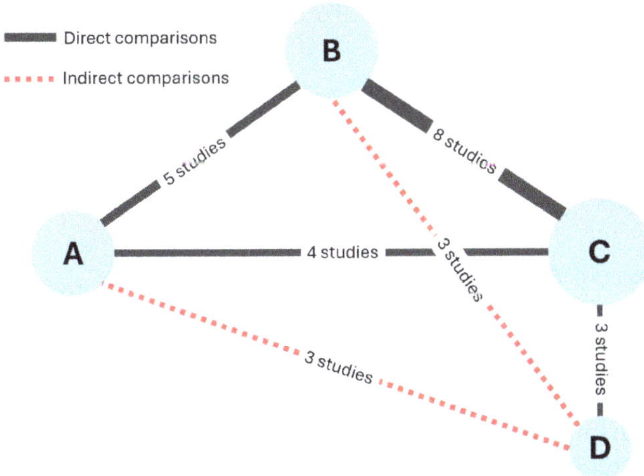

Figure 9.9 Example schematic network diagram for network meta-analysis. Nodes represent interventions and solid edges represent direct trial comparisons (thicker edges indicate more studies). Node size reflects the amount of evidence per treatment. Dotted edges are shown here only to illustrate indirect comparisons; most published NMA plots display direct comparisons only.

In practice, most NMA network diagrams display only direct comparisons; indirect evidence is inferred through the network structure.

Key elements of a network diagram are:

- **Nodes (circles):** represent the interventions being compared.
- **Edges (solid lines):** represent direct head-to-head trial comparisons.
- **Dotted lines (schematic only):** shown here to illustrate indirect comparisons inferred through shared comparators (most published NMA plots display direct comparisons only).
- **Line thickness:** proportional to the number of studies contributing to that particular comparison.
- **Node size:** may reflect the number of studies or participants contributing to each treatment.

Indirect comparisons are not usually drawn explicitly but are inferred through the connected structure of the network. Such diagrams help readers quickly visualize which treatments have been compared, how strong the evidence base is, and where indirect evidence is being used to inform the analysis. The following subsections discuss the key elements of a network diagram in relation to Figure 9.9.

Node Sizes

- **Node A:** represents 9 studies (5 from the A–B comparison and 4 from the A–C comparison), excluding indirect comparisons to avoid double-counting.
- **Node B:** represents 13 studies (5 from the A–B comparison and 8 from the B–C comparison), again excluding indirect links.
- **Node C:** represents 15 studies (8 from the B–C comparison, 4 from the A–C comparison, and 3 from the C–D comparison), making it the largest node.
- **Node D:** represents three studies, reflecting only the direct comparison between C and D.

Edges (Lines)

- **Solid grey lines:** direct comparisons, with labels indicating the number of studies supporting each link:

  A–B: 5 studies

  B–C: 8 studies

  C–D: 3 studies

  A–C: 4 studies.

- **Dotted red lines:** indirect comparisons, derived through a common comparator pathway:

  A–D: 3 studies (via A → C → D)

  B–D: 3 studies (via B → C → D).

Direct, Indirect, and Mixed Comparisons

- **Direct comparisons** are based on head-to-head clinical trials between two treatments.

- **Indirect comparisons** are estimated through shared comparators within the network when direct trials are unavailable.
- **Mixed comparisons** integrate both direct and indirect evidence, providing more precise and reliable estimates.

Steps in Performing NMA

Define the Research Question

- Formulate a PICO (population, intervention, comparison, outcome) question.
- Identify all relevant interventions for inclusion.

Conduct a Systematic Literature Search

- Search databases such as PubMed, Cochrane, Embase, and ClinicalTrials.gov.
- Apply inclusion/exclusion criteria to select appropriate studies.

Develop the Evidence Network

- Identify direct and indirect treatment comparisons.
- Construct a network diagram to visualize connections.

Assess Assumptions for NMA

Ensure the following key assumptions hold:

- **Transitivity:** studies must be similar in terms of population, settings, and outcome measurements.
- **Consistency:** effect sizes from direct and indirect comparisons should be statistically similar.
- **Homogeneity:** there should be low heterogeneity within direct treatment comparisons.

Perform Statistical Analysis

Use Bayesian or frequentist statistical models:

- Bayesian NMA (preferred approach): uses **Markov chain Monte Carlo (MCMC)** simulations.[18]
- Frequentist NMA: uses generalized linear models.

Software commonly used for these analyses include

- **R** (`gemtc, netmeta` packages)[19]
- **Stata** (`mvmeta`)[20]

---

[18] **Markov chain Monte Carlo (MCMC):** Posterior simulation (e.g. Gibbs/Metropolis). Check convergence (trace plots, R^≈1, effective sample size), allow burn-in, and use posterior-predictive checks before inference.

[19] **R** (`gemtc, netmeta`): gemtc performs Bayesian NMA via MCMC (commonly with JAGS/BUGS); netmeta implements frequentist graph-theoretic NMA with fixed/random-effects options and inconsistency checks.

[20] **Stata** (`mvmeta`): *mvmeta* fits multivariate meta-analytic models and underpins frequentist NMA workflows (with companion commands for network plots, inconsistency, and ranking).

- **WinBUGS**[21]
- **RevMan**[22]
- **JAGS.**[23]

Key outputs of the statistical analysis are:

- effect estimates (odds ratios, mean differences, etc.)
- Treatment rankings using surface under the cumulative ranking curve (**SUCRA**).[24] Treatment rankings should be interpreted cautiously, particularly when evidence is sparse or inconsistency is present.

Interpret Results

- **Forest plots and league tables:** show relative effect sizes across treatments.
- **SUCRA scores:** indicate which treatments are most effective.

Assess Confidence in the Evidence

The **CINeMA** (Confidence in Network Meta-Analysis)[25] framework evaluates confidence in network evidence. CINeMA provides a structured assessment of confidence in each network estimate, analogous to GRADE in pairwise meta-analysis. It assesses:

- risk of bias – limitations in the included trials (e.g. poor randomization or blinding)
- inconsistency – disagreement between direct and indirect evidence
- indirectness – differences between the evidence and the clinical question of interest
- imprecision – wide confidence intervals due to limited data or small sample sizes.

Overall confidence is rated as high, moderate, low, or very low for each network comparison.

Report Findings

- Follow the PRISMA extension for NMA guidelines.

Uses of NMA

- Enables comparisons across multiple treatments, even when no single trial compares all interventions.
- Provides a ranking of treatments based on effectiveness.
- Uses both direct and indirect evidence, improving decision-making.

---

[21] **WinBUGS:** Bayesian MCMC engine (BUGS language) for hierarchical/NMA models with flexible priors; frequently called from R scripts for custom models.

[22] **RevMan:** Cochrane's Review Manager for building reviews and pairwise meta-analyses (data entry, forest plots, RoB/ROBINS-I workflows); NMA generally run in R/Stata and is then reported in RevMan outputs.

[23] **JAGS:** Just Another Gibbs Sampler. Open-source Bayesian MCMC engine similar to BUGS; integrates tightly with R, widely used for hierarchical and network models.

[24] **SUCRA:** 'Surface under the cumulative ranking' (0–100%): summarizes how often a treatment ranks near 'best' in a network meta-analysis. Interpret with effect sizes, uncertainty (CIs/predictive intervals) and checks for heterogeneity/incoherence.

[25] **CINeMA:** Confidence in NMA via domains aligned to GRADE (within-study bias, reporting bias, indirectness, imprecision, heterogeneity, incoherence); yields transparent, domain-level judgements.

Limitations of NMA

- Assumptions may not always hold, affecting reliability.
- Complex to conduct and interpret, requiring statistical expertise.
- Limited by the quality and availability of indirect evidence.

Summary of NMA Steps

1. **Define the research question:** identify interventions and outcomes.
2. **Conduct systematic search:** find relevant studies for inclusion.
3. **Develop network diagram:** map direct and indirect treatment comparisons.
4. **Check assumptions:** ensure transitivity, consistency, and homogeneity.
5. **Perform statistical analysis:** use Bayesian/frequentist models to estimate effects.
6. **Interpret results:** use **league tables,**[26] SUCRA, and network plots.
7. **Assess confidence:** apply CINeMA framework for evidence quality.
8. **Report findings:** follow the PRISMA extension for network meta-analysis.

When to Use NMA

Network meta-analysis is particularly valuable when:

- comparing three or more treatments simultaneously
- no single trial directly compares all interventions of interest
- a ranking of treatments based on relative effectiveness or safety is required.

Chapter Summary

A systematic review is a structured synthesis of existing studies that answers a clinical question while minimizing bias. The key steps include:

1. Defining the research question using PICO (population, intervention, comparison, outcome).
2. Developing a protocol (e.g. PROSPERO registration) to ensure transparency.
3. Conducting a comprehensive literature search across multiple databases (PubMed, Cochrane, Embase, PsycINFO).
4. Screening and extracting data systematically.
5. Assessing risk of bias with tools like the Cochrane Risk of Bias Tool (for RCTs) and Newcastle–Ottawa Scale (for observational studies).
6. Evaluating publication bias using funnel plots, Egger's test, and trim-and-fill method.
7. Assessing heterogeneity using Cochran's Q test, I^2 statistic, and tau^2 (τ^2) variance.
8. Synthesizing findings via meta-analysis (when appropriate) or narrative synthesis.
9. Using statistical models such as fixed-effects (for low heterogeneity) and random-effects models (for substantial heterogeneity).
10. Interpreting results using the GRADE framework to assess certainty of evidence.

---

[26] **League tables:** Matrices listing all pairwise treatment comparisons (relative effects with CIs) and often rankings; aid cross-treatment interpretation at a glance.

11. Reporting findings in peer-reviewed journals in accordance with PRISMA reporting guidelines.

    Advanced techniques can help interpret systematic review findings, including:

    - Meta-regression analysis: examines whether study-level characteristics (e.g. sample size, intervention duration) influence effect sizes.
    - Sensitivity analysis: tests the robustness of findings by rerunning the meta-analysis under different conditions (e.g. excluding high-risk-of-bias studies).
    - Subgroup analysis: explores whether treatment effects differ across specific populations (e.g. age groups, disease severity).

The differences between these analyses can be summarized as:

- Regression: examines how study characteristics impact results.
- Sensitivity: checks the stability of the overall meta-analysis result.
- Subgroup analysis: evaluates how treatments work in different groups.

Network Meta-analysis

An NMA extends traditional meta-analyses by comparing multiple treatments in a single network, even when direct head-to-head trials are unavailable. The process includes:

1. Developing a network diagram to visualize treatment comparisons.
2. Assessing transitivity and consistency to ensure valid indirect comparisons.
3. Applying Bayesian or frequentist statistical models to estimate and rank treatments.
4. Interpreting results using league tables, SUCRA scores, and the CINeMA framework.

Practice Questions

For Q1–Q8: Researchers conducted a meta-analysis to assess the effectiveness of local anaesthesia for pain control during hysteroscopy. Randomized controlled trials were included if they compared local anaesthesia with no intervention, placebo, oral analgesics, or conscious sedation. Participants were women undergoing diagnostic or operative hysteroscopy as outpatients without general anaesthesia. The primary outcome measured was the level of pain associated with the procedure.

A total of 15 trials was included in the analysis, identifying four methods of local anaesthesia administration: intracervical, paracervical, and transcervical injections, as well as topical application. Given that different studies used various pain assessment scales, including continuous visual analogue scales and numerical scales, the standardized mean difference (SMD) in pain scores between treatment groups (local anaesthesia vs control) was calculated for each trial. The results of the meta-analysis are presented in Figure 9.10.

Q1. Which of the following statements is true for the subgroup of paracervical injection of local anaesthesia?

   A. For each trial, the standard error of the mean difference was used to calculate the SMD.

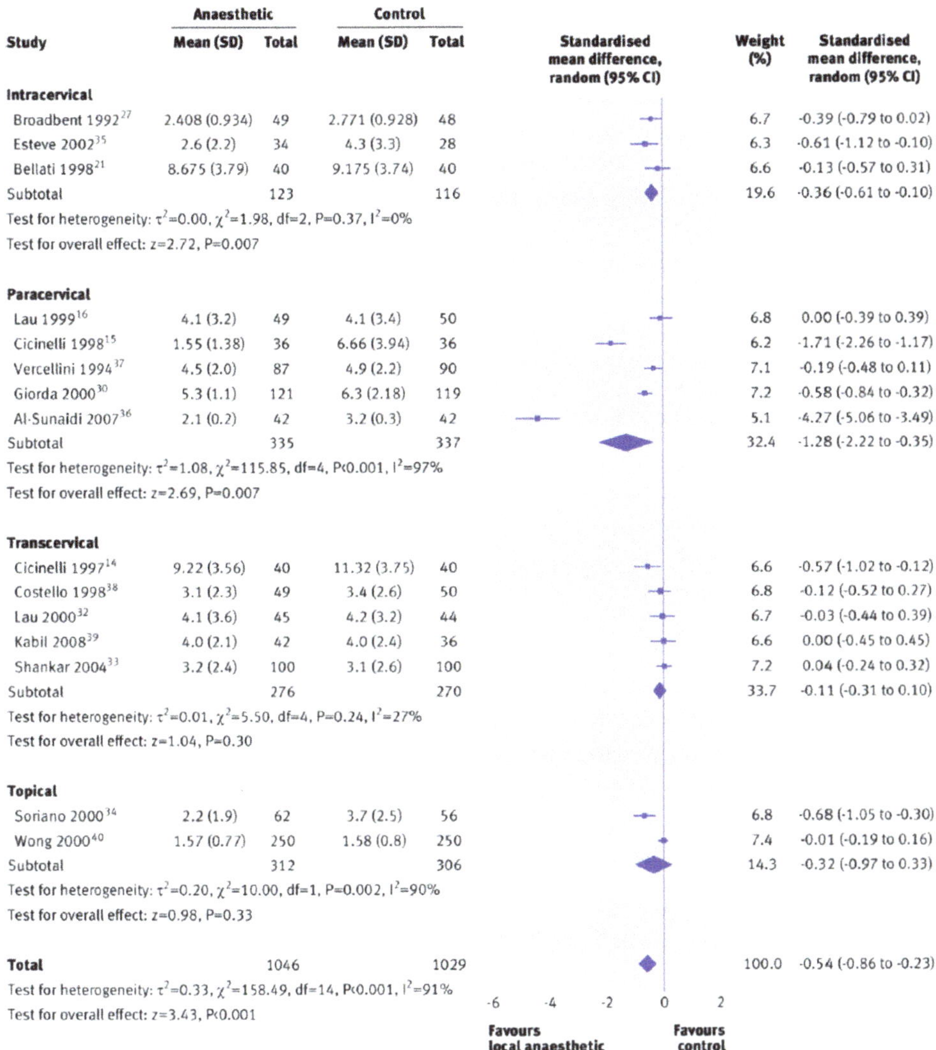

Study	Anaesthetic Mean (SD)	Anaesthetic Total	Control Mean (SD)	Control Total	Weight (%)	Standardised mean difference, random (95% CI)
Intracervical						
Broadbent 1992[27]	2.408 (0.934)	49	2.771 (0.928)	48	6.7	-0.39 (-0.79 to 0.02)
Esteve 2002[35]	2.6 (2.2)	34	4.3 (3.3)	28	6.3	-0.61 (-1.12 to -0.10)
Bellati 1998[21]	8.675 (3.79)	40	9.175 (3.74)	40	6.6	-0.13 (-0.57 to 0.31)
Subtotal		123		116	19.6	-0.36 (-0.61 to -0.10)
Test for heterogeneity: τ^2=0.00, χ^2=1.98, df=2, P=0.37, I^2=0%						
Test for overall effect: z=2.72, P=0.007						
Paracervical						
Lau 1999[16]	4.1 (3.2)	49	4.1 (3.4)	50	6.8	0.00 (-0.39 to 0.39)
Cicinelli 1998[15]	1.55 (1.38)	36	6.66 (3.94)	36	6.2	-1.71 (-2.26 to -1.17)
Vercellini 1994[37]	4.5 (2.0)	87	4.9 (2.2)	90	7.1	-0.19 (-0.48 to 0.11)
Giorda 2000[30]	5.3 (1.1)	121	6.3 (2.18)	119	7.2	-0.58 (-0.84 to -0.32)
Al-Sunaidi 2007[36]	2.1 (0.2)	42	3.2 (0.3)	42	5.1	-4.27 (-5.06 to -3.49)
Subtotal		335		337	32.4	-1.28 (-2.22 to -0.35)
Test for heterogeneity: τ^2=1.08, χ^2=115.85, df=4, P<0.001, I^2=97%						
Test for overall effect: z=2.69, P=0.007						
Transcervical						
Cicinelli 1997[14]	9.22 (3.56)	40	11.32 (3.75)	40	6.6	-0.57 (-1.02 to -0.12)
Costello 1998[38]	3.1 (2.3)	49	3.4 (2.6)	50	6.8	-0.12 (-0.52 to 0.27)
Lau 2000[32]	4.1 (3.6)	45	4.2 (3.2)	44	6.7	-0.03 (-0.44 to 0.39)
Kabil 2008[39]	4.0 (2.1)	42	4.0 (2.4)	36	6.6	0.00 (-0.45 to 0.45)
Shankar 2004[33]	3.2 (2.4)	100	3.1 (2.6)	100	7.2	0.04 (-0.24 to 0.32)
Subtotal		276		270	33.7	-0.11 (-0.31 to 0.10)
Test for heterogeneity: τ^2=0.01, χ^2=5.50, df=4, P=0.24, I^2=27%						
Test for overall effect: z=1.04, P=0.30						
Topical						
Soriano 2000[34]	2.2 (1.9)	62	3.7 (2.5)	56	6.8	-0.68 (-1.05 to -0.30)
Wong 2000[40]	1.57 (0.77)	250	1.58 (0.8)	250	7.4	-0.01 (-0.19 to 0.16)
Subtotal		312		306	14.3	-0.32 (-0.97 to 0.33)
Test for heterogeneity: τ^2=0.20, χ^2=10.00, df=1, P=0.002, I^2=90%						
Test for overall effect: z=0.98, P=0.33						
Total		1046		1029	100.0	-0.54 (-0.86 to -0.23)
Test for heterogeneity: τ^2=0.33, χ^2=158.49, df=14, P<0.001, I^2=91%						
Test for overall effect: z=3.43, P<0.001						

Figure 9.10 Forest plot of anaesthetic versus control across different administration routes (Source: Cooper NAM, Khan KS, Clark TJ. Local anaesthesia for pain control during outpatient hysteroscopy: systematic review and meta-analysis. *BMJ* 2010;340:c1130. doi: https://doi.org/10.1136/bmj.c1130).

B. For each trial, the SMD was on the same scale as the original measurement of pain.

C. The SMDs allowed direct comparison of treatment effects across trials that used different pain scales.

D. Local anaesthesia resulted in significantly increased pain compared with the control group.

E. The SMD expresses the difference between treatment groups in the assessment of pain as multiples of the observed standard error.

Q2. Which of the following statements is true?

A. The confidence interval of the pooled estimate for the paracervical subgroup is smaller than that of the intracervical subgroup.
B. The intracervical subgroup is given a higher percentage weight than the topical subgroup because it includes more studies.
C. Soriano 2000 is likely a larger study than Wong 2000 as it shows a statistically significant result.
D. Giorda 2000 is given more weight than Vercellini 1994 because it is more statistically significant.
E. The weight assigned to an SMD for a trial was determined by the precision of the estimate of the treatment effect.

Q3. What type of bias is meta-analysis particularly prone to?

A. Attrition bias
B. Funding bias
C. Measurement bias
D. Publication bias
E. Hawthorne bias

Q4. Which of the following statements is false regarding heterogeneity in this study?

A. The topical subgroup has less heterogeneity than the paracervical subgroup.
B. The overall heterogeneity of all the studies is low.
C. The intracervical subgroup has no heterogeneity.
D. The transcervical subgroup has low heterogeneity.
E. The overall heterogeneity estimate indicates that a random-effects model should be used to calculate the total pooled effect.

Q5. Based on the forest plot, which method of local anaesthesia shows the largest pooled reduction in pain score compared with control?

A. Intracervical injection
B. Paracervical injection
C. Topical application
D. Transcervical injection
E. Cannot be determined from the information provided

Q6. What is a potential limitation of using SMDs in this meta-analysis?

A. SMDs do not account for differences in sample size between studies.
B. SMDs may obscure clinically important differences between treatments if the underlying scales have different measurement properties.
C. SMDs cannot be used when studies use different types of outcome measures (e.g. continuous vs categorical).
D. SMDs are not appropriate for meta-analyses with high heterogeneity.
E. SMDs overemphasize the results of smaller studies.

Q7. What does the I^2 statistic indicate in this meta-analysis?

A. The extent of variability in treatment effects due to chance.
B. The proportion of total variation in study results due to heterogeneity rather than chance.
C. The number of studies included in the meta-analysis.
D. The confidence level of the overall pooled effect estimate.
E. The probability of publication bias affecting the results.

Q8. Based on the forest plot, which statement best describes the overall effect of local anaesthesia on pain reduction?

A. Local anaesthesia has no effect on pain control as the overall standardized mean difference crosses zero.
B. The overall standardized mean difference is statistically significant, favouring local anaesthesia for pain reduction.
C. The effect of local anaesthesia is only significant for the intracervical subgroup.
D. The results indicate that control interventions (placebo or no intervention) provide better pain relief than local anaesthesia.
E. The overall effect is influenced primarily by the paracervical subgroup.

Q9. What is the primary reason for using a random-effects model in the meta-analysis?

A. It assumes that all studies are estimating the exact same treatment effect.
B. It accounts for variability among studies beyond chance, allowing for differences in effect sizes.
C. It is used only when there is no heterogeneity in the included studies.
D. It ensures that larger studies have equal weight to smaller studies.
E. It forces the confidence interval to be wider, making results appear less significant.

Q10. Which pattern in a funnel plot would suggest the presence of publication bias?

A. A symmetric funnel shape, with studies evenly distributed around the pooled estimate.
B. An asymmetrical funnel shape, with fewer studies showing non-significant results.
C. A funnel plot with all studies clustered tightly around the pooled effect size.
D. A funnel plot with wider dispersion of points at the top than at the bottom.
E. A random distribution of points without any discernible pattern.

Q11. Which of the following best describes the purpose of the GRADE framework in systematic reviews?

A. To detect publication bias using funnel plot asymmetry.
B. To rank treatments using SUCRA scores in network meta-analysis.
C. To assess the certainty (quality) of evidence across outcomes in a review.
D. To calculate heterogeneity using Cochran's Q test.
E. To determine whether a fixed-effects model should be used.

For Q12–Q13: A systematic review examines the effectiveness of screening for intimate partner violence (IPV) in healthcare settings. The goal is to determine whether screening increases identification and referral to support services, improves women's wellbeing, reduces further violence, or causes harm. Figure 9.11 presents the meta-analysis results.

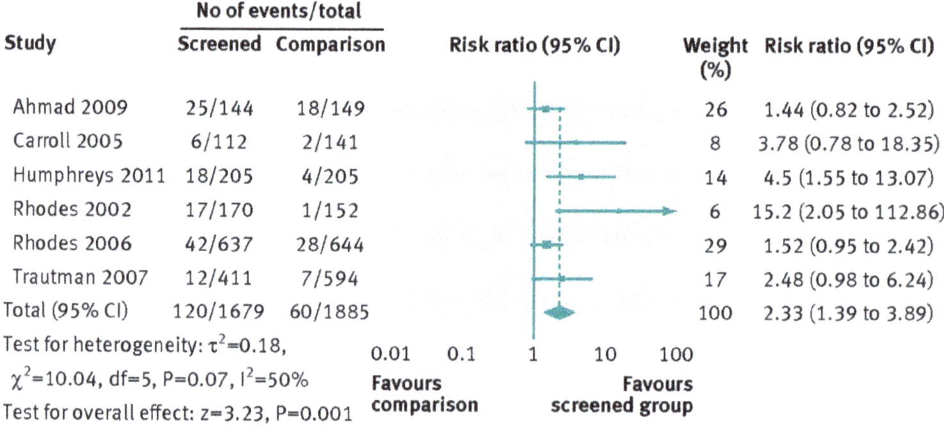

Figure 9.11 Forest plot of screening for intimate partner violence versus comparison group with risk ratios (95% CI) (Source: Doherty LJ, Taft A, Hegarty K, et al. Screening women for intimate partner violence in healthcare settings: abridged Cochrane systematic review and meta-analysis. *BMJ* 2014;348:g2913. doi: https://doi.org/10.1136/bmj.g2913).

Q12. What is the relative risk of the pooled data?

A. 1.39
B. 1.75
C. 2.25
D. 0.85
E. 3.02

Q13. In the forest plot, the CI for the Rhodes 2002 study is indicated by an arrow. What does this represent?

A. The confidence interval of Rhodes 2002 is so wide that its upper bound extends beyond the plotted range on the logarithmic scale.
B. Rhodes 2002 provided the most precise estimate in the meta-analysis.
C. The study's relative risk (RR) is exactly 1, meaning screening had no effect.
D. The confidence interval was incorrectly plotted.
E. The study was excluded from the pooled estimate due to high uncertainty.

Q14. Which tool is commonly used to assess the risk of bias in studies included in a systematic review?

A. Newcastle–Ottawa Scale
B. Cochrane Risk of Bias Tool

C. Egger's test
D. I^2 statistic
E. GRADE framework

Q15. What is the key advantage of an NMA over a traditional meta-analysis?
A. It includes only RCTs.
B. It allows for indirect comparisons of treatments not directly compared in trials.
C. It does not require assessing transitivity and consistency.
D. It eliminates publication bias completely.
E. It can only compare two interventions at a time.

Q16. In an NMA, what assumption must be met for valid indirect comparisons?
A. The assumption of transitivity
B. The assumption of normality
C. The assumption of linearity
D. The assumption of uniformity
E. The assumption of randomness

Answers

Q1. Correct answer: C. The SMDs allowed direct comparison of treatment effects across trials that used different pain scales. Standardized mean differences are used in meta-analyses when studies report outcomes using different measurement scales. Since the trials used various pain scales, SMDs enables direct comparisons by expressing results in a uniform metric (i.e. standard deviations).

Why other options are incorrect:

A. SMD is calculated using the standard deviation, not the standard error.
B. SMD is not on the original pain scale but a standardized scale.
D. The results suggest a reduction in pain (not an increase) with local anaesthesia.
E. SMD expresses the difference in terms of standard deviations, not standard errors.

Q2. Correct answer: E. The weight given to an SMD for a trial was determined by the precision of the estimate of the treatment effect. The weight assigned to each study in a meta-analysis depends on the inverse variance of the effect estimate, meaning studies with greater precision (smaller variance) are given more weight.

Why other options are incorrect:

A. The CI for the paracervical subgroup is wider than the intracervical subgroup, meaning more heterogeneity and lower precision.
B. The topical subgroup has more studies but was given less weight than intracervical because study size and variance also matter.
C. Statistical significance does not reliably indicate a larger study; it depends on both sample size and variance, not simply the *p*-value.
D. A study's weight is determined by its sample size and variance, not just statistical significance.

Q3. Correct answer: D. Publication bias. Publication bias occurs when studies with positive or significant results are more likely to be published than studies with negative or non-significant results. This is a common issue in meta-analyses because unpublished studies with null or negative findings are often missing, leading to an overestimation of treatment effects.

Why other options are incorrect:

A. Attrition bias occurs when there is a high dropout rate in studies, but meta-analyses focus on published results.
B. Funding bias: no evidence suggests industry sponsorship affected the study.
C. Measurement bias: differences in pain assessment methods could introduce variability, but SMD adjusts for this.
E. Hawthorne bias occurs when participants modify their behaviour due to being observed, which is unlikely in this study.

Q4. Correct answer: B. Overall heterogeneity of all the studies is low. Overall heterogeneity is high ($I^2 = 91\%$), not low, meaning substantial variability exists among studies.

Why other options are incorrect:

A. True: The topical subgroup ($I^2 = 90\%$) has slightly lower heterogeneity than the paracervical subgroup ($I^2 = 97\%$).
C. True: the intracervical subgroup has no heterogeneity ($I^2 = 0\%$), meaning results are consistent across these studies.
D. True: the transcervical subgroup has low heterogeneity ($I^2 = 27\%$), suggesting minimal variation between studies.
E. True: since heterogeneity is high, a random-effects model is appropriate.

Q5. Correct answer: B. The paracervical subgroup has the most negative pooled standardized mean difference (SMD), indicating the largest reduction in pain compared with the control group. Therefore, it shows the largest pooled effect size in the forest plot. Although the paracervical subgroup shows the greatest reduction, it also has very high heterogeneity ($I^2 \approx 97\%$), meaning results vary substantially across studies. Therefore, the estimate should be interpreted cautiously and does not necessarily indicate the most reliable or consistent method.

Q6. Correct answer: B. SMDs may obscure clinically important differences between treatments if the underlying scales have different measurement properties.

This is a key limitation of using SMDs. Even though they allow for comparison across different scales, they might not capture the full clinical significance if the scales have different properties (e.g. one scale is more sensitive to change than another).

Q7. Correct answer: B. The proportion of total variation in study results due to heterogeneity rather than chance. The I^2 statistic quantifies the percentage of variability in study results due to true differences between studies rather than random chance.

Why other options are incorrect:

A. Variability due to chance is measured by the *p*-value for heterogeneity.
C. The number of studies does not determine heterogeneity.

D. Confidence levels relate to precision, not heterogeneity.
E. I^2 does not measure publication bias.

Q8. Correct answer: B. The overall SMD is statistically significant, favouring local anaesthesia for pain reduction. The pooled effect size (SMD = −0.54, 95% CI −0.86 to −0.23, $p < 0.001$) shows a statistically significant reduction in pain with local anaesthesia.
Why other options are incorrect:

A. The confidence interval does not cross zero, meaning the effect is significant.
C. Other subgroups contribute to the overall effect, not just intracervical.
D. Local anaesthesia reduces pain rather than increasing it.
E. The effect is seen across all subgroups, not just paracervical.

Q9. Correct answer: B. It accounts for variability among studies beyond chance, allowing for differences in effect sizes. The random-effects model assumes that true effects vary between studies, accounting for heterogeneity.
Why other options are incorrect:

A. It describes a fixed-effects model.
C. A random-effects model is used specifically when heterogeneity exists.
D. Larger studies still contribute more weight.
E. Random-effects models adjust for heterogeneity but do not artificially widen confidence intervals.

Q10. Correct answer: B. An asymmetrical funnel shape, with fewer studies showing non-significant results. Publication bias occurs when studies with negative or non-significant results are missing, causing asymmetry in the funnel plot.
Why other options are incorrect:

A. Symmetry suggests no bias.
C. It describes normal patterns, not publication bias.
D. It describes normal patterns, not publication bias.
E. A random distribution would not indicate bias.

Q11. Correct answer: C. To assess the certainty (quality) of evidence across outcomes in a review. The GRADE framework (Grading of Recommendations, Assessment, Development, and Evaluation) is used in systematic reviews to rate the certainty of evidence for each outcome. Evidence is graded as: high, moderate, low, very low. GRADE considers factors such as risk of bias, inconsistency, indirectness, imprecision, publication bias.

A. Refers to funnel plots and Egger's test, not GRADE.
B. Relates to treatment ranking in network meta-analysis, not evidence certainty.
D. Refers to statistical heterogeneity testing, not overall evidence grading.
E. Concerns model choice (fixed vs random effects), not GRADE assessment.

Q12. Correct answer: C. 2.25. Draw a 2×2 table for the IPV screening study (Table 9.8).

Table 9.8 The 2 × 2 table for IPV screening study for calculation of relative risk

Group	Events (IPV identified)	No events (IPV not identified)	Total
Screened group	120	1,559	1,679
Comparison group	60	1,825	1,885

$$\text{EER} = \frac{120}{1,679} = 0.0714,$$

$$\text{CER} = \frac{60}{1,885} = 0.0318,$$

$$\text{RR} = \frac{\text{EER}}{\text{CER}} = \frac{0.0714}{0.0318} = 2.25.$$

Q13. Correct answer: A. The confidence interval of Rhodes 2002 is so wide that its upper bound extends beyond the plotted range on the logarithmic scale. The forest plot shows a CI extending beyond the plotted range, which is represented by an arrow instead of displaying the full interval. This occurs when the upper confidence limit is extremely large, meaning high uncertainty in the study's RR estimate. Possible reasons for a wide CI: small sample size because the study had only one event in the comparison group (1/152), leading to an unstable estimate; high variability – a large CI indicates that the effect size is not precisely estimated.

Why other options are incorrect:

B. A wide CI means low precision, not high.
C. If RR = 1, it would mean no effect, but the study's RR is uncertain, with a large possible range.
D. The CI is correctly plotted, with the arrow indicating an upper limit exceeding the scale.
E. Despite high uncertainty, Rhodes 2002 is included in the meta-analysis.

Q14. Correct answer: B. Cochrane Risk of Bias Tool. The Cochrane Risk of Bias Tool assesses bias in RCTs. Why other options are incorrect:

A. Newcastle–Ottawa Scale is used for observational studies.
C. Egger's test detects publication bias.
D. I^2 statistic measures heterogeneity.
E. GRADE framework evaluates quality of evidence, not bias.

Q15. Correct answer: B. It allows for indirect comparisons of treatments not directly compared in trials. Network meta-analysis enables the comparison of multiple treatments by using direct and indirect evidence. Transitivity and consistency must be assessed to ensure valid comparisons. Publication bias remains a challenge in all meta-analyses.

Q16. Correct answer: A. The assumption of transitivity. Transitivity ensures that the included trials are similar in terms of population, outcome, and methodology, allowing for valid indirect comparisons.

Further Reading

Begg CB, Mazumdar M. Operating characteristics of a rank correlation test for publication bias. *Biometrics*. 1994;**50**(4):1088–101. doi: https://doi.org/10.2307/2533446.

Cooper NAM, Khan KS, Clark TJ. Local anaesthesia for pain control during outpatient hysteroscopy: systematic review and meta-analysis. *BMJ*. 2010;**340**:c1130. doi: https://doi.org/10.1136/bmj.c1130.

DerSimonian R, Laird N. Meta-analysis in clinical trials. *Control Clin Trials*. 1986;**7**(3):177–88. doi: https://doi.org/10.1016/0197-2456(86)90046-2.

Duval S, Tweedie R. Trim and fill: a simple funnel-plot-based method of testing and adjusting for publication bias in meta-analysis. *Biometrics*. 2000;**56**(2):455–63. doi: https://doi.org/10.1111/j.0006-341X.2000.00455.x.

Egger M, Davey Smith G, Schneider M, Minder C. Bias in meta-analysis detected by a simple, graphical test. *BMJ*. 1997;**315**(7109):629–34. doi: https://doi.org/10.1136/bmj.315.7109.629.

Galbraith RF. A note on graphical presentation of estimated odds ratios from several clinical trials. *Stat Med*. 1988;**7**(8):889–94. doi: https://doi.org/10.1002/sim.4780070807.

Guyatt GH, Oxman AD, Vist GE, et al. GRADE: an emerging consensus on rating quality of evidence and strength of recommendations. *BMJ*. 2008;**336**(7650):924–6. doi: https://doi.org/10.1136/bmj.39489.470347.AD.

Higgins JPT, Thomas J, Chandler J, et al. (eds). *Cochrane Handbook for Systematic Reviews of Interventions*. 2nd ed. Chichester: Wiley; 2019. doi: https://doi.org/10.1002/9781119536604.

Higgins JPT, Thompson SG, Deeks JJ, Altman DG. Measuring inconsistency in meta-analyses. *BMJ*. 2003;**327**(7414):557–60. doi: https://doi.org/10.1136/bmj.327.7414.557.

Hutton B, Salanti G, Caldwell DM, et al. The PRISMA extension statement for reporting of systematic reviews incorporating network meta-analyses of health care interventions: checklist and explanations. *Ann Intern Med*. 2015;**162**(11):777–84. doi: https://doi.org/10.7326/M14-2385.

Nikolakopoulou A, Higgins JPT, Papakonstantinou T, et al. CINeMA: an approach for assessing confidence in the results of a network meta-analysis. *PLoS Med*. 2020;**17**(4):e1003082. doi: https://doi.org/10.1371/journal.pmed.1003082.

O'Doherty LJ, Taft A, Hegarty K, Ramsay J, Davidson LL, Feder G. Screening women for intimate partner violence in healthcare settings: abridged Cochrane systematic review and meta-analysis. *BMJ*. 2014;**348**:g2913. doi: https://doi.org/10.1136/bmj.g2913.

Page MJ, McKenzie JE, Bossuyt PM, et al. The PRISMA 2020 statement: an updated guideline for reporting systematic reviews. *BMJ*. 2021;**372**:n71. doi: https://doi.org/10.1136/bmj.n71.

Page MJ, Moher D, Bossuyt PM, et al. PRISMA 2020 explanation and elaboration: updated guidance and exemplars for reporting systematic reviews. *BMJ*. 2021;**372**:n160. doi: https://doi.org/10.1136/bmj.n160.

Richardson WS, Wilson MC, Nishikawa J, Hayward RS. The well-built clinical question: a key to evidence-based decisions. *ACP J Club*. 1995;**123**(3):A12–A13.

Salanti G, Ades AE, Ioannidis JPA. Graphical methods and numerical summaries for presenting results from multiple-treatment meta-analysis: an overview with suggestions for practice. *J Clin Epidemiol*. 2011;**64**(2):163–71. doi: https://doi.org/10.1016/j.jclinepi.2010.03.016.

Sutton AJ, Duval SJ, Tweedie RL, Abrams KR, Jones DR. Empirical assessment of effect of publication bias on meta-analyses. *BMJ*. 2000;**320**(7249):1574–7. doi: https://doi.org/10.1136/bmj.320.7249.1574.

Thompson SG. Why sources of heterogeneity in meta-analysis should be investigated. *BMJ*. 1994;**309**(6965):1351–5. doi: https://doi.org/10.1136/bmj.309.6965.1351.

Wells GA, Shea B, O'Connell D, et al. *The Newcastle–Ottawa Scale (NOS) for Assessing the Quality of Nonrandomised Studies in Meta-Analyses*. Ottawa: Ottawa Hospital Research Institute; 2011.

Chapter 10

Network Analysis

Introduction

Network analysis is an advanced analytical approach used to study complex relationships in healthcare, disease progression, and biological systems. It helps in understanding disease mechanisms, patient interactions, drug interactions, and healthcare networks by mapping and analysing the connections between various medical entities.

Network analysis is increasingly used in mental health to explore psychopathology, symptom interactions, treatment effects, and healthcare systems. Unlike traditional methods that view mental disorders as single constructs, network analysis examines how individual symptoms and factors interact, leading to a more nuanced understanding of mental illnesses. Figure 10.1 shows a network plot for depressive and anxiety symptoms in relation to COVID-19 status.

Building Blocks of Network Analysis

Nodes and edges are the building blocks of network analysis and 'centrality' represents the importance, influence, or prominence of a node within a network.

Nodes

Nodes represent the entities being studied and are chosen on the basis of the research question. These can be symptoms, individuals, organizations, or biological entities (e.g. genes, proteins, or cells). These are chosen on the basis of:

- **Relevance:** nodes should directly relate to the research question.
- **Availability:** data should exist for selected entities.
- **Granularity:** nodes should be at an appropriate level of detail – for example, 'depression' vs individual depression symptoms.
- **Non-redundancy:** avoid duplicate or highly similar nodes that do not add value.

Edges (Connections)

Edges represent how nodes are related. The type of edges chosen depends on the nature of interactions in the network:

- **Symptom networks:** edges represent statistical associations between symptoms, such as co-occurrence in surveys or correlations in time series data. For example

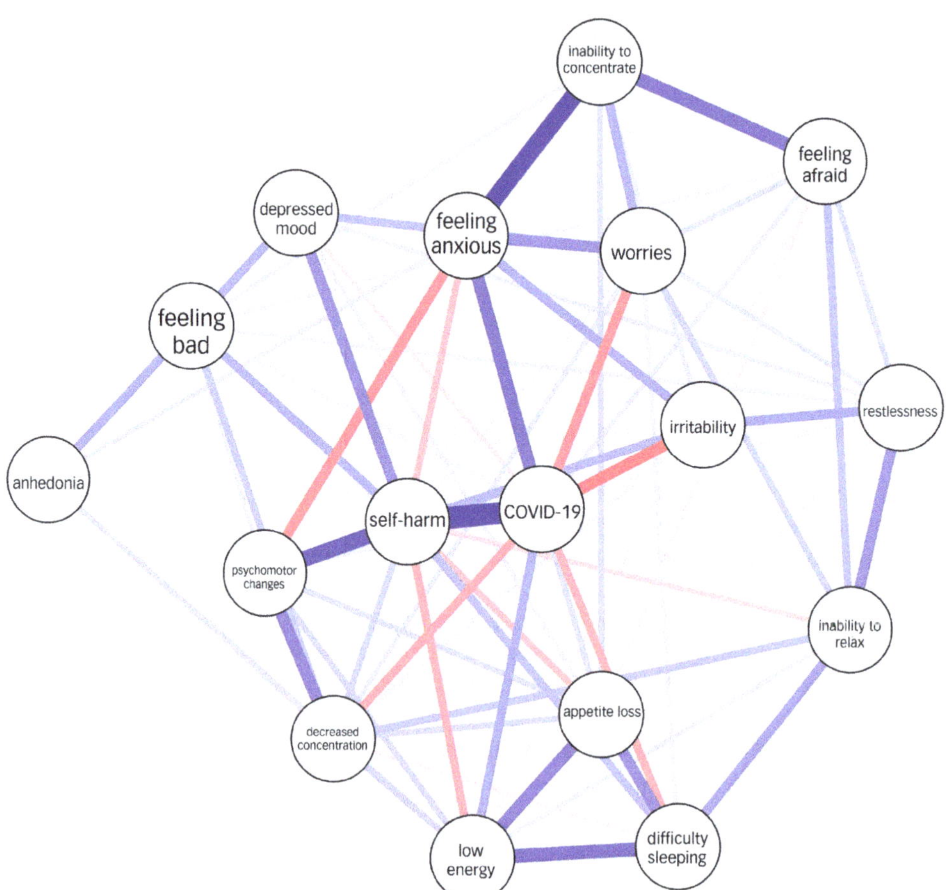

Figure 10.1 Network plot for depressive and anxiety symptoms in relation to COVID-19 status. Blue lines indicate positive correlations and red lines indicate negative correlations. The thickness of each line (or edge) represents the strength of the correlation. COVID-19 refers to COVID-19 status (positive polymerase chain reaction test result) (Source: Abdul Karim M, Ouanes S, Reagu SM, Alabdulla M. Network analysis of anxiety and depressive symptoms among quarantined individuals: cross-sectional study. *B J Psych Open*. 2021;7(6):e222. doi: https://doi.org/10.1192/bjo.2021.1060).

if insomnia frequently co-occurs with fatigue, an edge will connect these symptoms.

- **Comorbidity networks:** edges represent disease co-occurrence in patients. For example, if hypertension and diabetes are frequently diagnosed together, they are linked.
- **Social networks in medicine:** edges may represent social ties, patient referrals, or online interactions. For example, if two doctors frequently collaborate, they are connected in a healthcare network.

- **Biological networks:** edges represent physical interactions between proteins, genes, or neural connections. For example, if two proteins interact in a biochemical pathway, they are linked.

Centrality in Network Analysis

Centrality refers to measures that quantify the importance, influence, or prominence of a node within a network. It helps identify which nodes (e.g. symptoms in mental health or proteins in a biological network) play the most significant roles or are highly connected. Centrality measures try to capture the idea that some nodes are more influential, connected, or important than others.

Key Centrality Measures

Degree Centrality

This is the simplest measure, counting the number of direct connections (edges) a node has. A node with a high degree has many direct neighbours. It is useful for identifying highly connected nodes.

Betweenness Centrality

This measure quantifies how often a node lies on the shortest path between other pairs of nodes. Nodes with high betweenness act as 'bridges' or 'gatekeepers' in the network, controlling the flow of information. It is useful for identifying nodes that connect different parts of the network.

Closeness Centrality

This measure calculates the average shortest path length from a node to all other nodes in the network. Nodes with high closeness are 'close' to all other nodes, meaning they can quickly reach or be reached by others. It is useful for identifying nodes that can efficiently spread information.

Eigenvector Centrality

This measure considers not only the number of connections a node has but also how influential its connected neighbours are. A node with high eigenvector centrality is connected to other highly connected nodes. It is useful for identifying nodes that have influence over the entire network.

Centrality Plot in Network Analysis

A centrality plot is a visual representation of centrality measures for nodes in a network. It helps compare the importance of different nodes based on their degree, betweenness, closeness, eigenvector centrality, or other centrality metrics. Figure 10.2 shows centrality plots of the network analysis diagram in Figure 10.1.
Figure 10.3 shows a symptom network model.

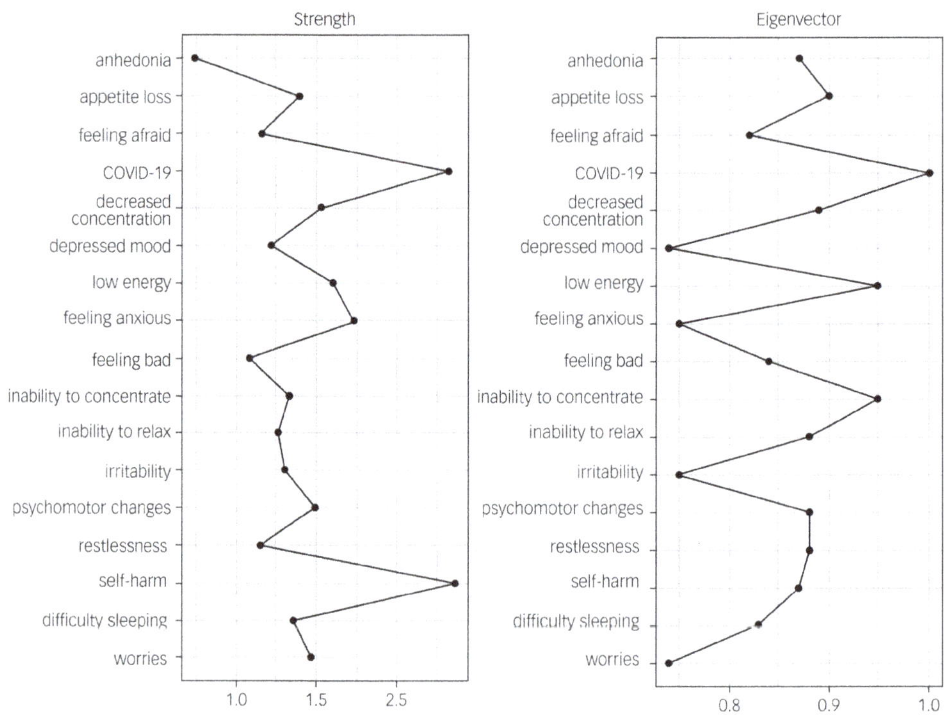

Figure 10.2 Centrality plots for the network of depressive and anxiety symptoms in relation to COVID-19 status (Source: Abdul Karim M, Ouanes S, Reagu SM, Alabdulla M. Network analysis of anxiety and depressive symptoms among quarantined individuals: cross-sectional study. *B J Psych Open*. 2021;7(6):e222. doi: https://doi.org/10.1192/bjo.2021.1060).

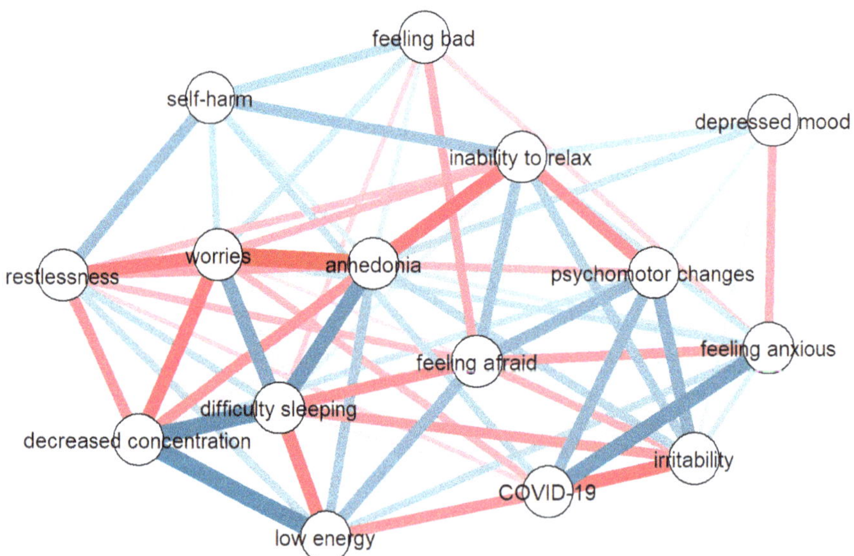

Figure 10.3 Symptom network model linking psychiatric symptoms and COVID-19. Abdul Karim M, Ouanes S, Reagu SM, Alabdulla M (Source: Abdul Karim M, Ouanes S, Reagu SM, Alabdulla M. Network analysis of anxiety and depressive symptoms among quarantined individuals: cross-sectional study. *B J Psych Open*. 2021;7(6):e222. doi: https://doi.org/10.1192/bjo.2021.1060).

Steps in Conducting a Network Analysis

Conducting a network analysis involves a series of steps, and the specifics can vary depending on the field of application. The following is a general overview of the process.

Define Objectives and Questions

Clearly state the purpose of the analysis. For example, are you trying to identify influential individuals in a social network, or understand how diseases spread through a population?

Data Collection

Identify the nodes (entities) and edges (relationships) of your network. Data is gathered according to type of network analysis. Data collection can be done by surveys and questionnaires, medical records or observational studies.

Data Preparation

Organize the data into a format suitable for network analysis. This often involves creating an adjacency matrix or an edge list. Clean and preprocess the data to handle missing values or inconsistencies.

Network Construction

Construct the network using appropriate software. Nodes are represented as points, and edges as lines connecting them. Various software tools and programming languages (e.g. **Gephi**, R (with packages like igraph) and Python (with packages like **NetworkX**)) are used.

Network Analysis

Once the network is constructed, various metrics help interpret the structure and relationships.

Symptom networks are often estimated using Gaussian graphical models with regularization techniques such as the graphical LASSO, which help reduce spurious connections in complex datasets.

Centrality Measures (Identifying Key Nodes)

- **Degree centrality** measures how many connections a node has.
- **Betweenness centrality** identifies nodes that act as bridges between different network parts.
- **Closeness centrality** measures how easily a node can reach others.
- **Eigenvector centrality** identifies influential nodes based on their connections to other important nodes.

This helps to identify symptoms with the highest centrality – for example, anhedonia in depression might be a prime target for treatment.

Clustering and Community Detection

Modularity analysis[1] helps to identify groups of nodes that are more strongly connected to each other than to the rest of the network, while **clustering coefficient**[2] measures how interconnected neighbouring nodes are. The **Louvain algorithm**[3] is used to detect sub-networks within larger systems. For example, in comorbidity networks, clustering might show that anxiety and depression share common symptoms.

Network Density and Connectivity

- **Density** measures how connected the overall network is (i.e. the proportion of all possible edges that are present).
- **Shortest path length** is the minimum number of edges needed to connect the two nodes.
- **Bridge nodes** help to identify critical connections between different network sections.

Visualization of the Network

Network visualization helps interpret complex relationships using software tools:

- `qgraph` **(R)**[4] is popular for mental health symptom networks.
- **Gephi**[5] is used for large-scale social and biological networks.
- **Cytoscape**[6] is common in bioinformatics and neuroscience.
- `NetworkX` **(Python)**[7] is used in statistical and computational modelling.

Interpretation and Clinical Application

Network findings can be used to inform clinical hypotheses. After analysing the network, findings can be used to improve treatment strategies by targeting key symptoms or to predict disorder progression.

Statistical Validation and Sensitivity Analysis

Network models should be assessed for stability and robustness. Common approaches include:

- **Bootstrapping** can be used to ensure the stability of estimated edges and centrality measures. Bootstrapping is a resampling technique used to estimate the sampling distribution of a statistic by repeatedly drawing random samples (with replacement)

---

[1] **Modularity (community detection):** Quality measure comparing within-community vs between-community connections; higher modularity (Q) indicates clearer community structure.

[2] **Clustering coefficient:** Proportion of a node's neighbour pairs that are also connected (local transitivity); the network average reflects overall 'cliquishness'.

[3] **Louvain algorithm:** Fast, greedy heuristic that optimizes modularity via node moves and community aggregation; scalable but non-deterministic across runs.

[4] **qgraph (R):** R package for estimating and visualizing psychometric/symptom networks; supports partial-correlation/graphical models, centrality plots, and bootstrapping.

[5] **Gephi:** Open-source, interactive platform for large-graph layout, filtering, and clustering (e.g. ForceAtlas, Louvain) used for exploratory visualization.

[6] **Cytoscape:** Open source environment widely used in bioinformatics/neuroscience for complex biological network visualization and plug-in-based analysis.

[7] **NetworkX (Python):** Python library for constructing and analysing networks (paths, centrality, communities) in computational/statistical workflows; integrates with NumPy/Pandas.

from the original dataset. It is commonly used to assess statistical accuracy, confidence intervals, and model stability.

- **Permutation** tests are used to check whether observed network patterns are different from what would be expected by chance. A permutation test is a non-parametric statistical method that assesses whether an observed result is significantly different from what would be expected by chance.
- **Robustness analysis** tests how removing certain nodes affects the network.

Applications of Network Analysis in Mental Health

Networks may be cross-sectional (single time-point) or dynamic/temporal, where symptom relationships are examined across time.

Symptom Network Analysis

Understanding Mental Disorders as Networks of Symptoms

Traditional models treat mental disorders as unified constructs – for example, depression as a sum of symptoms. In contrast, network analysis sees disorders as interconnected symptoms, where some symptoms reinforce others – for example, insomnia → fatigue → concentration issues → depressed mood (in a depression network).

Identifying Central Symptoms

Some symptoms act as key nodes driving the disorder – for example, 'anhedonia' in depression. Treating central symptoms may represent a promising intervention target, although centrality does not necessarily imply causality.

Comorbidity Networks

How Mental Disorders Occur Comorbidly

Many mental health conditions occur comorbidly, such as anxiety and depression or ADHD and autism. Network analysis helps identify shared symptoms or pathways linking disorders. For example, rumination may be identified as a key symptom linking depression and anxiety.

Predicting Disorder Progression

By examining symptom connections and bridging pathways, network approaches may help identify patterns that predict which disorders or symptom clusters are more likely to emerge over time in at-risk individuals.

Treatment Response and Personalized Interventions

Targeting Key Symptoms for Effective Treatment

Network analysis can guide psychotherapy and pharmacotherapy by identifying which symptoms to target first. For example, in personalized treatment, analysis of an individual's unique symptom network allows clinicians to identify the most influential symptoms to target with therapy. For example, if 'insomnia' is a major driver of depression, improving sleep could break the depressive cycle.

Assessing Therapy Effectiveness

Changes in network structure over time can indicate treatment success. For example, a study may show that symptom connections weaken after CBT, reducing disorder persistence.

Social Network Analysis in Mental Health

- **Patient support networks:** network analysis can inform how social connections affect mental wellbeing. For example, loneliness and lack of social ties can be risk factors for depression.
- **Therapist collaboration networks:** network analysis can show how mental health professionals collaborate to improve care delivery.
- **Online mental health support:** network analysis can inform interactions on online platforms or online therapy groups to understand emerging mental health trends.

Neurobiological and Cognitive Networks

Brain Network Analysis

Network analysis can be used with neuroimaging data (e.g. fMRI, EEG or diffusion MRI) to study patterns of brain connectivity in psychiatric disorders – for example, altered connectivity between the amygdala and prefrontal cortex has been linked to anxiety disorders.

Cognitive Networks in Mental Health

These networks allow studies of how thoughts, beliefs, and emotions interact in disorders such as OCD or psychosis.

Strengths and Weaknesses of Network Analysis

Strengths

- Identifies key nodes and relationships: helps detect the most influential nodes in a network.
- Captures interactions instead of just aggregates: examines relationships rather than overall averages.
- Works with large, high-dimensional data: can handle thousands of connections efficiently.
- Improves decision-making and targeted interventions: helps optimize treatment strategies and resource allocation.
- Versatile across disciplines: used in social networks, medicine, neuroscience, epidemiology, and finance.
- Analyses both static and dynamic networks: works with both fixed structures (e.g. hospital networks) and evolving systems (e.g. disease spread over time).

Weaknesses

- Requires high-quality data: incomplete or biased data can lead to inaccurate conclusions.
- Computationally intensive for large networks: networks with millions of nodes require significant processing power.

- Correlation does not imply causation: just because two nodes are connected does not mean one causes the other.
- Interpretation can be complex: large networks can be visually overwhelming and difficult to analyse.
- Results depend on node and edge definitions: the way connections are defined can significantly impact the network's structure and interpretation.
- Different centrality measures lead to different conclusions: a node can be important in one metric but not in another, leading to varying interpretations.

Chapter Summary

- Network analysis uses 'nodes' (entities) and 'edges' (connections) to map relationships.
- 'Centrality' measures (degree, betweenness, closeness, eigenvector) identify influential nodes.
- Process: the process involves defining objectives, data collection, preparation, network construction, analysis (centrality, clustering, density), visualization, interpretation, and statistical validation.
- Applications in mental health: symptom network analysis examines symptom interactions, identifying central symptoms. Comorbidity networks explore how mental disorders co-occur. Network analysis informs personalized treatment and therapy effectiveness. Social network analysis is used to understand patient support, therapist collaboration and online mental health. Neurobiological and cognitive networks are used to analyse brain activity and cognitive processes.
- Strengths: identifies key nodes, captures interactions, handles large data, improves interventions, and is versatile.
- Weaknesses: requires high-quality data, is computationally intensive, correlation doesn't equal causation, interpretation can be complex, and results depend on definitions and centrality measures.

Practice Questions

Q1. In network analysis, what do nodes represent?

A. The relationships between different entities
B. The individual entities being analysed
C. The size of the study population
D. The statistical methods used in analysis
E. The level of significance in hypothesis testing

Q2. Which centrality measure identifies the most directly connected nodes in a network?

A. Degree centrality
B. Betweenness centrality
C. Closeness centrality
D. Eigenvector centrality
E. Modularity score

Q3. What do edges represent in a network analysis?
A. The total number of participants in a study
B. The connections or relationships between nodes
C. The variance in statistical distributions
D. The standard deviation of data points
E. The control group in a randomized trial

Q4. Which centrality measure takes into account not just the number of connections but also the importance of those connections?
A. Degree centrality
B. Betweenness centrality
C. Closeness centrality
D. Eigenvector centrality
E. Louvain algorithm

Q5. Which of the following is *not* a method for collecting data in network analysis?
A. Surveys and questionnaires
B. Medical records
C. Randomized controlled trials
D. Observational studies
E. Social media interaction tracking

Q6. Which of the following is an example of a comorbidity network?
A. Examining online mental health support groups
B. Analysing co-occurring mental disorders such as anxiety and depression
C. Tracking genetic mutations in psychiatric disorders
D. Identifying the best medication for treating schizophrenia
E. Comparing different therapy methods for treating PTSD

Q7. Which of the following is a major limitation of network analysis?
A. It can only analyse small datasets.
B. It provides causal conclusions rather than associations.
C. It depends on the definition of nodes and edges.
D. It does not require computational resources.
E. It is only used in biological research.

Answers

Q1. Correct Answer: B. The individual entities being analysed. Nodes represent symptoms, individuals, diseases, or biological components in a network, depending on the research focus.

Q2. Correct answer: A. Degree centrality. Degree centrality counts the number of direct connections a node has, identifying highly connected elements in a network.

Q3. Correct answer: B. The connections or relationships between nodes. Edges define how nodes are related, such as correlations between symptoms, social connections, or interactions between proteins.
Q4. Correct answer: D. Eigenvector centrality. Eigenvector centrality evaluates not only how many connections a node has but also whether those connections are to other highly connected nodes.
Q5. Correct answer: C. Randomized controlled trials. Network analysis typically uses observational or relational data sources (e.g. surveys, records, social media). Randomized controlled trials are study designs for testing interventions, rather than a primary method for collecting network relationship data.
Q6. Correct answer: B. Analysing co-occurring mental disorders such as anxiety and depression. Comorbidity networks identify shared symptoms or risk factors between multiple disorders.
Q7. Correct answer: C. It depends on the definition of nodes and edges. The way nodes and edges are defined and measured can greatly impact network structure and interpretation.

Further Reading

Bastian M, Heymann S, Jacomy M. Gephi: an open source software for exploring and manipulating networks. In: *Proc Int AAAI Conf Weblogs Soc Media (ICWSM)*. 2009;361–2.

Blondel VD, Guillaume JL, Lambiotte R, Lefebvre E. Fast unfolding of communities in large networks. *J Stat Mech.* 2008;**10**:P10008.

Bonacich P. Power and centrality: a family of measures. *Am J Sociol.* 1987;**92**(5):1170–82.

Borsboom D, Cramer AOJ. Network analysis: an integrative approach to the structure of psychopathology. *Annu Rev Clin Psychol.* 2013;**9**:91–121. doi: https://doi.org/10.1146/annurev-clinpsy-050212-185608.

Borsboom D. A network theory of mental disorders. *World Psychiatry.* 2017;**16**(1):5–13. doi: https://doi.org/10.1002/wps.20375.

Epskamp S, Borsboom D, Fried EI. Estimating psychological networks and their accuracy: a tutorial paper. *Behav Res Methods.* 2018;**50**(1):195–212. doi: https://doi.org/10.3758/s13428-017-0862-1.

Epskamp S, Cramer AOJ, Waldorp LJ, Schmittmann VD, Borsboom D. qgraph: network visualizations of relationships in psychometric data. *J Stat Softw.* 2012;**48**(4):1–18.

Freeman LC. Centrality in social networks: conceptual clarification. *Soc Netw.* 1979;**1**(3):215–39.

Hagberg AA, Schult DA, Swart PJ. Exploring network structure, dynamics, and function using NetworkX. In: *Proc 7th Python in Science Conf (SciPy 2008)*. 2008. doi: https://doi.org/10.25080/TCWV9851.

Newman MEJ. Finding community structure in networks using the eigenvectors of matrices. *Phys Rev E.* 2006;**74**(3):036104. doi: https://doi.org/10.1103/PhysRevE.74.036104.

Newman MEJ. Modularity and community structure in networks. *Proc Natl Acad Sci U S A.* 2006;**103**(23):8577–82. doi: https://doi.org/10.1073/pnas.0601602103.

Newman MEJ. *Networks: An Introduction.* Oxford: Oxford University Press; 2010.

Shannon P, Markiel A, Ozier O, et al. Cytoscape: a software environment for integrated models of biomolecular interaction networks. *Genome Res.* 2003;**13**(11):2498–504.

Watts DJ, Strogatz SH. Collective dynamics of 'small-world' networks. *Nature.* 1998;**393**(6684):440–2.

Chapter 11

Descriptive Statistics

Introduction

Descriptive statistics focuses on summarizing and organizing data in a meaningful way. It simplifies large datasets, making them easier to understand, and helps to identify patterns, trends, and potential outliers. It provides valuable insights for decision-making without making predictions.

Displaying Data

Displaying data refers to presenting raw or processed data visually or in tabular form. It allows for a quick and intuitive grasp of data and is often key for hypothesis generation. Displaying summary statistics involves presenting key statistical measures that summarize and describe a dataset in an easy-to-understand format. This helps in understanding the central tendency, dispersion, and distribution of data. There are various ways to display data visually, including pie charts, bar charts, histograms, box plots, and scatter plots.

Graphical Methods for Displaying Data

- **Pie chart:** displays proportions of categorical, nominal, or dichotomous data. The area of each segment is proportional to the number or percentage in that group, ensuring that all data are represented (Figure 11.1).

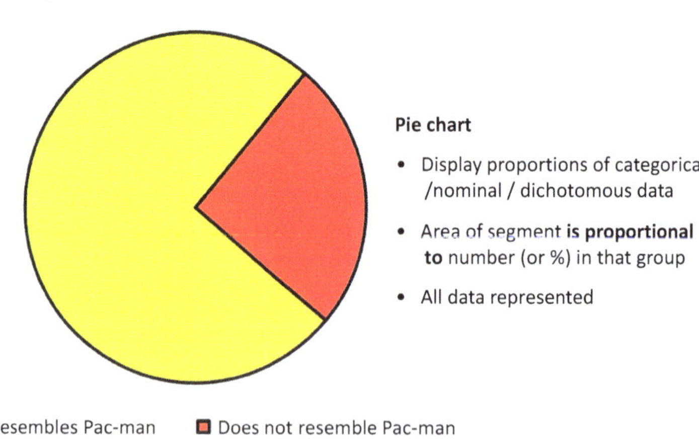

Figure 11.1 Example of a pie chart.

- **Bar chart:** represents categorical, nominal, or dichotomous variables using columns, where the height of each bar is dependent on frequency (Figure 11.2).

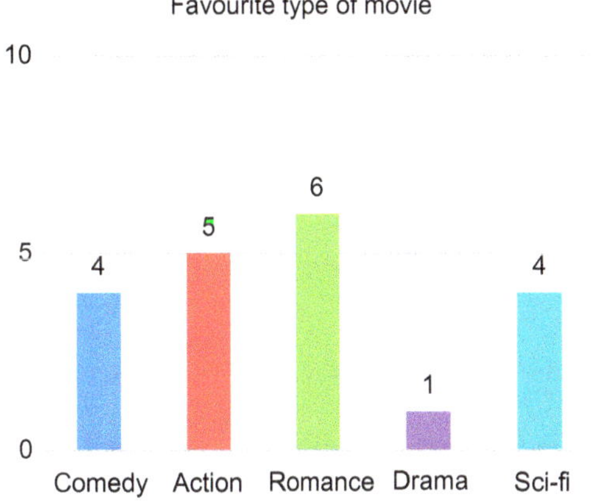

Bar chart

- Each column represents categorical / nominal / dichotomous data
- Arbitrary *x*-axis distribution
- Height of bars dependent on *y*-axis label (e.g. frequency)

Figure 11.2 Example of a bar chart.

- **Histogram:** displays numerical variables (interval or ratio) by splitting it into 'bins' and showing frequency density to illustrate the shape of the distribution (Figure 11.3).

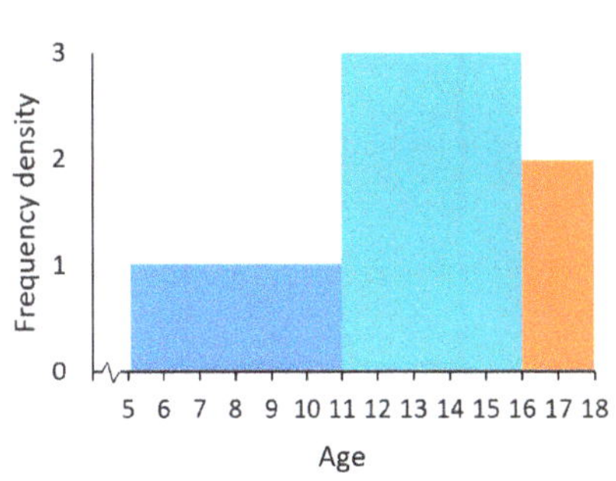

Histogram

- Numerical variables (interval or ratio) is split into 'bins'
- Area = frequency = frequency density * class width
- Can show the shape of the distribution

Age	Frequency
5-10	6
11-15	15
16-17	4
>18	0

Figure 11.3 Example of a histogram.

- Figure 11.4 shows the differences between a bar graph and a histogram.
- **Box (and whisker) plot:** summarizes numerical (continuous or ordinal) data distribution using quartiles, medians, and **outliers**,[1] highlighting dispersion and skewness (Figure 11.5).

[1] **Outlier:** An observation markedly distant from the bulk of the data. In box plots, points beyond 1.5 × IQR below Q1 or above Q3 are flagged. Outliers may reflect valid extreme values or data issues and should be interpreted in context.

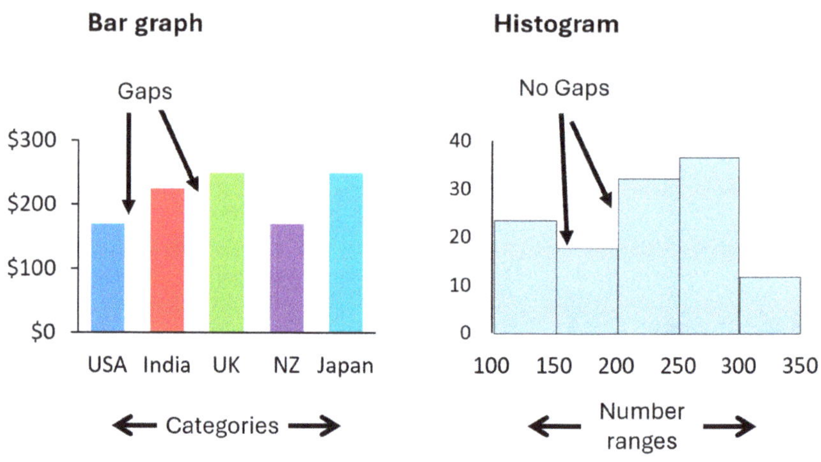

Figure 11.4 Bar graph vs histogram.

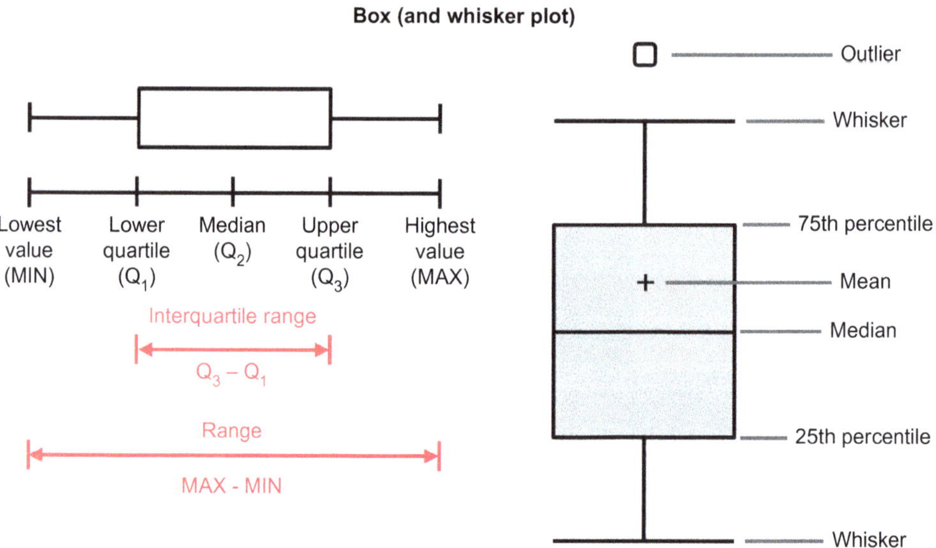

Figure 11.5 Box (and whisker) plots.

- **Scatter plot:** represents the relationship between two numerical variables, allowing visualization of correlations and regression lines. Each dot (or marker) represents one observation, with its position determined by two values:
  1. the value of one variable on the *x*-axis (horizontal)
  2. the value of another variable on the *y*-axis (vertical).
- The purpose of a scatter plot is to visually check whether the variables are related (positively, negatively, or not at all) and to detect patterns, clusters, or outliers in the data. For example:

- If you plotted study hours on the x-axis and exam score on the y-axis for 50 students, a scatterplot could reveal whether greater study time is generally associated with higher scores (Figure 11.6).

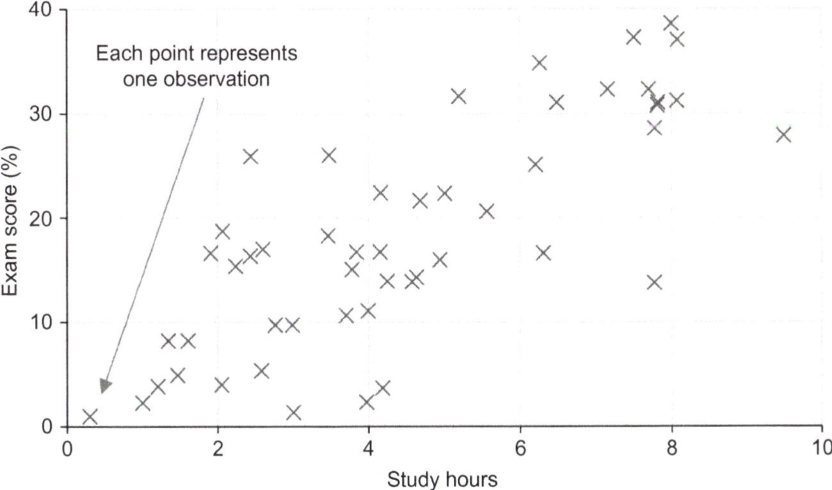

Figure 11.6 Example of a scatterplot.

The scatterplot in Figure 11.6 shows the relationship between study hours (x-axis) and exam score percentage (y-axis). Each point represents one observation, with its position determined by the values of the two variables. Scatterplots are used to assess correlation, trends, and potential outliers between two continuous variables. Figure 11.7 shows another example of a scatterplot, looking at the relationship between diligence and intelligence.

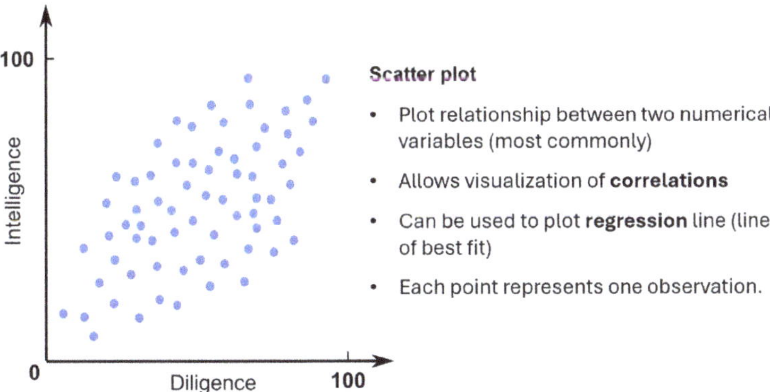

Figure 11.7 Scatter plot showing the relationship between diligence and intelligence.

Table 11.1 presents a summary of data types and display methods.

Table 11.1 Data types and recommended display methods

Data type	Examples	Best ways to display
Categorical (nominal and ordinal)	Gender, blood type, satisfaction level	Frequency table Bar chart Pie chart Stacked bar chart **Mosaic plot**[2]
Dichotomous (binary: 0/1, yes/no)	Pass/fail, male/female, presence/absence	Bar chart Pie chart Frequency table
Discrete numerical (counts)	Number of children, exam scores, hospital visits	Histogram Bar chart **Dot plot**[3] Box plot **Stem-and-leaf plot**[4]
Continuous numerical (measurements)	Height, weight, temperature, age	Histogram Box plot **Density plot**[5] Scatter plot Line graph
Time series (data over time)	Stock prices, sales trends, temperature changes	Line graph Area chart Time series scatter plot **Moving average** plot[6]
Relational data (two or more variables)	Age vs income, exercise vs weight loss	Scatter plot Bubble chart Heatmap **Pair plot**[7]

[2] **Mosaic plot:** Tiles encode a contingency table: typically, column widths reflect one variable's marginal proportions and tile heights reflect the conditional distribution of the second; tile area shows cell frequency, revealing association patterns.

[3] **Dot plot:** Displays each observation (or stacked duplicates) on a number line, preserving exact values without binning – useful for small to moderate sample sizes and for comparing groups side-by-side.

[4] **Stem-and-leaf plot:** A textual histogram that preserves the original numbers (stems = leading digits, leaves = trailing digits); quickly shows shape and outliers and can be 'back-to-back' for two groups.

[5] **Density plot (KDE):** A smoothed estimate of the distribution formed by summing kernels (often Gaussian) placed at each data point; the bandwidth controls smoothness. The curve integrates to 1 and approximates the probability density.

[6] **Moving average (time-series smoothing):** Mean of a sliding window to reduce short-term noise and highlight trend; longer windows smooth more but add lag. A centred window reduces lag compared with a trailing window.

[7] **Pair plot (scatter plot matrix):** Grid of scatter plots for all variable pairs; diagonals show each variable's distribution (histogram or KDE). Useful to spot linearity, clustering, and outliers before modelling.

Table 11.1 (cont.)

Data type	Examples	Best ways to display
Proportional data (percentages and ratios)	Market share, voter turnout, survey responses	Pie chart Stacked bar chart 100% stacked column chart **Treemap**[8]

Choosing the Right Statistical Test

Two critical factors influence the choice of statistical test are:

1. type of data
2. distribution of data.

Additional considerations will be discussed later.

Types of Data

Data in research can be broadly classified based on its nature, level of measurement, or collection methods. Understanding data types is crucial for choosing appropriate statistical analysis, data collection methods, and visualization techniques. The different types of data are described below

Binary Data

Binary data consists of two mutually exclusive categories (e.g. ill/not ill or dead/alive).

Nominal Data

Nominal data comprise three or more categories that have no mathematical relationship with one another (e.g. marital status, occupation, or ethnicity).

Ordinal Data

Ordinal data have inherent order but without consistent, quantifiable intervals. Examples include social class (I–V) and Likert scales. For example, the difference between social classes I and II cannot be assumed to be the same as the difference between social classes IV and V.

Interval Data

Interval data consist of numerical values with meaningful differences but lack a true zero that would indicate an absence of the measured attribute. For example, on the Fahrenheit scale (°F), a zero-degree temperature does not mean the absence of temperature.

Ratio Data

Ratio data are numerical, with meaningful intervals and a true zero that indicates the absence of the characteristic measured (e.g. Kelvin temperature scale (K), income, height, weight, unemployment rate). For example, zero weight would mean no weight.

[8] **Treemap:** Nested rectangles show hierarchical part-to-whole structure; area encodes magnitude and nesting reflects levels (e.g. category → subcategory). Good for many categories when pie/bar charts become crowded.

Quantitative vs Non-numerical

Data are also classified as quantitative (numerical) and qualitative or non-numerical. Non-numerical is a preferable term to qualitative, as it can misleadingly refer to qualitative research.

- Quantitative:
  - Interval: degrees Celsius
  - Ratio: height, income, degrees Kelvin
- Non-numerical:
  - Dichotomous/binary: dead/alive, male/female
  - Categorical/nominal: schizophrenia, bipolar disorder, blood types
  - Ordinal: social class (I, II, III, IV, V)

Interval and ratio data are quantitative, numerical, and measurable. They retain information about both the order and the magnitude of differences between observations, allowing a wider range of statistical analyses. Normally distributed numerical data form a Gaussian (bell-shaped) distribution and can be analysed with parametric tests. An example is IQ scores, which are normally distributed in the population. Gaussian distribution of IQ shown in Figure 11.8.

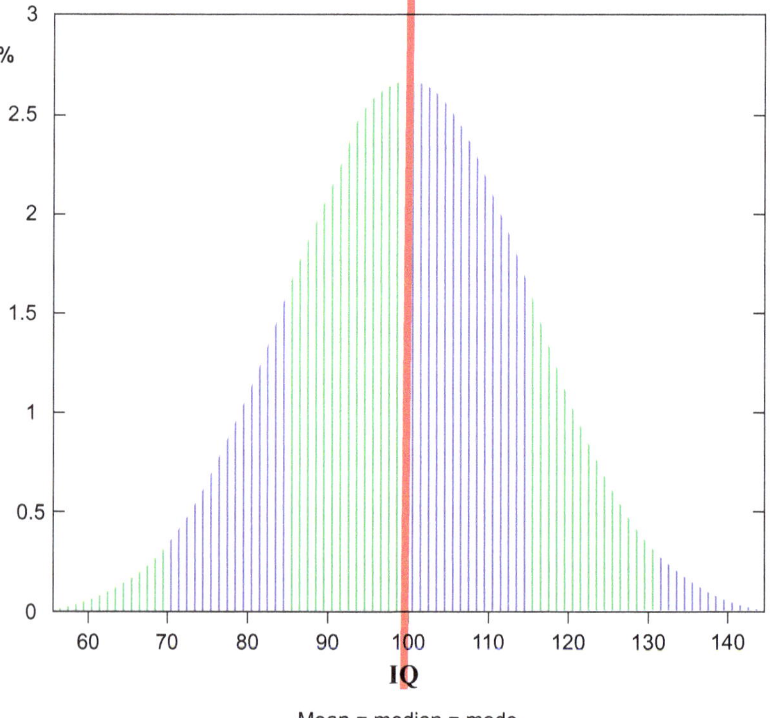

Figure 11.8 Normal (Gaussian) distribution for IQ.

Binary, ordinal, and nominal data are qualitative, non-numerical, and not normally distributed. They must be analysed using non-parametric tests, which focus on frequencies, ranks, or proportions rather than means and standard deviations.

Distribution of Data

For numerical data, it is important to distinguish between parametric and Gaussian (normal) concepts as these two terms are not synonyms. Parametric tests assume that data (or more precisely, the residuals) follow a particular distribution, most commonly the Gaussian (normal) distribution. Other possible distributions of parametric data include the exponential, Poisson, and binomial.

When numerical data do not follow a normal distribution, they are considered skewed and are better analysed using non-parametric tests. The direction of skewness (positive/right-skewed or negative/left-skewed) guides the choice of appropriate statistical methods.

In addition to skewness, another key feature of data that are not normally distributed is kurtosis, which describes the 'tailedness' or the sharpness of the peak of the distribution compared to a normal curve.

Leptokurtic distributions have heavier tails and a sharper peak, indicating more extreme values.

Platykurtic distributions have lighter tails and a flatter peak, suggesting fewer extreme values.

Mesokurtic distributions have a moderate peak and tails, closely resembling the normal distribution. The Gaussian distribution itself is the classic example of a mesokurtic distribution, with a kurtosis of 3 (excess kurtosis = 0). Excess kurtosis is calculated by subtracting 3 from the kurtosis value, so a normal distribution has an excess kurtosis of 0. However, mesokurtic is a broader category: any distribution with kurtosis equal or close to 3 can be called mesokurtic, even if it is not perfectly Gaussian in shape.

Skewness and kurtosis can be visualized graphically to provide an intuitive understanding of how a dataset departs from normality (Figure 11.9).

Skewness

The coefficient of skewness is a measure for the degree of symmetry in the variable distribution.

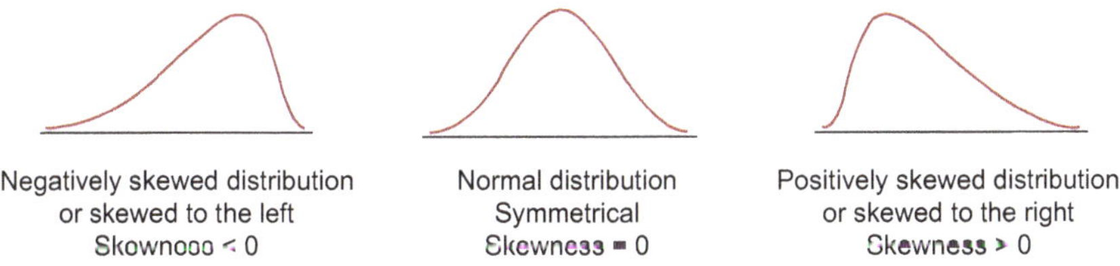

Kurtosis

The coefficient of kurtosis is a measure for the degree of peakedness/flatness in the variable distribution.

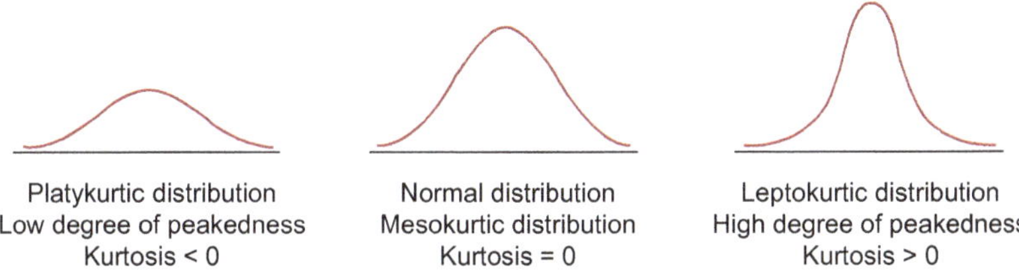

Figure 11.9 Skewness and kurtosis in distributions.

It is important to identify the most representative or typical value in a dataset (measure of central tendency) and how the rest of the data are distributed (measures of distribution). Most types of medical data tend to cluster around the centre of the distribution. The first step in examining a distribution is to look for the **central tendency** of the data.

Measures of Central Tendency

Measures of central tendency describe the centre or typical value of a dataset. The three main measures of central tendency are:

- **Mean:** the arithmetic average of all values, used for normally distributed numerical data (interval and ratio data).
- **Mode**: The most frequently occurring value in a dataset, used for categorical data.
- **Median:** the middle value when data are arranged in order, used when the data are skewed. Mean is not used as a measure of central tendency for skewed numerical data because it is highly sensitive to extreme values (outliers) and is pulled towards them. For example, consider the following right-skewed data:

  $\text{Data}: \ 9, \ 11, \ 15, \ 18, \ 97$

  $$\text{Mean} = \frac{9 + 11 + 15 + 18 + 97}{5} = 30$$

  $\text{Median} = 15$

- Therefore, the mean is much higher than the median because it is pulled towards the extreme value (97). In a positively skewed distribution (right-skewed), the mean is greater than the median because high values pull it to the right. In a negatively skewed distribution (left-skewed), the mean is smaller than the median because low values pull it to the left, as shown in Figure 11.10.

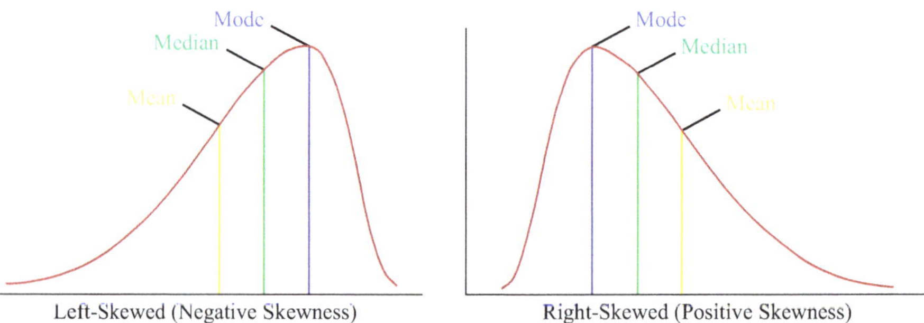

Figure 11.10 Negative and positive skewness.

Box 11.1 provides a brief summary of measures of central tendency.

Box 11.1 Measures of Central Tendency for Different Data Types

The central tendency is a number capturing the 'middle'.

- Dichotomous/categorical data (non-Gaussian distribution, no ordering):
  - mode = most frequent value
  - proportion = % of each group.
- Ordinal data (non-Gaussian distribution, ordering):
  - mode = most frequent value
  - median = middle value of ranked data.
- Interval/ratio data which is non-Gaussian (e.g. skewed):
  - mode or median
  - alternatively, data can be transformed to approximate a Gaussian distribution.
- Interval/ratio data (Gaussian):
  - mean = sum of all values / *n*.

Measures of Dispersion

After determining the central tendency, the next step is to assess how spread out (dispersed) the values are. Measures of dispersion describe variability in a dataset, indicating how much data deviate from the central value.

Dispersion is important because the data that are closer to the central value and are more compact are less likely to have error than the data that are widely spread around the measure of dispersion. For example, consider the following two continuous datasets:

- **Data 1:** 3, 3, 5, 6, 6, 5, 6, 6, 5, 5 → Mean = 50/10 = 5
- **Data 2:** 1, 10, 2, 9, 1, 1, 8, 8, 1, 9 → Mean = 50/10 = 5

Although the mean is the same for both datasets, Data 2 is much more widespread than Data 1, making it more likely to contain measurement variability or extreme values. This highlights the importance of dispersion measures in understanding the variability, reliability, and precision of a dataset.

Measures of Dispersion for Normally Distributed Data

Measures of dispersion for interval/ratio data that follow a Gaussian (normal) distribution include variance and standard deviation.

Variance

Variance measures how far each value in the dataset is from the mean. Variance is the sum of all the differences between all the values and the mean, squared (so that negative and positive deviations do not cancel each other out) and divided by the total number of observations minus 1 (degrees of freedom). In other words:

Variance = average squared deviation of values from the mean.

Sample variance is calculated as:

$$s^2 = \frac{\Sigma(x_i - \overline{x})^2}{(n-1)},$$

where s^2 is sample variance; Σ is summation (meaning you add up all the values); x_i is each individual data point in the sample; $\bar{x}$ is the sample mean; and n is the number of data points in the sample or sample size.

For example, consider the following simple values:

1, 3, 4, 3, 6, 7.

- mean = 4
- differences from mean:

  1 – 4 = –3

  3 – 4 = –1

  4 – 4 = 0

  3 – 4 = –1

  6 – 4 = 2

  7 – 4 = 3

- squaring the differences: 9, 1, 0, 1, 4, 9

  sum = 24

  variance $= \frac{24}{6-1} = 4.8$

It is important to note that degrees of freedom are applied when calculating the sample variance but not the population variance. Therefore, population variance is calculated as:

$$\sigma^2 = \frac{\Sigma(x_i - \mu)^2}{N}$$

where σ^2 is population variance; x_i is each individual data point; μ is the population mean; and N is the total number of data points in the population.

Degrees of Freedom

Degrees of freedom refer to the number of independent values in a dataset that are free to vary. A degree of freedom is lost every time a mean is calculated because mean becomes a fixed value around which other observations are free to vary. A helpful analogy is choosing which glove to put on first. You have two choices initially. Once you choose one, say the right, you lose that freedom, and the remaining choice is fixed – you must put on the left glove. If you have a sample of size n and you calculate the mean, then $(n - 1)$ values can vary freely, but the last value is constrained to make the sum equal to the total mean. Assume there are three values of the data set as below:

10, 15, 20,
Mean $= \overline{x} = 15.$

Variation from mean for the first two values is:

$10 - 15 = -5$ and $15 - 15 = 0.$

The third value must be 5 because the sum of all variations from the mean must be 0. Therefore, the third value is restricted from varying.

In hypothesis testing, degrees of freedom help to determine the shape of statistical distributions (e.g. *t*-distribution, chi-square distribution).

Standard Deviation

Standard deviation (SD) is simply the square root of variance. Taking the square root of the variance gives us the units used in the original data. Standard deviation is used more often as a measure of dispersion because variance tends to be large, and expressed in squared units. Therefore, standard deviation is more intuitive for describing the amount of spread in a dataset.

The formula, using the previous variance calculation is: $SD = \sqrt{variance}$.

Standard deviation provides significant information when describing a dataset. In a normal Gaussian distribution, it follows the empirical rule:

- 68% of values fall within ±1 SD of the mean
- 95% of values fall within ±2 SD of the mean
- 99.7% of values fall within ±3 SD of the mean.

For example, Figure 11.11 shows the standard deviation of IQ, which is normally distributed in the population.

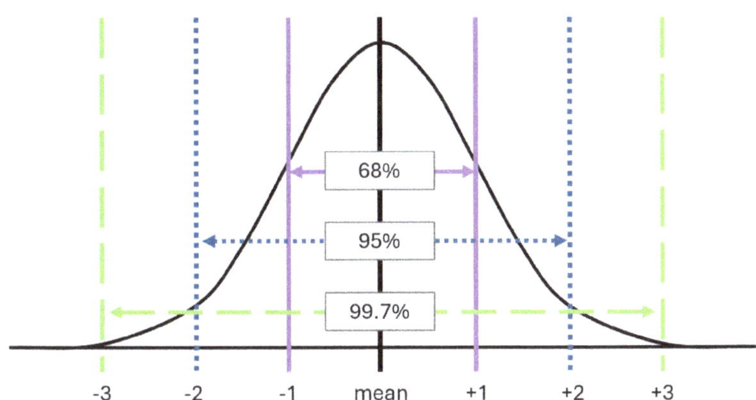

Figure 11.11 Normal distribution curve.

Standard Error of the Mean

The standard error of the mean (SEM) measures the variability of a sample mean in relation to the true population mean. Standard deviation shows the variability of the individual observations, whereas the SEM shows variability of means. It quantifies how much the sample mean is expected to vary if multiple samples are drawn from the same population. In other words, it gives an insight into how precise the sample mean is in estimating the population mean. Therefore, SEM rather than SD is used to calculate 95% confidence intervals.

It is not strictly a measure of dispersion, but rather a measure of the precision or uncertainty of the sample mean as an estimate of the population mean. However, it is closely related to measures of dispersion, as it is derived from the SD of the sample and is therefore described here for ease of understanding. It can be calculated from the SD by dividing it by the square root of the sample size using the formula:

$$\text{SEM} = \text{SD}\sqrt{n},$$

where SD is the standard deviation of the sample and n is the sample size (number of observations).

Using above example (values of 1, 3, 4, 3, 6, 7), the SEM will be calculated as follows:

$$\text{SD} = 2.19,$$
$$n = 6,$$
$$\text{Square root of the sample size}(\sqrt{n}) = \sqrt{6} = 2.449,$$
$$\text{SEM} = 2.19/2.449 \approx 0.894.$$

It can readily be seen that the SEM decreases as the sample size increases because larger samples provide more reliable estimates (i.e. the larger the sample size, the less the error).

A closely related concept is *standard error of the sample means*, which measures the variability in the means calculated from multiple samples drawn from the same population. It is essentially the standard deviation of the distribution of sample means around the true population mean. This distribution is also known as the sampling distribution of the mean.

The SEM describes how much variation there is between the means of multiple samples drawn from the same population. In practice, the SEM is the standard deviation of the sampling distribution of the mean; the distinction made here is for conceptual understanding. It is calculated as follows

$$\text{Standard error of sample means} = \text{population SD}/\sqrt{n},$$
$$\text{Population SD} = \text{standard deviation of the population},$$
$$n = \text{sample size (number of observations in each sample)}.$$

Table 11.2 lists the key differences between these two statistics.

Table 11.2 Key differences between the SEM and standard error of sample means

Aspect	Standard error of the mean	Standard error of the sample means
What it measures	Variability of the sample mean as an estimate of the population mean	Variability in means of multiple samples from the same population
Data source	Derived from a single sample	Derived from multiple samples
Formula	SEM = SD / √n	Standard error of sample means = population SD / √n
Sample size influence	Based on the sample size of a single sample	Based on the size of multiple samples and their variation
Use	Used for estimating the population mean from a single sample	Used for understanding the variation in sample means across multiple samples

Confidence Interval

The confidence interval (CI) provides an interval within which the true value of the population mean is expected to lie. A 95% confidence level means that if the study were repeated multiple times, 95% of the CIs would contain the true population parameter. The formula for a 95% CI is:

$$95\%\ \text{CI for the mean} = \text{sample mean} \pm 1.96 \times \text{SEM}.$$

For our above example, the CI is calculated as follows:

$$\begin{aligned} 95\%\ \text{CI} &= 4 \pm 1.96 \times 0.894 \\ &= 4 \pm 1.75 \\ &= (2.25, 5.75). \end{aligned}$$

Note: The value 1.96 is the standard normal multiplier for calculating 95% confidence intervals when sample sizes are large or when the population standard deviation is known. For small samples (commonly $n < 30$) where the population standard deviation is unknown, the t-distribution should be used to account for additional uncertainty. Here, the value 1.96 is used for illustrative purposes only.

Statistical formulas

- **Sample variance (s^2):** $s^2 = \Sigma(x_i - \bar{x})^2 / (n - 1)$
- **Standard deviation (SD):** SD = $\sqrt{\text{variance}}$
- **Standard error of the mean (SE):** SE = SD / $\sqrt{n}$
- **Confidence interval for the mean (CI):** CI = mean ± (1.96 × SE).

Measures of Dispersion for Skewed Numerical Data

When dealing with skewed numerical data, the measures of dispersion must account for the asymmetry of the distribution. Standard deviation may not fully capture the spread in such cases because it assumes a symmetric (normal) distribution.

For skewed data, **median**[9] is preferred as a measure of central tendency, and range and **interquartile range (IQR)**[10] are commonly used as measures of dispersion:

- **Range** is the simplest measure of spread, calculated as the difference between the maximum and minimum values. It reflects the total spread of the data but can be highly affected by extreme values (outliers).
- **Interquartile range** represents the spread of the central 50% of a dataset. It is calculated as the difference between the third quartile (Q3) and the first quartile (Q1):
  - IQR = Q3 − Q1
  - **first quartile (Q1):** the value below which 25% of the data falls (25th percentile)
  - **third quartile (Q3):** the value below which 75% of the data falls (75th percentile).

Because it focuses on the middle half of the data, the IQR is less sensitive to outliers than the full range.

---

[9] **Median:** The 50th percentile that splits ordered data in half. It is robust to skewness and outliers.

[10] **IQR (interquartile range):** The spread of the middle 50% of observations (Q3 − Q1). It is robust to skewness and outliers.

Example Calculation

Data: 6, 47, 49, 15, 43, 41, 7, 39, 43, 41, 36 (11 values)

Ordered data: 6, 7, 15, 36, 39, 41, 41, 43, 43, 47, 49

- Median (middle value): 41 (sixth value, at position $(n+1)/2$ in the ordered data)
- Range = 49 – 6 = 43
- Q1 = 15 (value at position $(n + 1)/4$ in the ordered data)
- Q3 = 43 (value at position $3(n + 1)/4$ in the ordered data)
- IQR = 43 – 15 = 28.

Calculation for Even Sample Size

Sample = 6, 7, 15, 36, 39, 41, 41, 43, 43, 47, 49, 52

- Median = 6, 7, 15, 36, 39, (41 + 41)/2, 43 43 47 49 52 = (41 + 41)/2 = 41
- $Q1 = \frac{15+36}{2} = \frac{51}{2} = 25.5$
- $Q3 = \frac{43+47}{2} = \frac{90}{2} = 45$
- $IQR = 45 - 25.5 = 19.5.$

Standard Error and Confidence Interval of Non-parametric Data

For non-parametric data, traditional formulas for calculating the standard error (SE) and CIs are often inappropriate because they rely on assumptions of normality. Instead, resampling-based methods are used.

- **Bootstrapping** is the most widely applied approach. In bootstrapping, repeated random samples (with replacement) are drawn from the observed dataset, and the statistic of interest (e.g. median) is recalculated for each resample. This process produces an empirical distribution of the statistic, from which variability and uncertainty can be estimated. In practice, bootstrapping is especially useful for estimating uncertainty around statistics such as the median, IQR, or correlation coefficients in non-parametric contexts, where classical formulas for SE and CI are not valid.
- **Bootstrapped standard error (SE):** the standard deviation of the bootstrapped distribution of the statistic provides an estimate of its standard error. This method avoids parametric assumptions and adapts to the actual shape of the data.
- **Percentile-based CIs:** after generating the bootstrapped distribution, the CI can be estimated by taking the appropriate **percentiles.**[11] For a 95% CI, the 2.5th and 97.5th percentiles of the bootstrapped distribution are used as the lower and upper bounds.
- **Bootstrapped CIs (bias-corrected and accelerated, BCa):**[12] more advanced bootstrap methods adjust for potential bias and skewness in the bootstrapped distribution, leading to more accurate confidence intervals, particularly for small or highly skewed samples.

[11] **Percentile:** The value at or below which a stated percentage of observations lie (e.g. 90th percentile is exceeded by 10%). For small samples it may be interpolated; the 50th percentile is the median.

[12] **Bootstrapped CI (BCa):** Bias-corrected and accelerated interval that adjusts for bias and skewness in the bootstrap distribution; typically more accurate than basic/percentile intervals – uses a large number of resamples (often thousands).

In bootstrapping, resampling is done *with replacement*. After each draw, the selected value is put back, and the next draw is made randomly from the *entire original dataset*. Each resample has the same size (n) as the original.

- On each of the n draws, one observation is chosen at random *from the original values only* (no new or 'nearest' values are created).
- Draws are *independent* and *equiprobable*: the same value can be picked again; others may not be picked at all.
- The *number of repeats and omissions varies randomly* from resample to resample – there is *no fixed number* of 'replacements'; it depends entirely on the random draws.

Example

- **Original dataset:** 110, 115, 120, 125, 160
- **Sample 2:** [120, 120, 125, 160, 160] → **110** and **115** omitted; **120** and **160** repeated
- **Sample 3:** [110, 110, 120, 115, 125] → **160** omitted; **110** repeated.

This randomness allows the bootstrap distribution to approximate the variability of repeated sampling from the population.

Worked Example: Bootstrapping the Median

Suppose we have a small dataset of systolic blood pressure readings (mmHg):

Dataset: [110, 115, 120, 125, 160]

- **Original statistic:** the median is 120 mmHg.
- **Bootstrap resampling:** we repeatedly draw samples *with replacement* of size 5. Example samples:

  Sample 1: [110, 115, 115, 160, 125] → Median = 115

  Sample 2: [120, 120, 125, 160, 160] → Median = 125

  Sample 3: [110, 110, 120, 115, 125] → Median = 115

  . . . continued for *at least 1,000 resamples* (5,000 is preferred in research for more stable results). For larger datasets use more resamples).

- **Bootstrap distribution:** the medians from all resamples form an empirical distribution.
- **Bootstrapped SE:** the standard deviation of this bootstrap distribution provides the SE.
- **Confidence interval:** the 2.5th and 97.5th percentiles of the bootstrap distribution form the 95% CI.

  Example: CI = 115–125 mmHg.

Bootstrapping uses the original data to generate a sampling distribution. Because resampling is random, repeating the process many times (≥1,000, ideally 5,000+) ensures stable estimates. This avoids assumptions of normality, making bootstrapping particularly useful for non-parametric data, small samples, and skewed distributions. Figure 11.12 shows the flow diagram for the bootstrapping process.

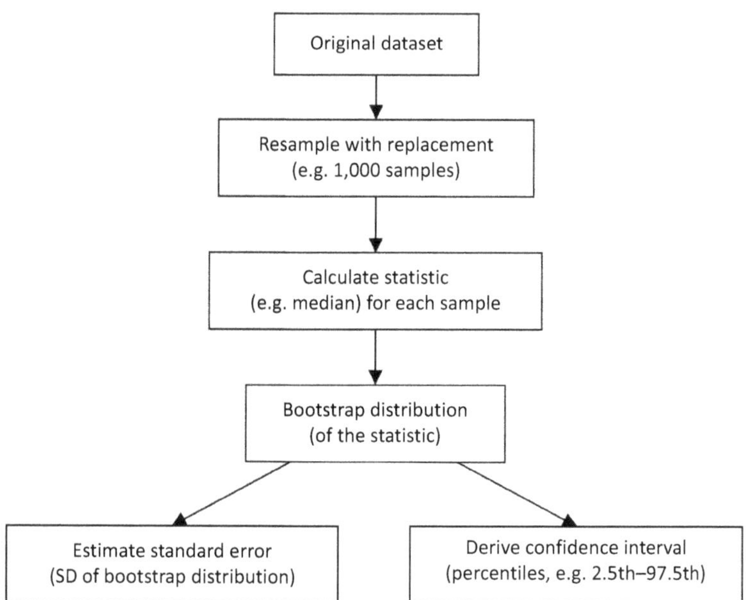

Figure 11.12 Flow diagram of the bootstrapping process.

Measures of Dispersion for Dichotomous and Categorical Data

For dichotomous, categorical, and ordinal data, standard deviation and variance are not always meaningful. Instead, dispersion is usually measured using proportions[13] or the **variation ratio (VR).**[14]

Proportion

A proportion expresses the fraction of observations in a particular category:

$$\mathrm{p} = \frac{x}{n},$$

where x is the number of observations in the category of interest and n is the total number of observations.

Example

In a group of 100 patients, 40 are smokers. The proportion of smokers is:

$$\mathrm{p} = \frac{40}{100} = 0.40 = 40\%.$$

[13] **Proportion:** The fraction of observations in a category: $p = x/n$, where x is the count in the category and n is the total. Example: for 40 smokers out of 100 patients, $p = 40/100 = 0.40$ (40%). Often reported with a 95% binomial CI (e.g. Wilson).

[14] **Variation ratio (VR):** A dispersion index for categorical data defined as 1 – (mode proportion). Higher values indicate greater heterogeneity across categories.

Variation Ratio

The VR measures the proportion of cases not in the modal category (the most frequent category). It reflects the degree of heterogeneity in categorical data:

$$VR = 1 - \frac{fm}{n},$$

where fm is the frequency of the modal category and n is the total sample size.

Example

In a sample of 100 people, if 60 prefer tea, 30 prefer coffee, and 10 prefer water, then:

$$VR = 1 - \frac{60}{100} = 0.40 = 40\%.$$

This means 40% of individuals do not belong to the modal category.

Standard Error and Confidence Interval for Dichotomous Data

For binary (yes/no) outcomes, the standard error of a proportion can be calculated as:

$$SE = \sqrt{\frac{p(1-p)}{n}}.$$

A 95% CI for the proportion is then:

$$CI = p \pm 1.96 \times SE.$$

Example

In a sample of 100 patients, 40 are smokers ($p = 0.40$):

$$SE = \sqrt{\frac{0.4\ (1 - 0.4)}{100}} = \sqrt{\frac{0.4(0.6)}{100}} = \sqrt{0.0024} = 0.049,$$

$$95\%\ CI = 0.40 \pm 1.96 \times 0.049 = (0.304,\ 0.496).$$

So, the true proportion of smokers in the population lies between 30.4% and 49.6%, with 95% confidence.

Confidence Intervals for Ordinal Data

The choice of method depends on whether interest lies in category-specific proportions or in the overall central tendency of the ordered outcome. There are two main approaches, depending on how ordinal data are treated:

1. Treat as categorical (nominal-like): you can calculate proportions and CIs for each category (mild, moderate, severe), using the same binomial formula as for nominal data.

   - Example: In 100 patients, 30 mild, 50 moderate, 20 severe → calculate SE and CI for each proportion separately.

2. Treat as numerical (using ranks): if ordinal data are coded numerically (e.g. mild = 1, moderate = 2, severe = 3), you can use non-parametric statistics:

   - median and IQR (instead of mean/SD)
   - confidence intervals for medians are estimated using bootstrapping since no closed-form analytic formula exists.

Example: Ordinal Data (Pain Severity)

Out of 100 patients:

- mild = 30
- moderate = 50
- severe = 20.

  Categorical (binomial) approach:
  For mild pain ($p = 0.30$):

$$SE = \sqrt{\frac{0.3 \times 0.7}{100}} = \sqrt{0.0021} = 0.0458,$$
$$CI = 0.30 \pm 1.96 \times 0.0458 = (0.211, 0.389).$$

  In the median approach (bootstrapping):

- If pain severity is coded 1–3, median = 2 (moderate).
- Bootstrapping generates a sampling distribution of medians, from which a Cl can be estimated.
- Ordinal data should not be analysed using parametric confidence intervals for the mean, as equal spacing between categories cannot be assumed.

Box 11.2 Measures of Dispersion (Spread) for Different Data Types

For dichotomous/categorical/ordinal data (non-Gaussian, no *equal* relationship between levels):

- proportion: used to describe how observations are distributed across categories.

For ordinal data, state the spread across ordered categories (e.g. concentration at lower vs higher levels). For non-Gaussian (e.g. skewed) interval/ratio data:

- range = highest – lowest value (100% spread)
- interquartile range= Q3 – Q1 values (spread of the central 50% of the data)
- alternatively, data may be transformed to approximate a Gaussian distribution.

For Gaussian (normal) interval/ratio data:

- variance = sum(difference between individual values and the mean)^2/(n – 1)
- standard deviation = sqrt(variance).

Chapter Summary

Descriptive statistics simplifies large datasets by summarizing and organizing data to enable easier interpretation. It helps identify patterns, trends, and outliers, but does not involve making predictions or inferences beyond the data observed.

Types of Data

- **Binary data:** consists of two mutually exclusive categories (e.g. ill/not ill, dead/alive).
- **Nominal data:** comprises three or more categories with no inherent order (e.g. marital status, occupation).
- **Ordinal data:** has a meaningful order but unequal intervals between values (e.g. social class I–V, Likert scales).
- **Interval data:** includes numerical values with meaningful differences but lacks a true zero (e.g. temperature in Fahrenheit).
- **Ratio data:** similar to interval data but includes a true zero (e.g. income, height, weight, temperature measured in Kelvin).

Displaying Data

Presenting data visually or in tabular form allows for quick interpretation and aids hypothesis generation.

Graphical Methods for Displaying Data

- **Pie chart:** represents proportions of categorical or dichotomous data, with segment areas proportional to group sizes.
- **Bar chart:** displays categorical variables using bars where height reflects frequency.
- **Histogram:** used for numerical data, dividing values into bins to show the distribution shape.
- **Box plot:** summarizes data distribution using quartiles, medians, and outliers, highlighting variability and skewness.

Distribution of Data

Measures of Central Tendency

Central tendency describes the typical value of a dataset.

- **Mean:** the arithmetic average, used for normally distributed numerical data.
- **Median:** the middle value in ordered data, preferred for skewed distributions as it is less affected by outliers.
- **Mode:** the most frequently occurring value, mainly used for categorical data.

Measures of Dispersion

Dispersion quantifies how spread-out data points are around the central value, affecting reliability and precision.

Measures for Normally Distributed Data

- **Variance (s^2):** Measures how much values deviate from the mean, squared to avoid cancelling out positive and negative differences: $s^2 = \Sigma(x_i - \bar{x})^2 / (n - 1)$.
- **Standard deviation:** the square root of variance, indicating spread in the same units as the original data. Empirical rule for normal distributions:
  - 68% of values fall within ±1 SD
  - 95% of values fall within ±2 SD
  - 99.7% of values fall within ±3 SD.

Degrees of Freedom

- Indicates the number of independent values in a dataset that can vary while satisfying statistical constraints.
- When calculating a mean, one degree of freedom is lost because the final value is constrained by the total.

Standard Error of the Mean

- Measures the precision of the sample mean as an estimate of the population mean: SEM = SD / $\sqrt{n}$.
- SEM decreases as sample size increases, improving precision.

Confidence Interval

A confidence interval provides a range within which the true population mean is expected to lie: 95% CI = sample mean ± 1.96 × SEM.

Measures of Dispersion for Skewed Data

When data is skewed, the interquartile range is preferred over standard deviation.

Interquartile Range

Measures the spread of the middle 50% of a dataset, reducing the impact of outliers:

- IQR = Q3 – Q1.
- **Q1 (first quartile):** the value below which 25% of the data falls.
- **Q3 (third quartile):** the value below which 75% of the data falls.

Standard Error and Confidence Interval for Non-parametric Data

For skewed (non-parametric) data, standard error and confidence intervals require alternative methods:

- **Bootstrapped standard error:** uses resampling to estimate standard error.
- **Percentile-based confidence intervals:** use percentiles rather than normal distribution assumptions.
- **Bootstrapped confidence intervals:** estimate variability by drawing repeated random samples from the dataset.

Measures of Dispersion for Categorical and Ordinal Data

For categorical and ordinal data, dispersion is measured using:

- **proportion:** the percentage of individuals in a specific category.
- **variation ratio:** the proportion of data that does not belong to the modal category.

Practice Questions

Q1. A psychiatrist notices that several patients with psychosis who started a new mindfulness programme report a significant reduction in their symptoms. The psychiatrist concludes that mindfulness is an effective treatment for all psychotic disorders. This is an example of:

A. Deductive reasoning
B. Controlled experimentation
C. Inductive reasoning
D. Statistical analysis
E. Placebo effect

Q2. Which of the following statements about interval data is true?

A. It has an absolute zero point.
B. It can only be analysed using non-parametric tests.
C. It consists of ordered categories with unequal intervals.
D. It has equal intervals but no true zero.
E. It is always normally distributed.

Q3. Which of the following types of data is most suitable for a pie chart?

A. Ordinal
B. Nominal
C. Interval
D. Ratio
E. Time series

Q4. Which type of data is best visualized using a scatter plot?

A. Ordinal
B. Nominal
C. Binary
D. Interval
E. Dichotomous

Q5. Social class rankings (I–V) are an example of which type of data?

A. Binary
B. Nominal
C. Ordinal
D. Ratio
E. Interval

Q6. Which of the following best describes the characteristics of a left-skewed (negatively skewed) distribution?

A. The mean is greater than the median, and the tail is longer on the right side.
B. The mean is less than the median, and the tail is longer on the left side.
C. The mean, median, and mode are always equal.
D. The median is always the largest value in the dataset.
E. The mode is always greater than both the median and mean in a right-skewed distribution.

For Q7–Q10: A study measures the anxiety levels of 15 participants before a public-speaking event. Their anxiety levels are rated on an ordinal scale from 1 (no anxiety) to 5 (extreme anxiety). The ratings are as follows:

2, 3, 1, 4, 3, 3, 5, 2, 4, 3, 2, 1, 5, 4, 3

Q7. Which of the following is the most appropriate measure of central tendency for this data?

A. Mean
B. Median
C. Mode
D. Variance
E. Standard deviation

Q8. What is the median anxiety level rating for this group of participants?

A. 1
B. 2
C. 3
D. 4
E. 5

Q9. Which of the following is the most appropriate measure of dispersion for this data?

A. Variance
B. Standard deviation
C. Interquartile range
D. Range
E. Confidence interval

Q10. What is the IQR of the anxiety level ratings?

A. 1
B. 2
C. 3
D. 4
E. 5

For Q11–Q12: A psychiatrist assesses the severity of depressive symptoms in eight patients using a standardized rating scale of non-parametric data. The scores are: 75, 88, 92, 68, 80, 85, 78, 90 (higher scores indicate more severe symptoms).

Q11. What is the median score on the depression rating scale?

A. 78
B. 80
C. 81.5
D. 82.5
E. 85

Q12. What is the IQR of the depression rating scale scores?

A. 8
B. 10.5
C. 13
D. 15.5
E. 18

Q13. A psychiatrist is studying the variability in the number of therapy sessions attended by patients diagnosed with generalized anxiety disorder (GAD). The number of sessions attended by six randomly selected patients is: 4, 6, 8, 6, 8, 10. What is the variance of this dataset?

A. 3.2
B. 4.0
C. 4.4
D. 5.6
E. 6.8

Q14. A psychiatrist is studying the effects of a new medication on cognitive function in patients with schizophrenia. A sample of 10 patients is assessed using a cognitive test before and after starting the medication. The mean improvement in cognitive scores after taking the medication is 8 points, and the variance of the differences is 4. Assuming the data are normally distributed and the population standard deviation (σ) is 2, what is the 95% confidence interval for the mean improvement in cognitive scores in the population?

A. (6.76, 9.24)
B. (5.7, 10.3)
C. (7.2, 8.8)
D. (7.6, 8.4)
E. (4.6, 11.4)

Answers

Q1. Correct answer: C. Inductive reasoning. Inductive reasoning is a logical process where you move from specific observations to a broader, general conclusion. The conclusions reached through inductive reasoning are probabilistic, meaning they are likely but not guaranteed to be true Why the other options are incorrect:

A. Deductive reasoning: deductive reasoning moves in the opposite direction (i.e. from general premise to specific cases) to reach a logically certain conclusion.
B. Controlled experiment: the scenario in the question describes an observation, not a controlled experiment.
D. Statistical analysis: while statistical analysis could be used to evaluate the effectiveness of mindfulness, the scenario described in the question is a simple observational generalization, not a formal statistical analysis of data.
E. Placebo effect: while the placebo effect could be a factor in the patients' reported improvement, the question is specifically asking about the type of reasoning used by the psychiatrist.

Q2. Correct answer: D. It has equal intervals but no true zero. Interval data has equal intervals (e.g. temperature in Celsius), but zero does not indicate an absence of the characteristic.

Q3. Correct answer: B. Nominal. Pie charts are best suited for categorical (nominal) data, where proportions or percentages are compared.

Q4. Correct answer: D. Interval. Scatter plots are used for continuous numerical data (interval or ratio) to explore relationships between two variables.

Q5. Correct answer: C. Ordinal. Social class rankings have an order but do not have equal intervals, making them ordinal data.

Q6. Correct answer: B. The mean is less than the median, and the tail is longer on the left side. In a left-skewed (negatively skewed) distribution, the data is asymmetrically distributed with a longer tail on the left side (towards lower values). This happens because extreme low values pull the mean downward more than they affect the median or mode.

Key relationships in a left-skewed distribution: mean < median < mode (since the mean is more affected by extreme values). The tail extends towards the left (negative direction). Most values cluster towards the higher end of the distribution.

Why the other options are incorrect:

A. The mean is greater than the median, and the tail is longer on the right side. This describes a right-skewed (positively skewed) distribution, not a left-skewed one.

C. The mean, median, and mode are always equal. This is only true for a perfectly symmetrical (normal) distribution.

D. The median is always the largest value in the dataset. The median is a central value but not necessarily the largest. The mode is often the largest in a left-skewed distribution.

E. The mode is always greater than both the median and mean in a right-skewed distribution. This statement confuses the distributions. In a right-skewed distribution, the correct order is mode < median < mean.

Q7. Correct answer: B. Median. Ordinal data: The anxiety levels are measured on an ordinal scale. This means that the data can be ordered (from low anxiety to high anxiety), but the differences between the levels may not be equal. For example, the difference between 'no anxiety' and 'mild anxiety' might not be the same as the difference between 'moderate anxiety' and 'severe anxiety'.

Median as the appropriate measure: the median is the middle value when the data is arranged in order. It is a good measure of central tendency for ordinal data because it is not affected by the potentially unequal intervals between the levels. The mean, on the other hand, can be influenced by extreme values and is more suitable for interval or ratio data where the intervals are equal.

Q8. Correct answer: C. 3. To find the median, we first need to order the data:

1, 1, 2, 2, 2, 3, 3, 3, 3, 3, 4, 4, 4, 5, 5

Since there are 15 data points, the median is the eighth value in the ordered list, which is 3.

Q9. Correct answer: C. Interquartile range. Variability for ordinal data: when dealing with ordinal data, we need a measure of variability that doesn't rely on the assumption of equal intervals.

The IQR is a non-parametric measure of variability. It is calculated as the difference between the third quartile (Q3) and the first quartile (Q1). The IQR represents the spread of the middle 50% of the data and is not affected by extreme values.

Why the other options are incorrect:

A. Variance is a parametric measure that assumes equal intervals between data points.
B. Standard deviation is a parametric measure that assumes equal intervals between data points.
D. Range is sensitive to extreme values.
E. Confidence intervals are used to estimate population parameters, not to describe the variability in a sample.

Q10. Correct answer: B. 2. To calculate the IQR, we first need to find Q1 and Q3:
Q1: the median of the lower half of the data (1, 1, 2, 2, 2, 3, 3) is 2.
Q3: the median of the upper half of the data (3, 3, 4, 4, 4, 5, 5) is 4.
Therefore, the IQR is: Q3 – Q1 = 4 – 2 = 2.

Q11. Correct answer: D. 82.5. Order the data: 68, 75, 78, 80, 85, 88, 90, 92.
Median for even data: the median is the average of the fourth and fifth values (80 + 85) / 2 = 82.5.

Q12. Correct answer: C. 13.
Find Q1: the median of the lower half (68, 75, 78, 80) is (75 + 78) / 2 = 76.5.
Find Q3: the median of the upper half (85, 88, 90, 92) is (88 + 90) / 2 = 89.
Calculate IQR: IQR = Q3 – Q1 = 89 – 76.5 = 12.5. Since we are dealing with a discrete scale, we round 12.5 to the nearest whole number, which is 13.

Q13. Correct answer: C. 4.4.
Step 1: calculate the mean (average) $= \frac{4+6+8+6+8+10}{6} = \frac{42}{6} = 7.$
Step 2: compute each deviation from the mean and square it:

$4 - 7 = -3^2 = 9$
$6 - 7 = -1^2 = 1$
$8 - 7 = 1^2 = 1$
$6 - 7 = -1^2 = 1$
$8 - 7 = 1^2 = 1$
$10 - 7 = 3^2 = 9$

Step 3: sum of squared deviations: 9 + 1 + 1 + 1 + 1 + 9 = 22.
Step 4: compute sample variance. Since this is a sample variance (not population), we divide by $n - 1$ (degrees of freedom):

$$\text{Variance} = \frac{22}{6-1} = \frac{22}{5} = 4.4.$$

Thus, the variance is 4.4.

Q14. Correct answer: A. (6.76, 9.24).
Standard deviation = square root of variance = $\sqrt{4} = 2$.
Standard error (SE) = standard deviation / $\sqrt{n} = 2/\sqrt{10} = 0.63$.
CI for mean = mean ±1.96 × SE = 8 ± (1.96 × 0.63) = 8 ± 1.24 = (6.76, 9.24).

Further Reading

Altman DG. *Practical Statistics for Medical Research*. London: Chapman & Hall/CRC; 1990.

Bland M. *An Introduction to Medical Statistics*. 4th ed. Oxford: Oxford University Press; 2015.

Brown LD, Cai TT, DasGupta A. Interval estimation for a binomial proportion. *Stat Sci.* 2001;**16**(2):101–33. doi: https://doi.org/10.1214/ss/1009213286.

Cleveland WS. *Visualizing Data.* Summit, NJ: Hobart Press; 1993.

Davison AC, Hinkley DV. *Bootstrap Methods and Their Application.* Cambridge: Cambridge University Press; 1997.

Efron B, Tibshirani RJ. *An Introduction to the Bootstrap.* New York: Chapman & Hall/CRC; 1993.

Freedman D, Diaconis P. On the histogram as a density estimator: L2L_2L2 theory. *Probab Theory Relat Fields.* 1981;**57**(4):453–76.

Joanes DN, Gill CA. Comparing measures of sample skewness and kurtosis. *J R Stat Soc Ser D (The Statistician).* 1998;**47**(1):183–9. doi: https://doi.org/10.1111/1467-9884.00122.

Kirkwood BR, Sterne JAC. *Essential Medical Statistics.* 2nd ed. Oxford: Blackwell Science; 2003.

Newcombe RG. Two-sided confidence intervals for the single proportion: comparison of seven methods. *Stat Med.* 1998;**17**(8):857–72. doi: https://doi.org/10.1002/(SICI)1097-0258(19980430)17:8<857::AID-SIM777>3.0.CO;2-E.

Silverman BW. *Density Estimation for Statistics and Data Analysis.* London: Chapman & Hall; 1986.

Tukey JW. *Exploratory Data Analysis.* Reading, MA: Addison-Wesley; 1977.

Chapter 12

Analytic or Inferential Statistics

Introduction

Inferential statistics allow researchers to generalize findings from a sample to a larger population using statistical methods (Figure 12.1). This process relies on **inductive reasoning,**[1] moving from specific observations (sample data) to general conclusions about the population. For example, researchers may measure the blood pressure of a sample of 500 patients and use these data to make inferences about blood pressure levels in the wider population. This contrasts with deductive reasoning, which moves from general principles to specific cases such as calculating medication dosage of an individual patient when dose per kilogram of body weight and the patient's weight are known.

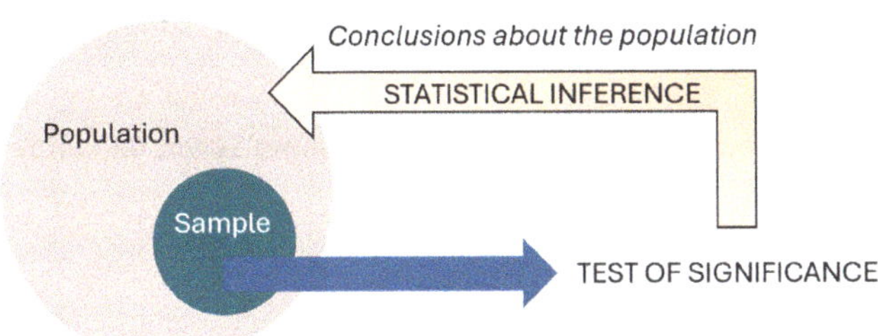

Figure 12.1 Inferential statistics: drawing conclusions about a population from a sample through statistical inference and tests of significance

There are two commonly used methods of hypothesis testing:

1. Baycsian hypothesis testing
2. frequentist hypothesis testing.

These methods provide different approaches to evaluating hypotheses and drawing conclusions from data.

---

[1] **Inductive reasoning (qualitative):** Bottom-up inference where codes, categories and themes are derived from the data rather than imposed a priori; patterns are refined iteratively (e.g. constant comparison) until saturation.

Bayesian Hypothesis Testing

Bayesian hypothesis testing focuses on the **probability**[2] of a hypothesis being true given the data, rather than the probability of observing the data given a hypothesis (as in frequentist methods). It incorporates prior knowledge into analyses. This will be discussed in more detail later on in the chapter.

Frequentist Hypothesis Testing

In frequentist hypothesis testing, analysis begins with the null hypothesis, which is specific, testable, and grounded in the principle of falsification.

Frequentist hypothesis testing involves the following key components:

- **Null hypothesis (H_0)**: Assumes no difference, association, or effect.
- **Alternative hypothesis (H_1)**: Represents a competing claim that contradicts the null hypothesis.
- **Falsification principle**: Introduced by Karl Popper, this principle states that scientific theories cannot be proven true, only falsified. According to Popper, falsifiability distinguishes scientific theories from non-scientific claims, such as storytelling.
- ***p*-Value:**[3] probability of observing data as extreme as, or more extreme than, those observed, assuming that the null hypothesis (H_0) is true. Conventionally, if $p < 0.05$, the null hypothesis is rejected.

Frequentist hypothesis testing does not provide the probability that the null hypothesis H_0 is true. Instead, it evaluates whether the observed data provide sufficient evidence to reject the null hypothesis under the assumption that it is true. The key idea is to determine the probability of observing data as extreme as ours under the assumption that the null hypothesis is true.

An example is provided to illustrate the principle of single group research using frequentist hypothesis testing.

Single Group Analysis: How Much Do Psychiatry CT Trainees Spend on Coffee in One Month?

Sample data (*n* = 4): £115, £85, £125, £75

- Mean $= \frac{£115 + £85 + £125 + £75}{4} = £100$
- Variance:

$115 - 100 = 15^2 = 225$

$85 - 100 = -15^2 = 225$

$125 - 100 = 25^2 = 625$

$75 - 100 = -25^2 = 625$

Variance = difference between all values and means, squared and added / n − 1

$$= \frac{225 + 225 + 625 + 625}{3} = 566.66$$

- Standard deviation (SD) = √variance = √566.66 ≈ 24

---

[2] **Probability:** The likelihood of an event occurring (0–1 or 0–100%). Always report the time horizon and baseline risk; derive NNT/NNH = 1/|RD| (round NNT up).

[3] ***p*-Value:** The probability of observing data as or more extreme than those observed, assuming the null hypothesis is true. It is not the probability the null is true and should be interpreted with effect sizes and CIs.

- Standard error (of mean) = $\frac{SD}{\sqrt{n}} = \frac{24}{2} = 12$
- 95% confidence interval (CI) = sample estimate (e.g. mean) ± 1.96 × SEM = (100) ± 1.96 × 12 = 76–124 (approximately)
- Note: The value 1.96 is the standard normal multiplier for calculating 95% confidence intervals when sample sizes are large or when the population standard deviation is known. For small samples (commonly $n < 30$) in which the population standard deviation is unknown, the *t*-distribution should be used to account for additional uncertainty. In this example, the value 1.96 is used for illustrative purposes only, to demonstrate the fundamental relationship between the mean, the standard error of the mean, and the width of the confidence interval.

With larger sample sizes, confidence intervals become narrower due to the standard error decreasing, as visualized in Figure 12.2. This is because sample size is in the denominator in the calculation of standard error.

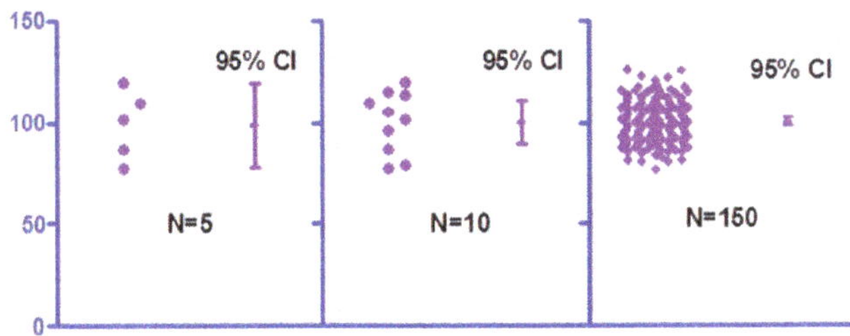

Figure 12.2 Effect of sample size on the width of 95% confidence intervals.

Comparing Two Groups: Frequentist Hypothesis Testing

The results above are from a single group study. To compare two groups using frequentist hypothesis testing, we ask a different question: 'Is there a difference between the average amount of money CT and ST trainees spend on coffee every month?'. In order to conduct research on this question we can set the null hypothesis and alternate hypothesis and run the research as follows:

Null hypothesis (H_0): no difference between mean monthly coffee expenditure between CT and ST trainees.

Alternative hypothesis (H_1): there is a difference in mean monthly coffee expenditure between CT and ST trainees.

A *one-tailed test* assumes one group spends *more than the other*; a *two-tailed test* tests whether there is any difference between groups, regardless of direction. Unless there is a strong a priori reason to specify direction, a two-tailed test is generally preferred.

We can obtain data from both groups in the same way as in the previous example. The results for the CT trainees:

- mean = £100
- 95% confidence interval = (76–124).

Suppose for ST trainees we get results as follows:

- mean = £115
- 95% confidence interval = (110–120).

These confidence intervals summarize the uncertainty around each group's mean but do not, by themselves, constitute a formal statistical test of difference between groups.

A statistical test determines how surprising the observed data is, assuming the null hypothesis (H_0) is true. The statistical test will also provide a ***p*-value** to estimate the probability of error as follows:

***p*-value** = $P(X \geq x \mid H_0)$ [one-sided, right-tailed test].

This is the probability of observing a test statistic (X) that is greater than or equal to a specific value (x), given that the null hypothesis (H_0) is true.

- **X:** the test statistic, which is a value calculated from the data to summarize the evidence against the null hypothesis. Common test statistics include the *t*-statistic, *z*-statistic, or chi-squared statistic, depending on the type of data, which will be discussed later in this chapter.
- **x:** the specific value of the test statistic observed in the data.
- **H_0:** the null hypothesis.
- **Alpha (α):** the pre-specified probability cut-off value, below which we reject the null hypothesis (conventionally set at 5% or 0.05).

The worked examples above illustrate how sample means and confidence intervals can be used to summarize data and quantify uncertainty within and between groups. However, confidence intervals alone do not provide a formal rule for deciding whether an observed difference is statistically meaningful under a specified assumption about the population. To address this, frequentist inference proceeds by explicitly testing a null hypothesis using a statistical test. This approach asks how likely the observed data would be if there were truly no difference between groups. The following section outlines the general process of null hypothesis significance testing that underpins the statistical methods introduced in this chapter.

Process for Testing Null Hypothesis for Statistical Significance

Box 12.1 summarizes the process of testing a null hypothesis for statistical significance, and the following text goes into greater detail.

Box 12.1 Process for Testing a Null Hypothesis for Statistical Significance

1. Develop the null and alternative hypotheses.
2. Establish an appropriate alpha level.
3. Perform a suitable test of statistical significance on appropriately collected data.
4. Compare the *p*-value from the test with the alpha level.
5. Reject or fail to reject the null hypothesis.

Develop Null/Alternative Hypothesis

- **Null hypothesis** (H_0)**:** States that there is no real (true) difference between the means (or proportions) of the groups being compared.
- **Alternative hypothesis (**H_1**):** states that there is a true difference between the groups being compared.

Establish Alpha Level

Before testing the hypothesis, an alpha level is established. This represents the highest risk of false positives (type I error) that investigators are willing to accept. By convention, alpha is set at 0.05 ($p = 0.05$), meaning we are willing to accept a *5% risk of error* when rejecting the null hypothesis.

Perform Tests of Significance

Once the alpha level is set, researchers perform statistical significance tests to calculate the *p*-value and estimate the difference between groups (means or proportions). These tests calculate the *critical ratio* against background noise (variability); for example:

- **Critical ratio (*t*-statistic):** t = (difference between two means) / (standard error of the difference between two means)
- **Critical ratio (*z*-statistic):** z = (difference between two means) / (standard error of the difference between two proportions)

The calculated *t*- or *z*-value is then compared with values from appropriate statistical tables to determine the significance.

Tests for Numerical Data

The appropriate test to use depends on whether the data is *normally distributed* or *skewed* (Table 12.1).

Table 12.1 Tests for numerical continuous data

	Parametric tests (normally distributed)	Non-parametric tests (non-normal (e.g. skewed) data)
One sample	One-sample *t*-test	Wilcoxon signed-rank test (sign test as a less powerful alternative)
Two paired samples	Paired *t*-test	Wilcoxon matched pairs signed test (sign test as a less powerful alternative)
Two unpaired samples	Unpaired *t*-test	Mann–Witney U test (or Wilcoxon rank-sum test)
More than two paired samples	ANOVA (repeated measures)	Friedman's test
More than two unpaired samples	ANOVA	Kruskal–Wallis ANOVA

The sign test is a distribution-free alternative for one-sample and paired non-parametric data that uses only the direction of change and not the magnitude. It is therefore less powerful than the Wilcoxon signed-rank test and is not appropriate for independent (unpaired) samples.

t-Statistic

When data are normally distributed in two groups, the difference in means is calculated using **Student's *t*-test**:

- **Independent *t*-test:** used when the two groups are different subjects (independent).
- **Paired *t*-test:**[4] used when the same subjects are measured at different points in time (paired).

The formula for the independent *t*-test is:

$$t = \frac{\overline{x}1 - \overline{x}2}{\sqrt{\frac{s1}{n1}^2 + \frac{s2^2}{n2}}},$$

where $\bar{x}_1$, $\bar{x}_2$ are the means of groups 1 and 2; s_1, s_2 are the standard deviations of groups 1 and 2; and n_1, n_2 are the sample sizes of groups 1 and 2.

The formula for the **paired *t*-test** is:

$$t = \frac{\overline{d}}{\frac{s\_d}{\sqrt{n}}},$$

where $\bar{d}$ is the mean difference between pairs; *s_d* is the standard deviation of the differences; and *n* is the number of pairs.

In both tests, *t* is calculated by taking the observed differences between the means of the two groups and dividing this difference by the standard error of the difference between the means of the two groups. The standard error of the difference between the means is the square root of the sum of the respective population variances, each divided by their own sample size.

The assumptions of the *t*-test are:

- The data are normally distributed.
- The two groups have *equal variances* (homogeneity of variance). **Levene's test**[5] can be used to assess this assumption.
- The data are *continuous*.

Tests of Normality

Before performing a *t*-test, it is important to assess whether the data follow a normal distribution. Table 12.2 summarizes commonly used tests of normality.

---

[4] **Paired *t*-test:** A parametric test comparing means of two related measurements (e.g. before and after). Assumes approximately normal differences.

[5] **Levene's test (homogeneity of variance):** Test for equal variances across groups; robust to non-normality (uses absolute deviations from group medians/means); commonly checked before *t*-tests/ ANOVA.

Table 12.2 Comparison of tests of normality

Test	Best for sample size	Key feature	Strengths	Limitations
Shapiro–Wilk test	Small to medium ($n < 50$)	Most powerful for detecting normality	High power for small samples	Sensitive to minor deviations
Kolmogorov–Smirnov test	Large ($n > 50$)	Compares dataset with normal distribution	Works for large samples	Low sensitivity for small samples
Anderson–Darling test	Small to medium	Focuses on tails of the distribution	More sensitive than Kolmogorov–Smirnov test	Conservative, requires larger sample
Lilliefors test	Small to medium	Modification of Kolmogorov–Smirnov test	Works when population parameters are unknown	Less commonly used
D'Agostino–Pearson test	Medium to large	Based on skewness and kurtosis	Robust for large datasets	Less effective for small samples

Which Test to Use?

- For small samples ($n < 50$): Shapiro–Wilk test
- For large samples ($n > 50$): Kolmogorov–Smirnov test
- For detecting deviations in tails: Anderson–Darling test
- For checking skewness and kurtosis: D'Agostino–Pearson test
- If population parameters are unknown: Lilliefors test

F-Statistic

When there are three or more groups and the data is normally distributed, the appropriate test is **ANOVA (analysis of variance).**[6] This method seeks to determine why groups are different and how much of the total variation is explained by the variables defining the groups.

Understanding ANOVA

(With permission from Jekel J. *Epidemiology, Biostatistics, and Preventative Medicine.* Amsterdam: Elsevier Health Sciences; 2007.)

Consider the example of heights of men and women. We know that, on average, men are taller than women. However, if we ask why the shortest woman is shorter than the tallest man, statistically, two factors explain this variation:

1. **Intergroup variation:** women, as a group, have a shorter mean height than men.
2. **Intragroup variation**: within each group (men and women), individuals vary in height.

[6] **ANOVA (analysis of variance):** A family of tests comparing means across three or more groups by partitioning variance into between- and within-group components. Significant results typically require post hoc tests to identify which groups differ.

The greater the distance between the group means, the higher the proportion of variation explained by intergroup differences. Similarly, larger standard deviations within each group indicate greater intragroup variation. If all men were of equal height and all women were of equal height, all variation would be due to intergroup differences. Conversely, if men and women had the same mean height but varied widely within their groups, all variation would be due to intragroup differences and left unexplained by grouping.

How ANOVA Works

- **Between-group variability** is calculated as the sum of all the differences between each group mean and the overall mean, squared and multiplied by the number of observations in that group. This sum of squares is then divided by the appropriate **degrees of freedom.**[7]
- **Within-group variability** is calculated by multiplying each group's variance by the number of subjects in the group minus one, and summing the results.

The *F* ratio is defined as:

$$F \text{ ratio } = \frac{\text{Between-group variance}}{\text{Within-group variance}} = \frac{\text{Between-group mean square}}{\text{Within-group mean square}}.$$

If the *F* ratio is close to 1.0, the two estimates of variance are similar, suggesting that the group means are not significantly different, and the null hypothesis – that all means come from the same underlying population – is not rejected.

If the *F* ratio is much larger than 1.0, this suggests that the treatment or grouping variable has caused the means to differ, and the null hypothesis is rejected.

Types of ANOVA

- **One-way ANOVA:** used when comparing three or more independent groups.
- **Repeated measures ANOVA:** used when measuring the same group of individuals at multiple time points.

Post-hoc Analysis

ANOVA only identifies whether a significant difference exists between groups but does not specify which groups differ, the direction of those differences, or the magnitude of the effect. In other words, ANOVA tells us that the players on a football field are not all the same height, but it would not tell us who is taller or by how many centimetres. For this reason, ANOVA is described as an omnibus test, as it evaluates the entire dataset all at once. *Post-hoc significance tests*, such as the **Bonferroni correction,**[8] are used to determine specific group differences while controlling for type I error. Table 12.3 summarizes common post-hoc tests.

---

[7] **Degrees of freedom (df):** Number of independent pieces of information available to estimate a parameter (e.g. two-sample *t*-test, df $\approx n_1 + n_2 - 2$ when variances are pooled).

[8] **Bonferroni correction (multiple comparisons):** Controls family-wise error rate by testing each comparison at α/m (m = number of comparisons); it is simple but conservative.

Table 12.3 Summary of post-hoc tests

Post-hoc test	Best used when . . .	Controls type I error?	Pairwise or complex comparisons?
Bonferroni	Few planned comparisons	Yes (strict)	Pairwise
Tukey's HSD[9]	All pairwise comparisons	Yes	Pairwise
Dunnett's	Comparing multiple treatments to a single control	Yes	Control vs treatment
Scheffé's	Any linear combination of means	Yes (very conservative)	Complex contrasts
Fisher's LSD[10]	ANOVA is significant and few comparisons needed	No	Pairwise

Non-parametric Tests

Non-parametric tests are used to compare skewed data. These include *Wilcoxon signed-rank test*, *Wilcoxon matched pairs signed test*, *sign test*, *Mann–Whitney U test*, *Friedman's test*, and *Kruskal - Wallis ANOVA*, depending on the number and types of groups being compared.

In non-parametric tests, data is ranked or ordered. The ranks are then summed in each group, and the test statistic derived from rank sums is compared with its sampling distribution.

It is important to note that these tests can also be used to compare parametric data, but parametric tests are generally more powerful and preferable when assumptions of normality are met.

Tests for Binary Data

Tests for binary (dichotomous) data are outlined in Figure 12.3.

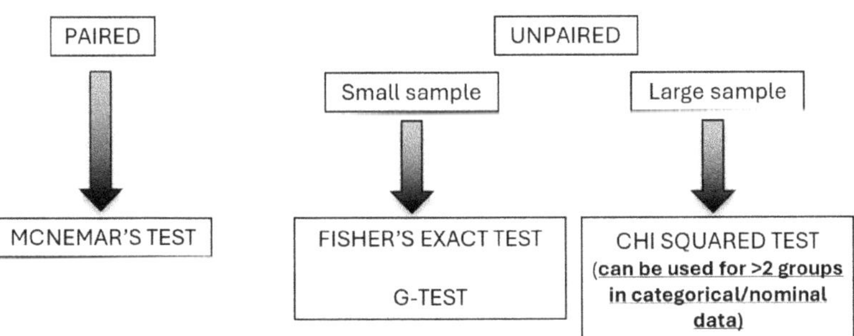

Figure 12.3 Tests for binary (dichotomous) data.

[9] **Tukey's HSD:** A post hoc test controlling familywise error while comparing all pairs of means after ANOVA. It balances type I error control and power.

[10] **Fisher's LSD:** A relatively liberal post hoc procedure following ANOVA for pairwise comparisons. It offers more power at the cost of higher type I error risk.

Chi-Squared Test

The chi-squared test is used to analyse whether there is an association between two or more categorical variables. The following steps outline the process:

1. **Setting up a contingency table:** data is arranged into a contingency table with rows and columns representing categories of each variable (e.g. admitted (yes/no) and compliance with medication (yes/no)).
2. **Calculating expected frequencies:** the test compares the observed frequencies to the expected frequencies under the assumption that there is no association between the variables.
3. **Calculating the chi-square statistic:** the formula for the chi-square statistic is:

$$\chi^2 = \sum \frac{(\text{Observed frequency} - \text{Expected frequency})^2}{\text{Expected frequency}}$$

4. **Determining degrees of freedom (df):** the degrees of freedom depend on the size of the contingency table.
5. **Finding the *p*-value:** the calculated chi-square statistic is compared to a chi-square distribution table to determine the *p*-value. If the *p*-value is less than the significance level (typically 0.05), the null hypothesis is rejected.

The chi-squared test can also be used to analyse subgroup differences in a stratified analysis. It can look into other variables for subgroup differences in a stratified analysis.

Adjustments for Small Sample Sizes

The following corrections and alternative tests are used to account for small sample sizes:

- **Yates' correction:**[11] applied when the total sample size is less than 100 or if any expected cell value is between 5 and 10 in a 2 × 2 table.
- **Fisher's exact test:** used when any expected frequency is less than 5.
- **McNemar's test:** a specialized chi-squared test used for matched data or paired groups.

Table 12.4 outlines commonly used statistical tests for categorical data and their appropriate applications, depending on sample size and expected frequencies.

Table 12.4 Comparison of tests for categorical data

Test	When to use	Best for
Chi-squared test	When all expected frequencies ≥5	Large samples ($n > 100$)
Yates' correction (chi-squared)	When expected frequencies are between 5 and 10	Moderate sample sizes
Fisher's exact test	When any expected frequency is <5	Small sample sizes ($n < 30$)

[11] **Yates' continuity correction (2 × 2 χ^2):** Continuity adjustment for small samples in Pearson χ^2 on 2 × 2 tables; reduces type I error but may be conservative.

Tests for Ordinal Data

Ordinal data is a type of data that falls between numerical and categorical data. Since it is not normally distributed, *parametric tests cannot be used*. Likewise, tests for categorical variables (like chi-squared, Fisher's exact test, G-test, or McNemar's test) are not appropriate because ordinal values have an inherent order.

To test hypotheses involving ordinal data, researchers typically use *non-parametric tests* designed for numerical data, such as:

- Mann–Whitney U test
- Wilcoxon signed-rank test
- Kruskal–Wallis ANOVA
- Friedman's test.

One-Tailed and Two-Tailed Tests

In statistical hypothesis testing, the choice between a *one-tailed test* and a *two-tailed test* depends on the specific research question being addressed.

- A one-tailed test is used when researchers have a clear, a priori hypothesis about the direction of an effect. This test evaluates whether an effect occurs in one specific direction only (either greater than or less than a given value). For example, if researchers are specifically investigating whether a new ADHD medication reduces hyperactivity, a one-tailed test would be appropriate.
- A two-tailed test assesses whether there is a statistically significant difference in either direction. It evaluates if an observed effect is significantly higher or lower than expected. For example, when comparing a new medication to a placebo or standard treatment, a two-tailed test is appropriate if the researchers are interested in detecting any difference, whether an increase or a decrease in effectiveness.

Illustrative Example

Consider researchers studying the effectiveness of a new antipsychotic medication in reducing hallucinations in patients with schizophrenia:

- If researchers are specifically interested in whether the new drug decreases hallucinations, they should use a one-tailed test.
- If the researchers aim to find whether the frequency of hallucinations differs in either direction (increase or decrease) compared to a standard antipsychotic medication, a two-tailed test is appropriate.

Important Considerations

- One-tailed tests allocate the entire significance level (alpha (α), typically set at 0.05) to one direction. While this increases statistical power, it also increases the risk of a type I error (false positive) if used without strong justification.

- Two-tailed tests divide the significance level between both directions, making them more conservative and generally preferable unless there is a clear theoretical or clinical rationale for predicting the direction of the effect.

The choice between a one-tailed and two-tailed test directly affects the resulting *p*-value, which represents the probability of obtaining results as extreme as (or more extreme than) those observed, assuming the null hypothesis is true. In a one-tailed test, the entire alpha level is allocated to a single tail of the sampling distribution. In contrast, a two-tailed test divides the alpha level equally between both tails.

Figures 12.4 and 12.5 offer flowchart guides to selecting tests for binary, nominal, ordinal, and numerical data means.

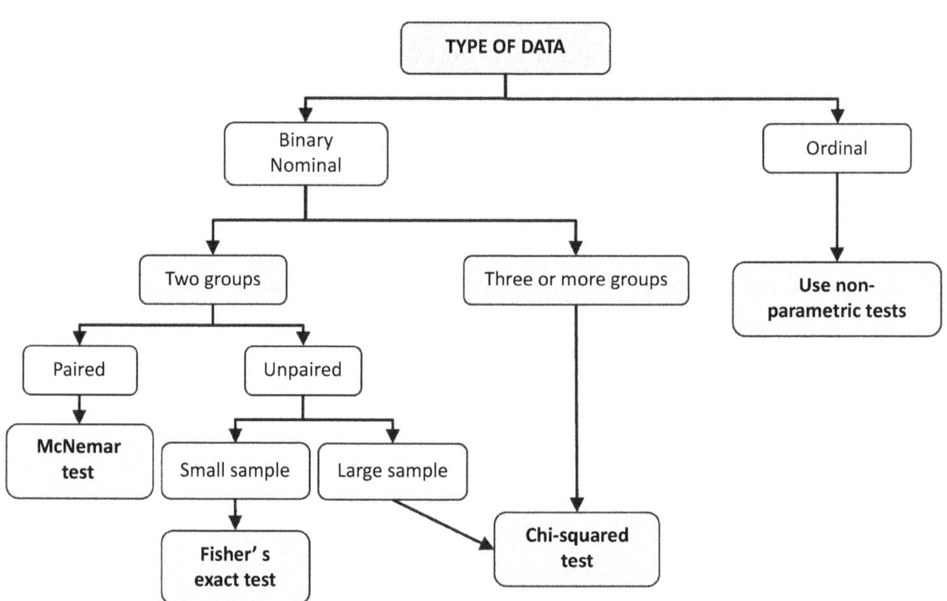

Figure 12.4 Categorical data: flowchart of statistical tests for comparing proportions.

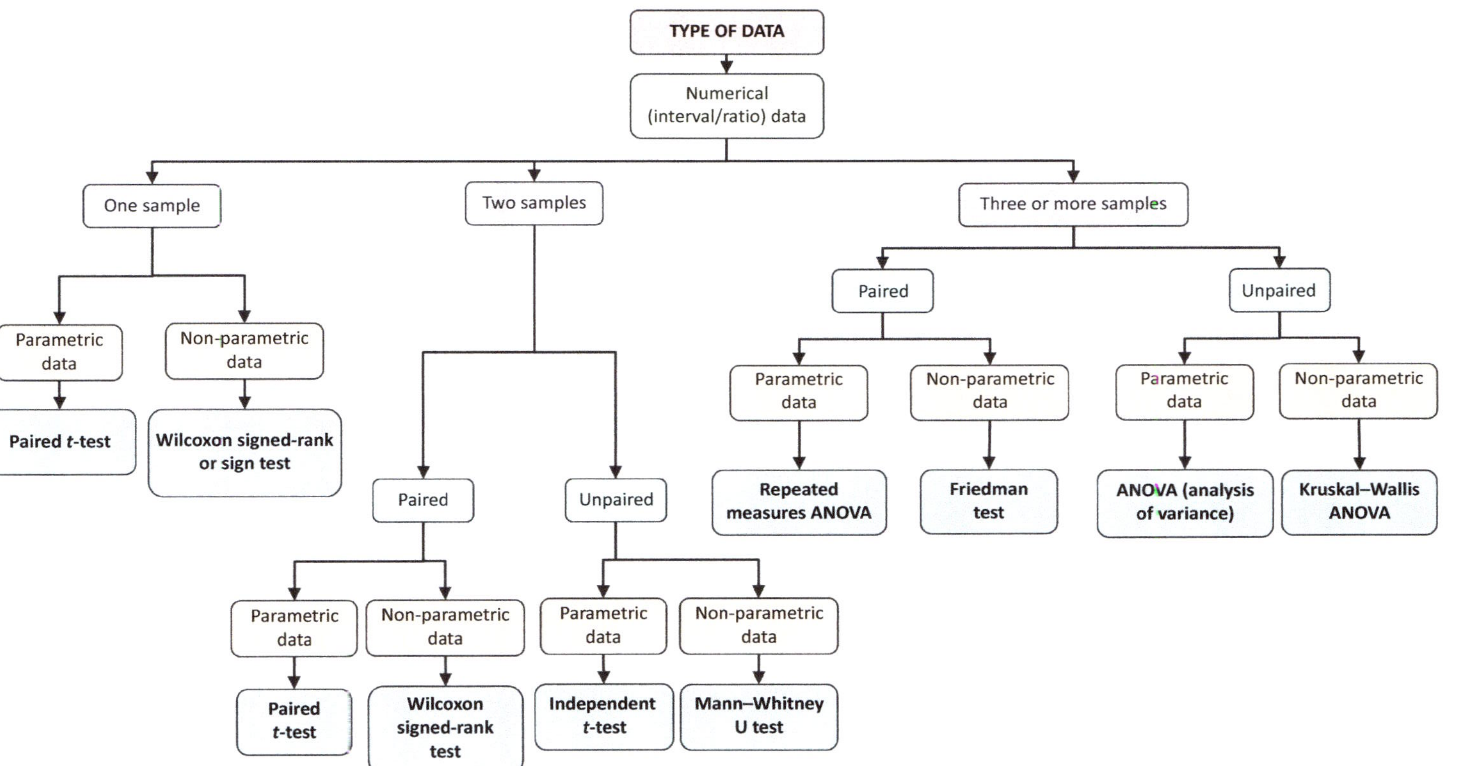

Figure 12.5 Numerical data: flowchart of statistical tests for comparing means.

Correlation Coefficient

The **correlation coefficient,**[12] denoted as r, is a statistical measure that quantifies the *strength and direction* of a linear relationship between two variables. However, correlation does not imply *causation* and does not indicate which variable influences the other. Figure 12.6 is a graph showing correlation between intelligence and diligence.

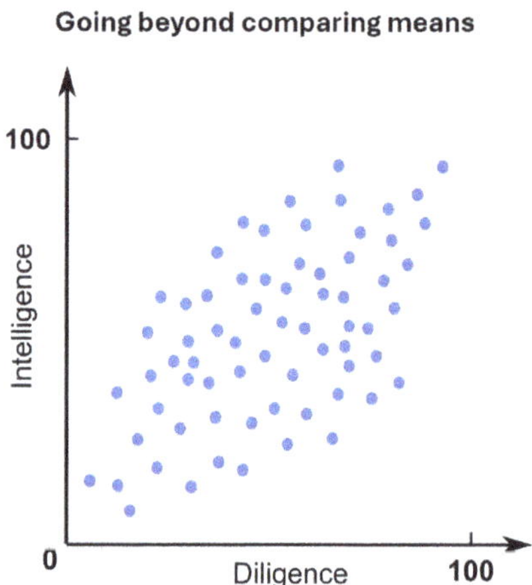

Is there a *relationship* between two variables?

(when one goes up, does the other go up... intrinsically linked to covariance)?

Null hypothesis: 'There is no relationship between diligence and intelligence'

Figure 12.6 Moving beyond comparing means: exploring relationships between variables.

Key Properties of the Correlation Coefficient

- **Unit-free measure:** The value remains consistent regardless of the units of measurement.
- **Range:** The correlation coefficient lies between −1 and 1:

  +1: perfect positive correlation – both variables move in the same direction (e.g. as study time increases, exam scores increase proportionally).

  0: no correlation – changes in one variable do not predict changes in the other.

  −1: perfect negative correlation – the variables move in opposite directions (e.g. as distance travelled increases, distance remaining decreases).

Types of Relationships

Linear Relationship

A linear relationship means that as one variable changes, the other changes at a constant rate. The relationship can be represented by a straight-line equation. For example, if one

---

[12] **Correlation coefficient:** A statistic (e.g. Pearson's r, Spearman's ρ) quantifying strength and direction of association between two variables. Values range from −1 (perfect negative) to +1 (perfect positive).

extra hour of study consistently increases a test score by five points, this is a linear increase (Figure 12.7).

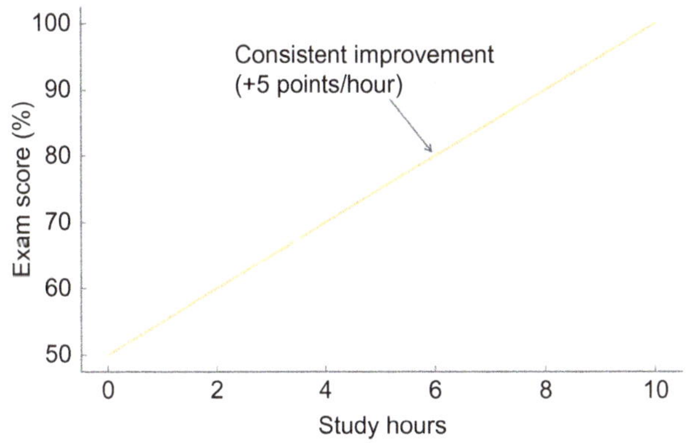

Figure 12.7 Example of a linear relationship.

Monotonic Relationship

In a monotonic relationship, as one variable increases, the other either always increases or always decreases. However, unlike a linear relationship, the rate of change does not need to be constant. The strength of the association may vary across the range of values, but the direction does not reverse. For example, initially increased study time significantly improves exam scores, but beyond a certain point additional study hours result in smaller improvements due to fatigue (Figure 12.8).

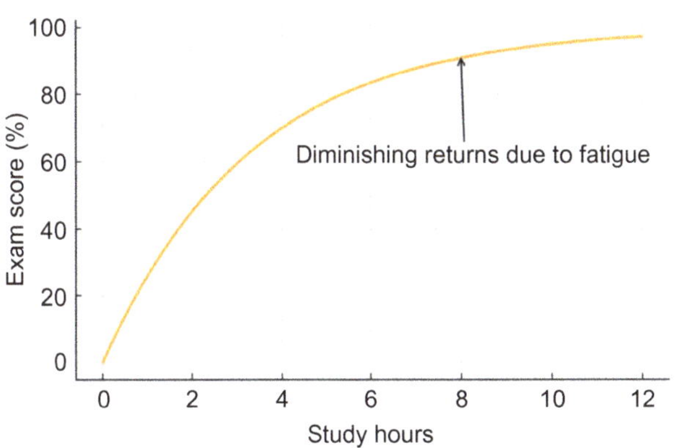

Figure 12.8 Example of a monotonic relationship.

Non-monotonic Relationship

In non-monotonic relationships, the direction of the association changes at some point. Key characteristics of non-monotonic relationships:

- A change in direction (e.g. positive to negative).
- The presence of an 'optimal zone' for performance or health outcomes.
- The need for non-linear models (e.g. quadratic regression) to analyse.

For example, moderate levels of anxiety may enhance performance in an exam, but excessive anxiety may impair concentration and reduce performance (Figure 12.9).

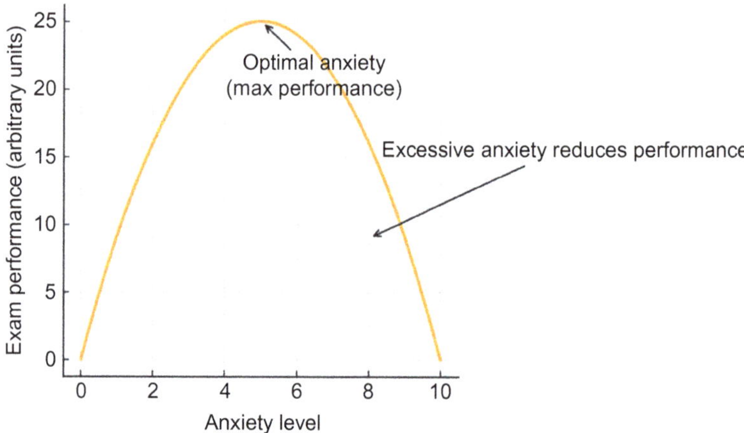

Figure 12.9 Example of a non-monotonic relationship.

This type of curve is often described as an inverted U-shaped relationship, commonly explained by the Yerkes–Dodson law in psychology. It highlights the principle that too little or too much of a variable can be detrimental, while a moderate amount is beneficial.

Correlation Levels

Figure 12.10 illustrates different levels of correlation, from perfect positive to perfect negative, with examples of how data points are distributed in each case.

Types of Correlation Coefficients

Different types of correlation coefficients are used, depending on the nature of the data and the type of relationship between variables.

Pearson's Correlation Coefficient (*r*)

Pearson's correlation cofficient is used when variables are continuous, approximately normally distributed, and linearly related (Figure 12.11). It measures the strength of association between two continuous variables, such as number of hours studied vs exam scores.

R^2 (coefficient of determination)[13] represents the proportion of variance in one variable explained by the other.

Spearman's Rank Correlation Coefficient (*ρ*)

Spearman's correlation is used when:

- Variables are ordinal or not normally distributed.
- The relationship is monotonic but not necessarily linear.
- Example: the relationship between physical activity levels and depression severity.

[13] **R^2 (coefficient of determination):** Proportion of variance in the outcome explained by the model (0–1); note: this is not the 'coefficient of variation'.

Correlation

- The strength of the ***relationship*** between two continuous variables
- Correlation coefficients range from –1 to 1
- 0 = no correlation
- +/–1 = perfect correlation
- **Says nothing about causation**

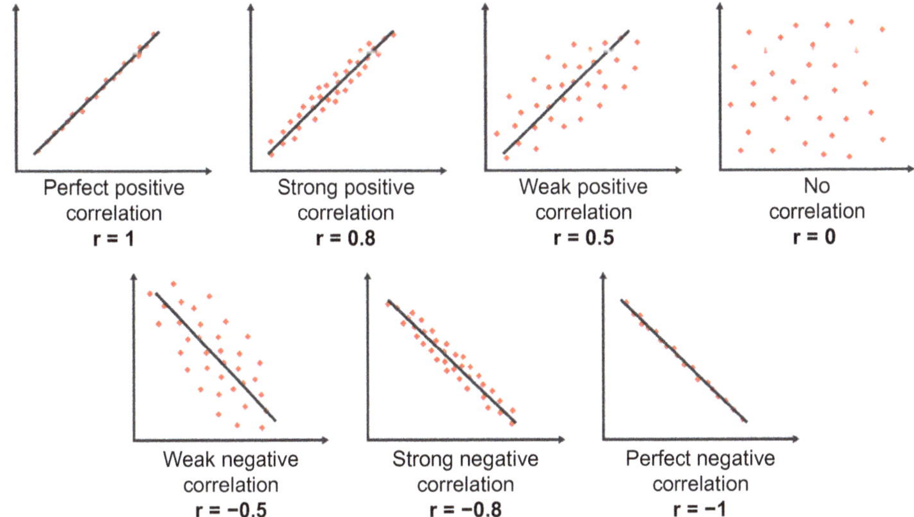

Figure 12.10 Correlation and the strength of relationships between variables.

A comment on 'r' and 'slope'

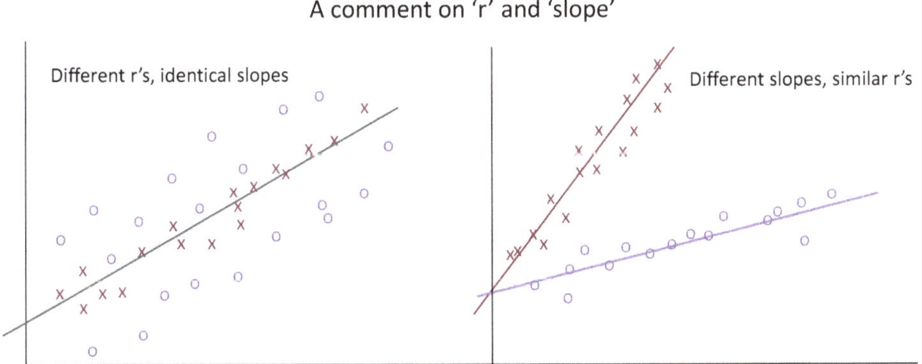

Pearson's correlation coefficient is the slope of a regression on standardized (z-scored) variables

Figure 12.11 Correlation coefficient (r) and regression slope.

Kendall's Correlation Coefficient (τ)

Kendall's correlation is an alternative to Spearman's correlation but differs in how it ranks and compares data:

- It is less sensitive to outliers than Spearman's correlation.
- It is used in small datasets or when ranks are tied.

Phi Coefficient (φ)

Phi correlation is a special case of Pearson's correlation used to measure the association between two binary (dichotomous) variables:

- It is computed using a 2×2 contingency table.
- Example: the relationship between attending MRCPsych course classes (yes/no) and passing the exam (yes/no).

Point-Biserial Correlation Coefficient

The point-biserial correlation measures the relationship between a *continuous* variable and a *dichotomous* variable:

- Example: the relationship between gender (male/female) and exam scores.

Cramér's V

Cramér's V measures the strength of association between two categorical variables with multiple categories:

- Example: the relationship between psychiatric diagnosis (e.g. depression, anxiety, bipolar disorder) and preferred therapy type (e.g. CBT, MBT, DBT).

Comparison

Table 12.5 compares commonly used correlation coefficients, the types of relationships they measure, and the data types for which they are suitable.

Table 12.5 Comparison of correlation coefficients

Correlation coefficient	Type of relationship	Data type
Pearson	Linear	Continuous
Spearman's rank	Monotonic	Continuous or ordinal
Kendall's rank	Monotonic	Continuous or ordinal
Point-biserial	Linear	Continuous and dichotomous
Cramér's V	Non-linear	Categorical

Figure 12.12 shows a flowchart to guide coefficient choice.

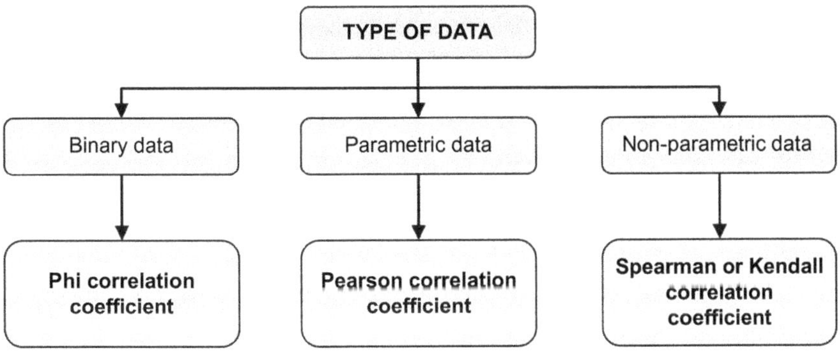

Figure 12.12 Exploring association flowchart outlining correlation methods according to data type.

Regression Analysis

Regression analysis is a statistical technique used to model the relationship between a **dependent variable** (outcome)[14] and one or more **independent variables** (predictors).[15] It helps determine how changes in one variable affect another, and is widely used for *prediction*, *hypothesis testing*, and *supporting causal inference when appropriate assumptions are met*. Regression models allow for:

- prediction (extrapolation and interpolation)
- assessing relationships between variables
- fitting an equation to data (line of best fit).

Key terminology related to regression analysis includes:

- **Dependent variable (*Y*):** the variable being predicted; also called the *outcome* or *target variable.*
- **Independent variable (*X*):** the variable that explains or influences the dependent variable; also called the *predictor* or *explanatory variable.*

Different types of regression analyses are used, depending on the nature of the data and the relationship between variables.

Simple Linear Regression

Simple linear regression (Figure 12.13) examines the relationship between one independent variable (X) and one dependent variable (Y). For example, predicting reduction in depression scores (Y) based on number of psychotherapy sessions (X). The formula for simple linear regression is:

$$Y = a + bX + \varepsilon,$$

[14] **Dependent variable (outcome):** The variable measured to assess the effect of the exposure or intervention. It is also called the response or outcome variable.

[15] **Independent variable:** A variable manipulated or classified to observe its effect on a dependent (outcome) variable.

where: Y is the dependent variable (outcome); X is the independent variable (predictor); a is the intercept (value of Y when $X = 0$); b is the slope (change in Y for a one-unit increase in X); and ε is the error term (unexplained variation). In figures and graphs, the regression line is often written as: $y = \beta_0 + \beta_1 X$ or $Y = mX + C$. These equations represent the estimated line of best fit and therefore omit the error term. Although the symbols differ, the equations describe the same linear relationship:

- a, β_0, C: intercept
- b, β_1, m: slope
- ε: random error (not shown in plots).

The difference reflects notation choice rather than a difference in meaning.

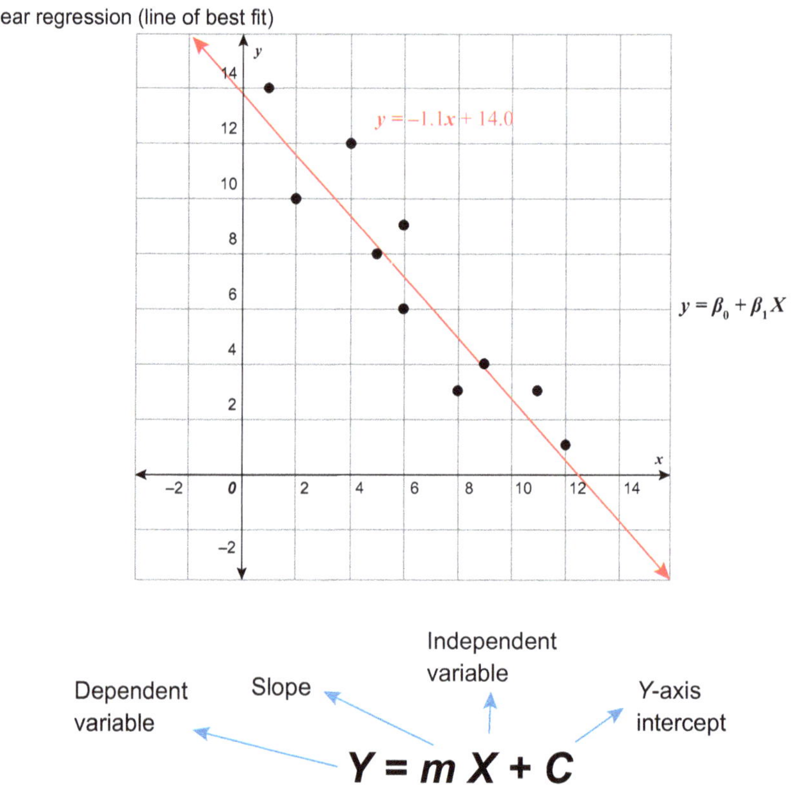

Figure 12.13 Simple linear regression (line of best fit).

Logistic Regression

Logistic regression[16] (Figure 12.14) is used when the dependent variable is binary (e.g. yes/no, 0/1). It predicts the **probability** of an outcome occurring based on independent

[16] **Logistic regression:** Models log-odds of a binary outcome as a linear function of predictors; coefficients exponentiate to odds ratios. Check linearity-in-the-logit for continuous predictors.

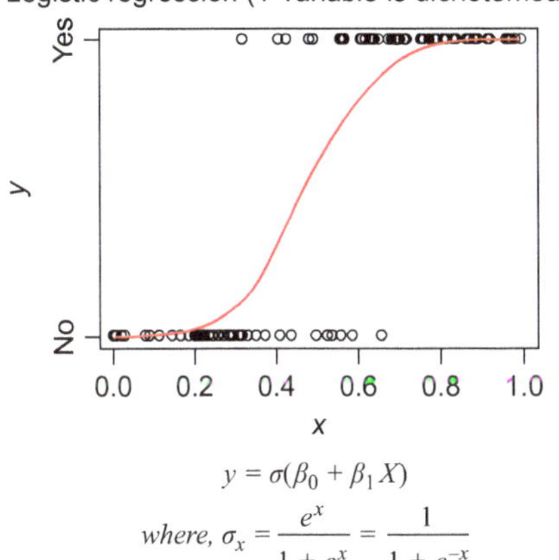

Figure 12.14 Logistic regression (dichotomous dependent variable).

variables. For example, predicting the presence of diabetes (yes/no) based on BMI scores. It can be exponentiated to yield odds ratios representing the change in the odds of Y for a one-unit change in X.

Multiple Regression

Multiple regression models the relationship between one dependent variable and two or more independent variables. For example, exam performance predicted by revision time, test anxiety, lecture attendance, and gender. A multivariate multiple regression extends this to cases with multiple dependent variables.

Assumptions of Multiple Regression

- **Linearity:** the relationship between X and Y is linear.
- **Independence:** observations are independent of each other.
- **Homoscedasticity:** residual errors have constant variance.
- **Normality:** residuals are approximately normally distributed.
- **Multicollinearity:** predictor variables should not be highly correlated.

Polynomial Regression

Polynomial regression[17] (Figure 12.15) is used when the relationship between X and Y is non-linear and follows a curved pattern. For example, study time vs test scores, where initially more study time improves scores, but excessive studying may lead to fatigue and reduced performance. The formula is:

$$\mathrm{Y} = a + b_1X + b_2X^2 + b_3X^3 + \cdots + \varepsilon,$$

[17] **Polynomial regression:** A regression that models non-linear relationships by including polynomial terms. It risks overfitting at high degrees.

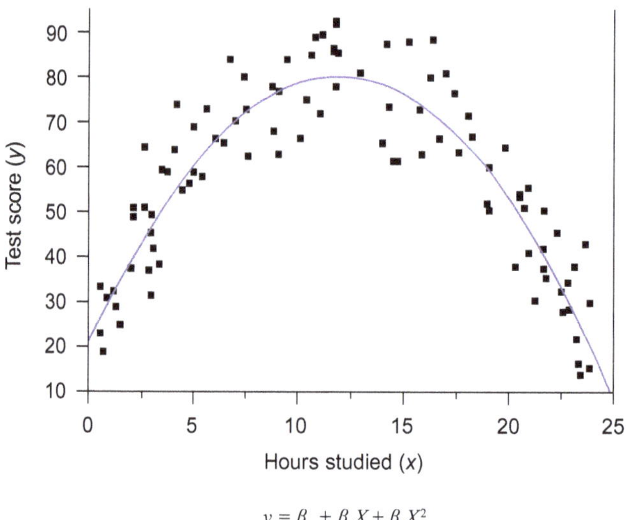

Figure 12.15 Non-linear relationship between variables (quadratic regression).

$$y = \beta_0 + \beta_1 X + \beta_2 X^2$$

where Y is the dependent (outcome) variable; X is the independent (predictor) variable; A is the intercept (the expected value of Y when $X = 0$); $b_1, b_2, \ldots, b_k$ are regression coefficients (weights) for $X, X^2, \ldots, X^k$; k is the degree (highest power) of the polynomial; and ε is the error term (unexplained variation).

Different texts use different notation for regression coefficients. In this chapter, a is equivalent to β_0, and $b_1, b_2, \ldots$ are equivalent to $\beta_1, \beta_2, \ldots$. The models are mathematically identical.

Ordinal Regression

Ordinal regression (also known as *ordinal logistic regression*) is used when the dependent variable is ordinal (i.e. has ordered categories). For example, predicting patient satisfaction on a **Likert scale**[18] based on treatment effectiveness.

Ridge and Lasso Regression (Regularized Regression)

Regularized regression techniques are used to address *multicollinearity* (high correlation between predictor variables) and **overfitting.**[19]

- **Ridge regression (L2 regularization):** a type of linear regression that prevents overfitting by adding a penalty to large regression coefficients, reducing their impact while retaining all variables.
- **Lasso regression (L1 regularization):** performs feature selection by shrinking less relevant coefficients to zero, effectively removing unimportant variables from the model.

[18] **Likert scale:** Ordered categorical response format (typically 5–7 points from 'strongly disagree' to 'strongly agree') for attitude or opinion items. Analyse single items as ordinal; summed/averaged multi-item scores are often treated as approximate intervals. Report number of points, anchors, direction, and check internal consistency.

[19] **Overfitting:** When a model captures noise instead of signal, harming generalizability. Cross-validation and regularization help prevent it.

- **Elastic net regression:**[20] A combination of ridge and lasso, balancing penalty-based regularization while also performing feature selection.

An example use case for ridge and lasso regression is predicting diabetes progression using multiple biomarkers, such as age, BMI, cholesterol levels, and blood pressure.

Poisson Regression

Poisson regression[21] is used to model count data, representing the number of times an event occurs within a fixed time period or space. It is particularly useful for analysing rare events where the outcome variable is a non-negative integer (0, 1, 2, etc.).

The model is based on the **Poisson distribution**, a probability distribution that describes the likelihood of a given number of events occurring within a fixed interval, assuming events occur independently and at a constant rate (λ). In a Poisson distribution, the mean and variance are equal.

- **Assumptions:** the mean and variance of the count variable are approximately equal (Poisson assumption).
- **Applications:** predicting event frequencies, such as disease occurrences, hospital admissions, or system failures.
- **Example:** predicting the number of asthma attacks per year based on air pollution levels.

Comparison of Regression Models

Table 12.6 provides a comparison of commonly used regression models, their best applications, the types of dependent variables they analyse, and example use cases in psychiatry and

Table 12.6 Comparison of regression models

Regression model	Best for	Dependent variable type	Example use case
Simple linear regression	Relationship between one predictor and outcome	Continuous	Predicting Beck Depression Inventory scores based on number of psychotherapy sessions
Multiple linear regression	Relationship between multiple predictors and outcome	Continuous	Predicting exam performance based on revision time, test anxiety, lecture attendance and gender
Logistic regression	Predicting binary outcomes (yes/no)	Binary (0/1)	Predicting likelihood of diabetes mellitus (yes/no) based on BMI
Polynomial regression	Modelling non-linear relationships	Continuous	Predicting marks in exam based on number of hours studied

[20] **Elastic net regression:** A penalized regression that blends L1 (lasso) and L2 (ridge) penalties. It handles correlated predictors and performs variable selection and shrinkage.

[21] **Poisson regression:** A loglinear model for count outcomes assuming a Poisson distribution. Offsets allow modelling of rates (events per person time).

Table 12.6 (cont.)

Regression model	Best for	Dependent variable type	Example use case
Ridge regression	Handling multicollinearity in multiple regression	Continuous	Predicting blood pressure based on age, BMI, cholesterol, sodium intake, and physical activity
Lasso regression	Feature selection in large datasets	Continuous	Predicting the progression of diabetes mellitus using multiple biomarkers, including age, BMI, blood glucose levels, cholesterol levels, blood pressure, and various genetic markers
Elastic net regression	Combination of ridge and lasso	Continuous	Predicting diabetes risk using genetic and lifestyle factors
Poisson regression	Modelling count data	Count data	Predicting asthma attacks per year based on air pollution exposure, smoking status and physical activity
Negative binomial regression[22]	Handling overdispersion in count data[23]	Count data	Predicting number of psychiatric relapses in patients with schizophrenia
Ordinal regression	Predicting ordered categorical outcomes	Ordinal	Predicting severity of depression (mild, moderate, severe) based on stress levels
Multinomial logistic regression	Predicting categorical outcomes with more than two categories	Categorical	Predicting preferred treatment method (psychotherapy, medication, combined) based on symptoms
Cox regression (survival analysis)	Predicting time-to-event outcomes	Survival time data	Predicting time until relapse in addiction recovery programmes

medical research. Figure 12.16 presents a flowchart of regression and modelling approaches for different data structures.

Type I Error, Type II Error, and Power Calculation

Type I Error (False Positive)

A type I error occurs when the null hypothesis (H_0) is falsely rejected, meaning a difference is found when none actually exists.

- It is also known as a false positive result.
- It can be caused by bias or confounding.
- The probability of making a type I error is equal to the *pre-specified significance level (alpha, α).*

[22] **Negative binomial regression:** Count outcome model for overdispersed data (variance > mean). It extends Poisson by adding a dispersion parameter; use when Poisson residuals show overdispersion or mean–variance equality is violated.

[23] **Overdispersion (counts):** When variance exceeds the mean (violating Poisson); handle with negative binomial or quasi-Poisson models and check a dispersion statistic.

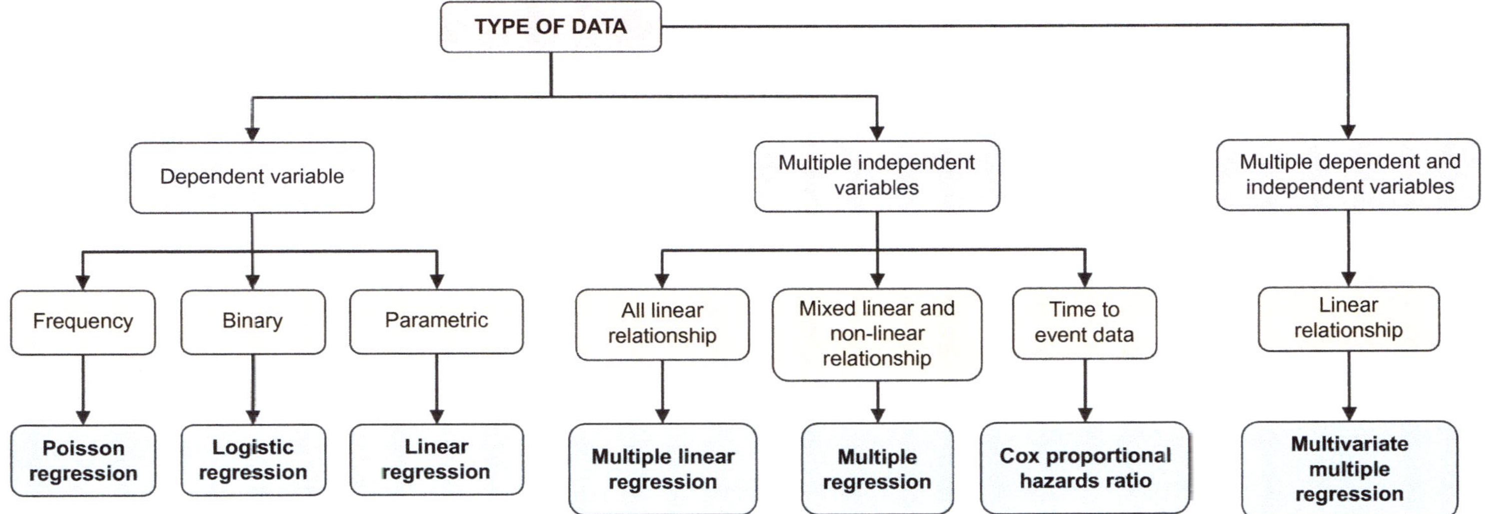

Figure 12.16 Exploring relationships: flowchart of regression and modelling approaches for different data structures.

- A *p*-value of 0.05 means there is a 5% chance of incorrectly rejecting H_0.
- The conventional threshold (α) for statistical significance is 0.05, but lowering alpha (e.g. to 0.01) reduces the risk of type I error.

Type II Error (False Negative)

A type II error occurs when the null hypothesis is falsely not rejected, meaning no difference is found when one actually exists.

- It is also known as a false negative result.
- The most common cause is small sample size.
- Represented by β (beta), which is typically set at 0.2 (20%).
- The power of a study is the probability of correctly rejecting the null hypothesis when a true difference exists, calculated as $1 - \beta$.
- A study with $\beta = 0.2$ has 80% power, meaning an 80% chance of detecting a real effect.

Effect Size

Effect size quantifies the *strength* or *magnitude* of a difference between two or more variables or the *impact of an intervention*. It provides a more practical interpretation of study results than statistical significance alone.

Common measures of effect size are:

- **Cohen's *d*:**[24] measures the difference between two means, divided by a pooled standard deviation.
- Pearson's *r*: measures the strength of correlation between two variables.
- Odds ratio (OR) and relative risk (RR): used in clinical studies to compare event probabilities.
- Eta squared (η^2): measures the proportion of variance explained by an independent variable in ANOVA.

Key considerations for effect sizes are:

- Unlike *p*-values, which indicate whether an effect exists, effect size measures how strong or meaningful the effect is, regardless of statistical significance.
- A statistically significant result ($p < 0.05$) does not necessarily indicate a clinically meaningful effect.
- *Example:* A new drug reduces blood pressure by 4 mmHg. While this result may be statistically significant, it could be clinically insignificant in real-world applications.

Power Calculation and Sample Size Estimation

Power calculations help estimate the sample size needed to detect a statistically significant effect if one exists.

- It ensures the study is not underpowered (risking type II error) or overpowered (excessively large sample).
- Required inputs for sample size estimation are:

---

[24] **Cohen's *d* (effect size):** Standardized mean difference = $(\text{mean}_1 - \text{mean}_2)$/pooled SD; Hedges' *g* applies a small-sample correction.

expected variance (s^2)

alpha level (z_α) (typically 0.05)

beta level (z_β) (typically 0.2)

smallest clinically significant difference (d)

mean proportion of success ($\overline{p}$) (for proportion-based studies).

Sample Size Formulas

For a paired *t*-test:

$$N = \frac{(z_\alpha + z_\beta)^2 \times 2 \times S^2}{d^2}.$$

For an independent *t*-test:

$$N = \frac{(z_\alpha + z_\beta)^2 \times 2 \times S^2}{d^2}.$$

For a proportion difference test:

$$N = \frac{(z_\alpha + z_\beta)^2 \times 2 \times \overline{p}(1 - \overline{p})}{d^2}.$$

where N is required sample size; $z\alpha$ = z-value for alpha (significance level); $z\beta$ = z-value for beta (power level); s^2 = variance; $\overline{p}$ = mean proportion of success; and d = minimal detectable difference. Please note that z_α is usually defined according to whether the test is one-tailed or two-tailed. For a two-tailed test at $\alpha = 0.05$, $z_\alpha/2$ is used, which has a value of 1.96. For a statistical power ($1 - \beta$) of 80%, the corresponding z_β is 0.84.

Survival Analysis

Survival analysis is a statistical method used to analyse time-to-event data, where the goal is to estimate the time until a specific event occurs. This event could be death, disease recurrence, treatment failure, or recovery.

Key Features of Survival Data

Time-to-Event (Survival Time)

- Time-to-event (or survival time) refers to the duration from the start of observation to the occurrence of a predefined event. The event may be adverse (e.g. death, relapse) or neutral (e.g. remission, service contact).
- Examples include:
  - time to death following a cancer diagnosis
  - time to relapse after remission in schizophrenia
  - time from discharge to readmission in psychiatric services.
- Unlike simple binary outcomes, survival analysis incorporates both whether and when an event occurs.

Censoring

Censoring occurs when the event of interest is not observed exactly for all individuals, either because it has not yet occurred, has already occurred before observation began, or occurs between observation points. In censored observations, individuals are included in the analysis, but the exact timing of the event is partially unknown. There are three main types:

- Right censoring occurs when the event has not occurred by the end of follow-up, or when an individual is lost to follow-up or withdraws before experiencing the event.
  - For example, in a study estimating time to relapse in major depressive disorder, a participant is followed for five years but does not relapse during the observation period. The relapse time is therefore right censored at five years.
  - Right censoring is the most common form of censoring in longitudinal psychiatric studies.
  - A related but distinct concept is left truncation (also known as delayed entry). Left truncation occurs when individuals only enter the study if they have survived event-free up to a certain time, meaning those who experienced the event earlier are never observed. For example, a study examining time from onset of psychosis to first hospital admission recruits participants only at first admission to psychiatric services. Individuals who developed psychosis but died, recovered, or disengaged from services before admission are never included. Only those who survived without admission long enough to be recruited enter the study.
- Left censoring occurs when the event has already occurred before the individual enters the study, but the exact timing of the event is unknown.
  - For example, in a study estimating age at first onset of major depressive disorder (MDD), a participant is assessed at age 35 and meets diagnostic criteria for MDD at their first assessment. They report that symptoms began several years earlier but cannot recall the exact age of onset. The onset of MDD is therefore left censored, as it occurred before study entry but at an unknown time.
  - A related but distinct concept is right truncation. Right truncation occurs when individuals are included in a study only if the event has already occurred by a specified time, so those whose event occurs later are never observed. For example, a study examining age at suicide using a coroner's database covering deaths between 2010 and 2020 includes only individuals who died by suicide during that period. Individuals who are alive or who die by suicide after 2020 are excluded, meaning later events are systematically missing.
- Interval censoring occurs when the exact time of the event is unknown, but it is known to have occurred within a specific time interval.
  - For example, a study examining time from study entry to first onset of psychotic disorder follows individuals at high risk of psychosis with structured assessments every six months. A participant does not meet criteria for psychosis at the 6-month assessment but does meet criteria at the 12-month assessment. The exact onset of psychosis is unknown, but it must have occurred between 6 and 12 months, resulting in interval-censored data.

Common Survival Analysis Methods

Median Survival Time (*X*, given *Y*)

- The time taken for 50% of participants to reach the event.
- Other survival percentiles may also be reported to describe the distribution of survival times. For example, the time at which survival probability falls to 5% indicates that 95% of participants have experienced the event. These measures provide summary descriptions but do not model group differences or covariates directly.

Survival Probability (*Y*, given *X*)

- The proportion of the population that has not yet reached the event at a given time. It allows comparison between groups (e.g. treatment vs placebo) at specific time points but does not adjust for multiple predictors simultaneously
- Both *median survival time* and *survival probability* can be used to compare groups (e.g. treated vs placebo).

Kaplan–Meier Estimator (KM Curve)

- A non-parametric method to estimate survival probability over time in the presence of censoring.
- It produces a stepwise survival curve, with downward steps occurring at observed event times (Figure 12.17). Kaplan–Meier curves are particularly useful for visualizing time-to-event distributions and comparing groups descriptively

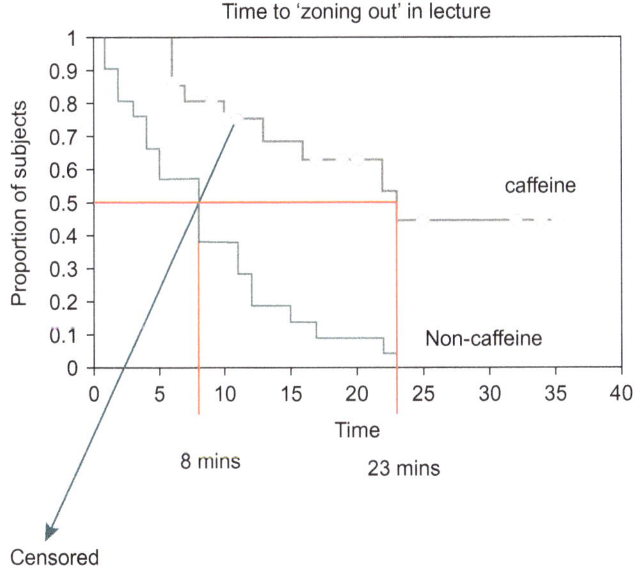

Figure 12.17 Kaplan–Meier survival curve.

- *Example:* in schizophrenia studies, a Kaplan–Meier Curve can show time until relapse after medication discontinuation (Figure 12.18).

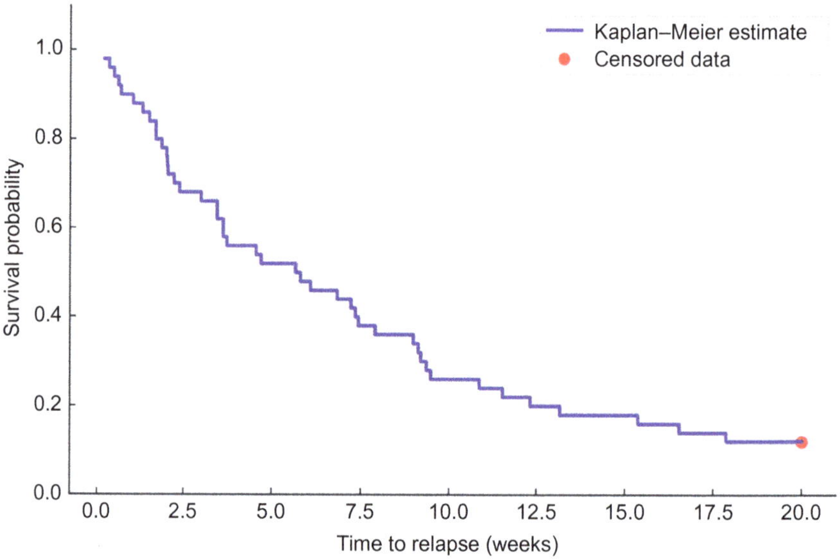

Figure 12.18 Kaplan–Meier survival curve.

Statistical Tests in Survival Analysis

Log-Rank Test

- Compares survival curves between two or more groups (Figures 12.19 and 12.20).

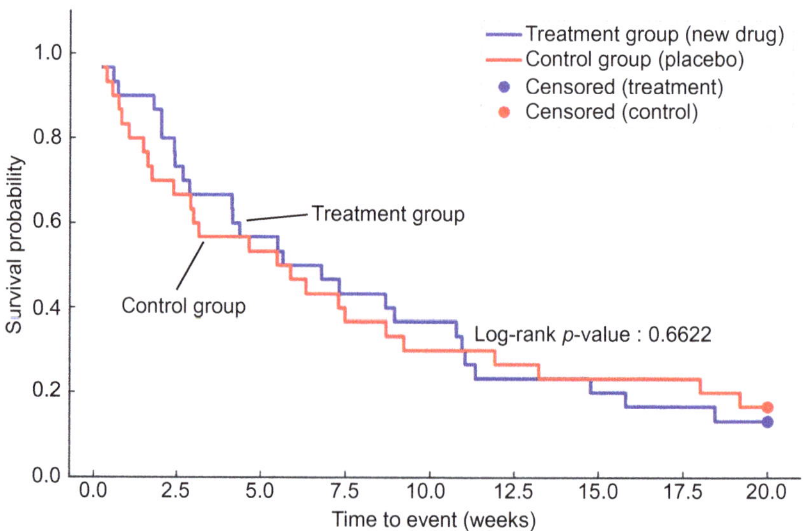

Figure 12.19 *Kaplan–Meier survival curves with log-rank test.*

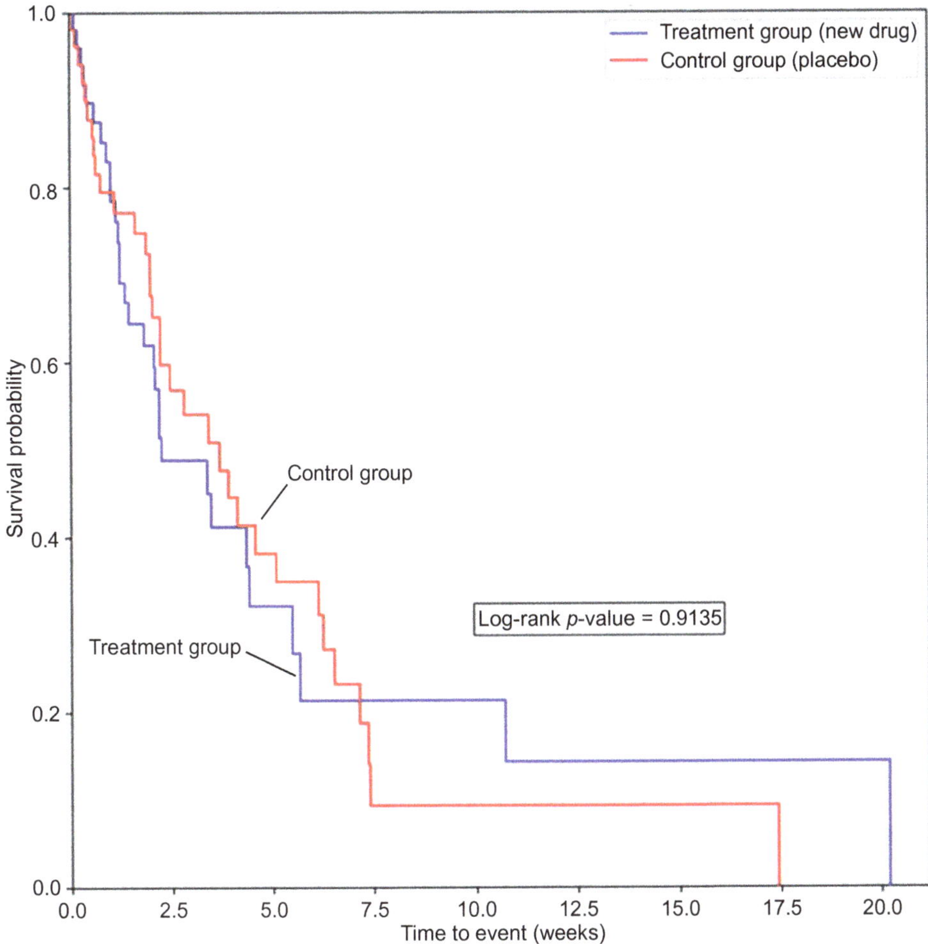

Figure 12.20 Kaplan–Meier survival curves with log-rank test (new drug vs placebo).

- Unlike median survival time, it considers the entire observation period.
- *Example:* do patients receiving antidepressants have a longer time before relapse than those receiving psychotherapy alone?

Cox Proportional Hazards Regression

- A multivariable regression model used to examine the effect of multiple predictors on survival time (Figure 12.21). Key features include:
  - no assumption about the baseline survival distribution.
  - adjustment for multiple covariates
- Produces a hazard ratio (HR) (similar to an odds ratio or risk ratio) which quantify the relative risk of the event occurring at any given time.
- *Example:* predicting risk of suicide relapse based on age, medication type, and past hospitalizations.

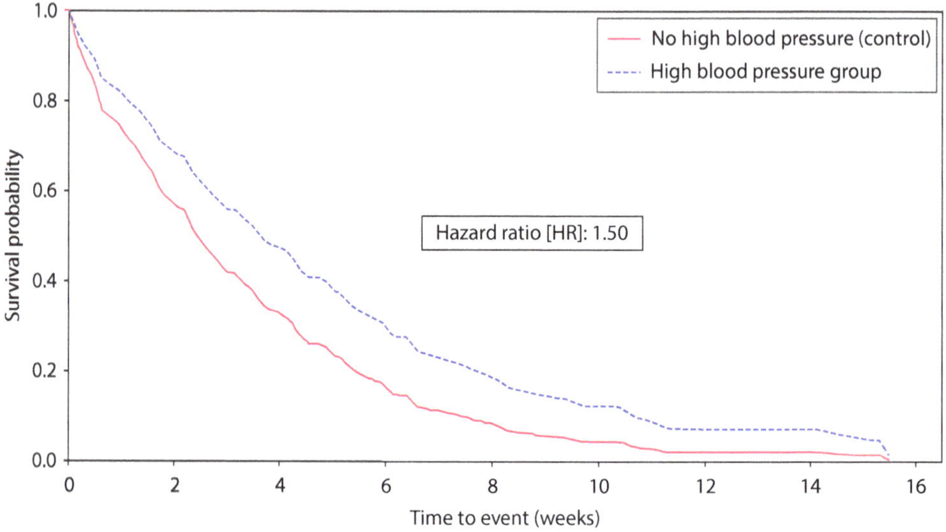

Figure 12.21 Cox proportional hazards regression – survival curve (high blood pressure).

Summary

- Kaplan–Meier analysis describes when events occur.
- Log-rank tests compare whether survival differs between groups.
- Cox regression explains why survival differs, by modelling predictors of risk.

Bayesian Statistical Analysis

Bayesian statistical analysis is a method of statistical inference that uses Bayes' Theorem to update the probability of a hypothesis as new evidence becomes available. It provides a framework for combining prior knowledge with new data to refine conclusions and improve accuracy.

At its core, Bayesian analysis continuously updates the probability of a hypothesis based on new evidence, making it particularly useful in scenarios with limited data or uncertainty.

Key Concepts in Bayesian Analysis

Bayes' Theorem

Bayes' Theorem describes how to update the probability of a hypothesis when new evidence is introduced:

$$P(A|B) = \frac{[P(B|A) \times P(A)]}{P(B)},$$

where:

- $P(A|B)$ = posterior probability (updated probability of hypothesis A given evidence B)

- $P(B|A)$ = likelihood (probability of observing evidence B if A is true)
- $P(A)$ = prior probability (initial belief about A before seeing the evidence)
- $P(B)$ = probability of observing the evidence B.

Components of Bayesian Analysis

Prior Probability

- The initial probability of a hypothesis before new data is considered.
- It is based on previous knowledge, beliefs, or assumptions.

Likelihood

- The probability of observing the new evidence, given the hypothesis, reflecting how well the hypothesis explains the data.

Posterior Probability

- The updated probability of the hypothesis after incorporating new evidence.
- Represents the revised belief in the light of the data.

Key Steps in Bayesian Analysis

1. **Define the prior:** establish the initial probability distribution for the hypothesis.
2. **Collect data:** gather new data or evidence relevant to the hypothesis.
3. **Calculate the likelihood:** determine how likely the observed data are, given the hypothesis.
4. **Apply Bayes' Theorem:** use the formula to compute the posterior probability.
5. **Interpret results:** analyse the posterior probability to make informed inferences.

Advantages of Bayesian Analysis

- **Incorporates prior knowledge:** allows for the integration of previous research, expert opinion, or real-world experience.
- **Intuitive interpretation:** provides probabilities that directly quantify belief in a hypothesis rather than a simple accept/reject decision.
- **Handles uncertainty well:** particularly useful when dealing with small samples or incomplete data.

Disadvantages of Bayesian Analysis

- **Subjectivity:** results may be influenced by the choice of prior, especially when data are sparse.
- **Computational complexity:** Bayesian methods require intensive calculations, especially for complex models.

Chapter Summary

Inductive vs Deductive Reasoning

- Inductive reasoning derives general conclusions from specific observations.
- Deductive reasoning applies general principles to specific cases.

Single-Group and Multi-Group Analysis

Single-Group Analysis (Normally Distributed Data)

- Variance, standard deviation, and standard error summarize data variability.
- 95% CI = sample estimate ± 1.96 × SEM.

Comparing Two or More Groups

1. Develop hypotheses: null (H_0) vs alternative (H_1).
2. Set alpha level (e.g. 0.05).
3. Perform tests of significance.

Statistical Tests

- Parametric tests: one-sample *t*-test, paired *t*-test, independent *t*-test, ANOVA
- Non-parametric tests: Wilcoxon signed-rank test, Mann–Whitney U test, Kruskal–Wallis ANOVA
- Tests for binary data: McNemar test, chi-squared test.

Correlation Analysis

- The correlation coefficient (r) quantifies the strength and direction of a relationship but does not imply causation.

Types of Correlation Coefficients

- Pearson's (r): measures linear association between two continuous, normally distributed variables. *Example:* hours studied vs exam scores.
- Spearman's rank (ρ): used for ordinal or non-normal data. *Example:* physical activity and depression severity.
- Kendall's (τ): alternative to Spearman's, better for small datasets or tied ranks.
- Phi coefficient (φ): measures binary variable correlation. *Example:* course attendance (yes/no) and exam pass rate (yes/no).
- Point-biserial correlation: used when one variable is continuous and the other binary. *Example*: gender and exam scores.
- Cramér's V: measures association between categorical variables. *Example:* psychiatric diagnosis and therapy preference.

Regression Analysis

Regression models assess relationships between a dependent variable (Y) and independent variables (X) for prediction and causal inference.

Types of Regression Models

- Simple linear regression: models a continuous outcome with one predictor. *Example:* depression score reduction based on psychotherapy sessions.
- The formula is $Y = a + bX + \varepsilon$.
- Logistic regression: used for binary outcomes (yes/no, 0/1). *Example:* predicting diabetes based on BMI.

- Multiple regression: analyses the effect of multiple predictors on a continuous outcome. *Example:* exam performance based on revision time, test anxiety, and gender.
- Polynomial regression: Captures non-linear relationships. *Example:* study time vs test scores.
- Ordinal regression: used for ordered categorical outcomes. *Example:* predicting patient satisfaction on a Likert scale.
- Ridge and lasso regression: prevents overfitting in complex models by penalizing large coefficients.
- Poisson regression: models count data. *Example:* number of asthma attacks per year based on air pollution levels.
- Cox regression: used in survival analysis to predict time-to-event outcomes. *Example:* time until relapse in addiction recovery programmes.

Type I and II Errors, Power, and Sample Size

- Type I error (false positive): incorrectly rejecting H_0 (controlled by alpha).
- Type II error (false negative): failing to reject H_0 when false (controlled by beta).
- Power calculation: ensures sample size is adequate to detect a real effect.

Survival Analysis

Survival analysis estimates the time until an event occurs (e.g. death, disease recurrence, treatment failure).

Key Features of Survival Data

- Time-to-event: measures duration from study entry until event occurs. *Example:* time to schizophrenia relapse after stopping medication.
- Censoring: accounts for incomplete observations:
  - Right censoring: event hasn't occurred before the study ends.
  - Left censoring: event happened before study inclusion.
  - Interval censoring: exact event time unknown but within a specific range.

Survival Analysis Methods

- Kaplan–Meier estimator (KM curve): stepwise survival curve showing event-free probability over time.
- Median survival time: the time at which 50% of participants have experienced the event.
- Survival probability: the proportion of individuals remaining event-free at different time points.

Statistical Tests in Survival Analysis

- Log-rank test: compares survival curves between two or more groups. *Example:* comparing relapse rates in antidepressant vs psychotherapy users.
- **Cox proportional hazards**[25] regression: a multivariate model estimating how risk factors influence survival. Produces a hazard ratio (HR) to quantify risk. *Example:* predicting suicide relapse risk based on age and medication type.

---

[25] **Proportional hazards (Cox):** Key assumption that the hazard ratio is constant over time; assess with Schoenfeld residuals or log-minus-log plots.

Bayesian Statistical Analysis

Bayesian statistical analysis updates the probability of a hypothesis as new evidence becomes available using Bayes' Theorem. It integrates prior knowledge with new data, making it useful for limited or uncertain datasets.

Key Concepts

- Bayes' Theorem: calculates the posterior probability by updating the prior probability based on new evidence (likelihood).
- Prior probability: the initial belief about a hypothesis before seeing data.
- Likelihood: the probability of observing the data if the hypothesis is true.
- Posterior probability: the revised probability after incorporating new evidence.

Steps in Bayesian Analysis

1. Define the prior probability.
2. Collect new data.
3. Calculate the likelihood of the data given the hypothesis.
4. Apply Bayes' Theorem to update the probability.
5. Interpret the posterior probability.

Advantages

- Incorporates prior knowledge for better inference.
- Intuitive probability-based interpretation rather than binary accept/reject decisions.
- Effective for small sample sizes and uncertain data.

Disadvantages

- Subjectivity in choosing prior probabilities.
- Computational complexity for large datasets.

Practice Questions

Q1. Which of the following statements best describes the difference between inductive and deductive reasoning?

A. Inductive reasoning moves from specific observations to general conclusions, whereas deductive reasoning moves from general premises to specific conclusions.
B. Deductive reasoning is always correct, while inductive reasoning is prone to errors.
C. Inductive reasoning is used exclusively in scientific research, while deductive reasoning is used in logic and mathematics.
D. Deductive reasoning involves making probabilistic conclusions, whereas inductive reasoning leads to certain conclusions.
E. Both inductive and deductive reasoning require empirical data to reach valid conclusions.

Q2. Which of the following is the primary purpose of a null hypothesis in hypothesis testing?

A. To prove that the alternative hypothesis is correct.
B. To minimize the risk of type I and type II errors.

C. To provide a baseline for determining statistical significance.
D. To ensure that the sample size is adequate for meaningful results.
E. To demonstrate the practical relevance of study findings.

Q3. In hypothesis testing, reducing the alpha (α) level primarily decreases the risk of:
A. Type II error
B. Type I error
C. False negative results
D. Confounding bias
E. Observer bias

Q4. Which of the following conditions must be met for a result to be considered statistically significant?
A. p-Value is greater than α.
B. p-Value is less than or equal to α.
C. Type I and type II errors are equal.
D. The null hypothesis is proven false.
E. The study has a large sample size.

Q5. Which of the following is *not* an assumption of parametric tests?
A. The data must be measured on an interval or ratio scale.
B. The samples must be drawn from populations with equal variances (homogeneity of variance).
C. The data must be positively skewed.
D. The observations must be independent.
E. The population distribution should be approximately normal.

Q6. Which of the following describes the primary difference between a one-tailed and two-tailed hypothesis test?
A. The type of data analysed
B. The sample size required
C. The directionality of the hypothesis
D. The statistical software used
E. The number of variables being tested

Q7. Which of the following research questions is best addressed using linear regression?
A. Is there a difference in the proportion of patients who respond to two different medications?
B. Does smoking status (smoker/non-smoker) predict the likelihood of developing lung cancer?
C. How does the amount of exercise (hours per week) influence weight loss (kilograms)?
D. What is the relationship between gender and preferred type of music?
E. Does the presence of a genetic marker predict the blood type of an individual?

Q8. Which of the following scenarios is best suited for linear regression?
A. Predicting the likelihood of developing diabetes based on BMI

B. Estimating a patient's heart rate based on their exercise duration
C. Classifying patients into high-risk and low-risk groups for cardiovascular disease
D. Identifying the best treatment for depression based on patient demographics
E. Determining whether a new drug is effective in reducing symptoms compared to a placebo

Q9. Which of the following correlation coefficients (r) value represents the weakest correlation between two variables?

A. −0.85
B. 0.12
C. 0.92
D. −0.67
E. 0.78

Q10. A researcher is designing a study to compare the effectiveness of two different antidepressant medications in reducing depression scores. To ensure the study has sufficient power, they conduct a power calculation. Which of the following factors will *not* directly affect the power of the study?

A. Sample size
B. Effect size
C. Significance level (α)
D. p-Value
E. Variability in the population

Q11. A researcher is designing a study to compare the effect of cognitive behavioural therapy (CBT) versus medication on anxiety symptoms. The power of the study is set at 80% (0.80). What does this mean in the context of the study?

A. There is an 80% chance of correctly rejecting the null hypothesis when there is truly no difference between the treatments.
B. There is an 80% chance of detecting a true difference between the treatments if one exists.
C. There is an 80% probability of making a type I error.
D. There is an 80% probability that the null hypothesis is true.
E. There is an 80% chance that the study results will be statistically significant.

Q12. Which of the following statements best distinguishes Bayesian hypothesis testing from frequentist hypothesis testing?

A. Frequentist methods calculate the probability of observing the data given that the null hypothesis is true, while Bayesian methods do not.
B. Bayesian methods incorporate prior knowledge into the analysis, whereas frequentist methods rely only on the data from the current study.
C. Frequentist methods update probabilities as new data becomes available, while Bayesian methods do not.
D. Bayesian methods determine the p-value, whereas frequentist methods use Bayes' theorem to update the probability of a hypothesis.
E. Frequentist and Bayesian approaches are identical in how they handle statistical inference, differing only in terminology.

Q13. Which post hoc test is most appropriate when comparing all possible pairs of means while controlling for type I errors?

A. Bonferroni correction
B. Tukey's honestly significant difference (HSD) test
C. Dunnett's test
D. Scheffé's test
E. Fisher's least significant difference (LSD) test

Q14. Which of the following statistical tests is most appropriate for assessing whether a dataset follows a normal distribution?

A. Kolmogorov–Smirnov (K-S) test
B. Shapiro–Wilk test
C. Levene's test
D. Bartlett's test
E. Wilcoxon signed-rank test

Q15. Theme: statistical tests in research. For each research study below, select the most appropriate hypothesis test from the option list that follows.

1. A study compares the mean PANSS scores in three groups of patients. The data is normally distributed.
2. An RCT assesses the difference in anxiety scores in a group of patients before and after a mindfulness-based therapy programme.
3. A study compares the proportion of patients with bipolar disorder who experience relapse when treated with lithium versus valproate.
4. A clinical trial compares the reduction in psychotic symptoms (measured by the PANSS scale) between a new antipsychotic medication and a standard antipsychotic medication, while controlling for the participants' baseline severity of psychosis.
5. A study evaluates the effect of childhood trauma on cortisol levels in patients with PTSD, comparing three trauma exposure groups. The data is not normally distributed.
6. A study compares the change in social functioning scores (measured on a Likert scale) between two independent groups: patients receiving a social skills training programme and those receiving standard care. The data is not normally distributed.
7. A study assesses the effectiveness of a public health campaign aimed at reducing smoking. Researchers ask participants whether they smoke (yes/no) before and after the campaign.

A. ANCOVA
B. ANOVA
C. Chi-square test
D. Kruskal–Wallis test
E. Mann–Whitney U test
F. McNemar's test
G. Paired *t*-test

H. Unpaired *t*-test
I. Wilcoxon matched pairs signed rank test

Q16. Theme: survival analysis tests. For each research study below, select the most appropriate hypothesis test from the option list that follows.

1. A clinical trial follows 200 patients with schizophrenia for 5 years, comparing the time until first relapse between those on clozapine versus those on risperidone. The researchers want to estimate the probability of remaining relapse-free over time.
2. A study compares the survival times of patients with treatment-resistant depression receiving electroconvulsive therapy (ECT) versus ketamine infusion. Researchers want to determine whether the survival curves differ significantly between the two treatment groups.
3. Researchers are analysing the effect of multiple risk factors (e.g. baseline depression severity, age, and medication adherence) on the time to relapse in patients treated for major depressive disorder. They aim to quantify the independent effect of each factor on survival time.
4. A study follows a cohort of patients with Alzheimer's disease to measure the time until nursing home admission. Some patients are lost to follow-up before admission, while others die from unrelated causes before needing nursing home care. The researchers need to classify these cases appropriately.
5. A psychiatric hospital is evaluating the effectiveness of a suicide prevention programme. They measure the time until the first suicidal attempt post-discharge and compare the median survival time before the attempt in patients receiving standard care versus the new intervention.
6. In a trial investigating the impact of a new antipsychotic on hospital readmission rates, researchers want to compare early and late differences in survival between groups, giving more weight to early events.
7. A study examines the risk of self-harm relapse in young adults with borderline personality disorder. The researchers report the likelihood of relapse per year based on demographic and clinical characteristics.

A. Kaplan–Meier estimator
B. Log-rank test
C. Cox proportional hazards regression
D. Wilcoxon (Breslow–Gehan) test
E. Life table method.
F. Median survival time calculation
G. Censoring identification

Q17. Theme: statistical tests. For each research study below, select the most appropriate statistical test from the option list.

A. Phi correlation coefficient
B. Pearson's correlation coefficient
C. Spearman's correlation coefficient
D. Poisson regression
E. Linear regression
F. Multiple linear regression
G. Cox proportional hazards model

H. Multiple logistic regression
I. Wilcoxon signed-rank test

1. A psychiatrist is studying the relationship between patient adherence to medication (yes/no) and relapse rates (yes/no) in schizophrenia patients.
2. A researcher wants to examine the association between daily caffeine intake (milligrams) and reaction time (milliseconds) in a group of medical students. The data is normally distributed and continuous.
3. A mental health researcher wants to assess the correlation between depression severity (mild, moderate, severe) and level of social support (low, moderate, high) in patients with major depressive disorder.
4. A study is conducted to examine the association between number of suicide attempts and severity of borderline personality disorder (BPD), measured using a validated rating scale.
5. A researcher analyses the relationship between age (independent variable) and PTSD score (dependent variable), assuming a linear relationship.
6. A team of epidemiologists is investigating the effect of early-life trauma on schizophrenia risk by analysing survival data over a 10-year period, with schizophrenia diagnosis as the outcome.
7. A study aims to predict whether a new antidepressant reduces depression relapse (yes/no) based on baseline depression severity, age, and medication adherence.
8. A study examines whether there is an association between childhood trauma (yes/no) and risk of developing depression (yes/no) in adulthood.
9. A researcher wants to predict the number of emergency room visits per year among patients with schizophrenia, based on symptom severity, medication adherence, and substance use history.

Answers

Q1. Correct answer: A. Inductive reasoning moves from specific to general, while deductive reasoning moves from general to specific.
Why the other options are incorrect:

B. Deductive reasoning is logically valid only if premises are true, but inductive reasoning can still be strong even if not absolute.
C. Inductive reasoning is commonly used in science, but deduction is also widely applied.
D. Inductive reasoning leads to probabilistic conclusions, while deductive reasoning provides certain conclusions if premises are true.
E. Deductive reasoning does not necessarily require empirical data; it can rely solely on logical premises.

Q2. Correct answer: C. To provide a baseline for determining statistical significance.
Why the other options are incorrect:

A. The null hypothesis is not used to prove the alternative hypothesis; rather, it is tested for possible rejection.

B. While hypothesis testing considers error control, the null hypothesis itself does not minimize these risks.
D. Sample size affects statistical power, but the null hypothesis does not ensure an adequate sample size.
E. The null hypothesis is a statistical tool and does not assess practical relevance directly.

Q3. Correct answer: B. Type I error.
Why the other options are incorrect:

A. Lowering alpha actually increases the risk of type II error (β), making it harder to detect a true effect.
C. False negative results are associated with type II error, not type I error.
D. Confounding bias is related to study design and is not controlled by alpha.
E. Observer bias is a systematic error in measurement and is not affected by statistical significance levels.

Q4. Correct answer: B. p-Value is less than or equal to α.
Why the other options are incorrect:

A. Statistical significance occurs when $p \leq \alpha$, not when $p > \alpha$.
C. Type I (α) and type II (β) errors do not need to be equal for significance.
D. Hypothesis testing does not 'prove' the null hypothesis is false; it only provides evidence to reject it.
E. A large sample size increases statistical power but does not guarantee significance.

Q5. Correct answer: C. The data must always be positively skewed.
Why the other options are incorrect:

A. Parametric tests require data on an interval or ratio scale (e.g. weight, height, temperature in Celsius).
B. Many parametric tests, such as the t-test and ANOVA, assume homogeneity of variance (Levene's test can check this).
D. Observations must be independent, meaning one data point should not influence another.
E. Most parametric tests assume normal distribution of the population, especially for small samples.

Q6. Correct answer: C. The directionality of the hypothesis. The key difference between one-tailed and two-tailed tests is whether the hypothesis is directional or non-directional. A one-tailed test is used when the hypothesis predicts a specific direction (e.g. 'Drug A will increase reaction time'). A two-tailed test is used when the hypothesis simply predicts a difference (e.g. 'Drug A will affect reaction time'). Therefore, the direction the hypothesis is aiming to prove is the primary difference.
Why the other options are incorrect:

A. The type of data analysed: the type of data (e.g. continuous, categorical) determines the type of statistical test used (e.g. t-test, chi-square), but it does not determine whether the test is one-tailed or two-tailed. Both one- and two-tailed tests can be used on the same types of data.

B. The sample size required: while sample size is crucial for statistical power, it does not dictate whether a test is one-tailed or two-tailed. The sample size affects the test's ability to detect a significant difference, but not the directional nature of the test.

D. The statistical software used: statistical software (e.g. SPSS, R) can perform both one-tailed and two-tailed tests. The user selects the appropriate test based on their hypothesis, not based on limitations or differences in statistical software.

E. The number of variables being tested: the number of variables is more relevant to the type of statistical test (e.g. *t*-test for comparing two groups, ANOVA for comparing multiple groups). It does not determine the one-tailed or two-tailed nature of the hypothesis test.

Q7. Correct answer: C. How does the amount of exercise (hours per week) influence weight loss (kilograms)? Linear regression is used to model the relationship between a continuous dependent variable (outcome) and one or more independent variables (predictors). It assumes a linear relationship between the predictor and the outcome. Why the other options are incorrect:

A. Is there a difference in the proportion of patients who respond to two different medications? This involves comparing proportions (categorical outcomes), making it more suitable for a chi-square test or logistic regression if controlling for confounders.

B. Does smoking status (smoker/non-smoker) predict the likelihood of developing lung cancer? The dependent variable (lung cancer: yes/no) is binary, making logistic regression a more appropriate method rather than linear regression.

D. What is the relationship between gender and preferred type of music? Gender (categorical: male/female/other) and preferred music type (categorical: rock, classical, jazz, etc.) suggest that chi-square test or multinomial logistic regression would be more appropriate.

E. Does the presence of a genetic marker predict the blood type of an individual? Blood type is categorical (A, B, AB, O), and a genetic marker is also categorical.

Q8. Correct answer: B. Estimating a patient's heart rate based on their exercise duration. Linear regression is used when the goal is to model the relationship between a continuous dependent variable (outcome) and one or more independent variables (predictors). It assumes a linear relationship between the predictor and the outcome. Why the other options are incorrect:

A. Predicting the likelihood of developing diabetes based on BMI. The dependent variable (diabetes: yes/no) is binary, meaning that logistic regression would be more appropriate.

C. Classifying patients into high-risk and low-risk groups for cardiovascular disease. The dependent variable (risk category: high/low) is categorical, making logistic regression (if binary classification) or multinomial logistic regression (if more than two categories) more appropriate.

D. Identifying the best treatment for depression based on patient demographics. This scenario likely involves categorical treatment options and multiple predictor variables, making it more suited for logistic regression or decision tree models rather than linear regression.
E. Determining whether a new drug is effective in reducing symptoms compared to a placebo. If the outcome is measured as symptom improvement on a continuous scale, an unpaired *t*-test or ANOVA would be appropriate. If multiple predictors are involved, ANCOVA could be used.

Q9. Correct answer: B. 0.12. (The closer *r* is to 0, the weaker the correlation.

Q10. Correct answer: D. *p*-Value. Power calculation determines the minimum sample size required to detect a statistically significant effect, given that a true effect exists. However, *p*-value is not a factor in power calculation. The *p*-value is the probability of observing the data (or more extreme data) if the null hypothesis is true. It is an outcome of statistical testing, not an input factor in power calculation. The factors that directly influence statistical power include the incorrect answers:

A. Sample size: a larger sample size increases power because it reduces random variation and increases the likelihood of detecting a true effect.
B. Effect size: a larger effect size increases power because bigger differences are easier to detect statistically.
C. Significance level (α): a lower α (e.g. 0.01 instead of 0.05) reduces power, making it harder to detect an effect, while a higher α increases power but also raises the risk of a type I error.
E. Variability in the population: higher variability (standard deviation) decreases power because greater spread in the data makes it harder to detect a true effect.

Q11. Correct answer: B. There is an 80% chance of detecting a true difference between the treatments if one exists. Statistical power refers to the probability of correctly rejecting the null hypothesis when a true effect exists. A power of 80% (0.80) means that if there is a real difference between the two treatments, the study has an 80% chance of detecting it.
Why the other options are incorrect:

A. Power is not related to rejecting the null hypothesis when there is no difference (that would be a type I error).
C. Type I error (false positive) is represented by α (e.g. 0.05 or 5%), not by power.
D. The probability of the null hypothesis being true is not related to power. Power is about detecting an effect when the null hypothesis is false.
E. Power does not guarantcc statistical significance in all cases – it only increases the likelihood of detecting a true effect if it exists.

Q12. Correct answer: B. Bayesian methods incorporate prior knowledge into the analysis, whereas frequentist methods rely only on the data from the current study. Bayesian hypothesis testing incorporates prior knowledge (prior probability distributions) and updates beliefs as new data are obtained. Frequentist hypothesis testing only uses the current dataset and does not incorporate prior beliefs.
Why the other options are incorrect:

A. Frequentist hypothesis testing does not calculate the probability that the null hypothesis is true; it calculates the probability of obtaining the observed data (or more extreme data) assuming the null hypothesis is true (i.e. p-value). Bayesian methods, on the other hand, allow for direct probability statements about the hypothesis.
C. Bayesian methods update probabilities as new data become available, while frequentist methods do not – they use fixed procedures that do not allow for such updates.
D. Frequentist methods rely on p-values and confidence intervals, whereas Bayesian methods use Bayes' Theorem to update probability estimates. Frequentists do not use Bayes' Theorem in hypothesis testing.
E. Frequentist and Bayesian approaches are fundamentally different in their treatment of probability. Frequentists interpret probability as long-run frequencies, whereas Bayesians interpret it as a degree of belief.

Q13. Correct answer: B. Tukey's HSD test. It is specifically designed for pairwise comparisons while maintaining control over type I errors. It assumes equal variances and normality.
Why the other options are incorrect:

A. Bonferroni correction is a conservative method that adjusts the significance level (α) by dividing it by the number of comparisons. It reduces type I error risk but increases type II error probability. Best used when only a few planned comparisons are needed.
C. Dunnett's test is used when comparing multiple treatment groups against a single control group (not for all pairwise comparisons). It is more statistically powerful than Tukey's HSD in control-group comparisons.
D. Scheffé's test is a very conservative post hoc test that allows comparisons among any linear combination of means (not just pairwise comparisons). It is less powerful for pairwise comparisons but useful for complex contrasts.
E. Fisher's LSD test does not control for type I errors when multiple comparisons are made. It is used only when ANOVA is significant to test differences without adjustment. It is considered the least conservative post hoc test.

Q14. Correct answer: B. Shapiro–Wilk Test. It is one of the most powerful tests for normality, particularly for small sample sizes.
Why the other options are incorrect:

A. Kolmogorov–Smirnov test is a general goodness-of-fit test for normality, but less powerful than Shapiro–Wilk for small samples.
C. Levene's test is used for testing homogeneity of variances, not normality.
D. Bartlett's test also tests homogeneity of variances, but assumes normality.
E. Wilcoxon signed-rank test is a non-parametric test used for paired data, not for normality testing.

Q15. The statements and options are paired as follows.

1. B. ANOVA. ANOVA is used to compare the means of more than two independent groups when the data is normally distributed.

2. G. Paired t-test. A paired t-test is used when comparing pre- and post-treatment scores in the same group of patients with normally distributed data.
3. C. Chi-square test. The Chi-square test is used to compare proportions in categorical variables (e.g. relapse: yes/no) between two independent groups (lithium vs valproate).
4. A. ANCOVA. ANCOVA is used when you want to compare the means of a continuous outcome variable (PANSS score reduction) between groups (new vs standard medication) while controlling for a continuous covariate (baseline psychosis severity).
5. D. Kruskal–Wallis test. The Kruskal–Wallis test is a non-parametric alternative to ANOVA when comparing more than two independent groups with non-normally distributed data.
6. E. Mann–Whitney U test. When comparing two independent groups with non-normally distributed data, the Mann–Whitney U test (a non-parametric test) is the appropriate choice. It compares the medians of the two groups.
7. F. McNemar test. McNemar's test is used for dichotomous data in paired groups. It will be used here to determine if there's a significant change in the proportion of smokers within the same individuals after the campaign.

Q16. The statements and options are paired as follows:

1. A. Kaplan–Meier estimator. The Kaplan–Meier (KM) estimator is used to estimate survival probabilities over time. It provides a stepwise survival curve, showing the probability of remaining event-free (e.g. relapse-free) at different time points. In this case, the KM estimator is appropriate because the study follows patients over time and estimates their probability of remaining relapse-free.
2. B. Log-rank test. The log-rank test is used to compare survival distributions between two or more groups. It determines whether the survival curves for different groups are significantly different. Since this study compares the survival times of patients receiving ECT versus ketamine and tests for differences in survival curves, the log-rank test is the best choice.
3. C. Cox proportional hazards regression. Cox regression (also called the Cox proportional hazards model) assesses the impact of multiple independent variables (e.g. age, depression severity, medication adherence) on time-to-event data. Since this study aims to identify how multiple factors influence time to relapse, Cox regression is the appropriate choice.
4. G. Censoring identification. Censoring occurs when the event of interest (e.g. nursing home admission) has not happened by the end of the study or the patient is lost to follow-up. Here, patients who drop out or die from unrelated causes before nursing home admission are considered censored observations, meaning their exact survival time is unknown.
5. F. Median survival time calculation. Median survival time is the time at which 50% of the study population has experienced the event (e.g. suicide attempt). Since this study compares the median survival time before suicide attempts in different treatment groups, the appropriate method is calculating the median survival time.

6. D. Wilcoxon (Breslow–Gehan) test. The Wilcoxon (Breslow–Gehan) test is a variation of the log-rank test that gives more weight to early events in survival analysis. It is useful when early differences in survival between groups are more important. Since this study compares early and late differences in survival (hospital readmission), the Wilcoxon test is the best choice.
7. C. Cox proportional hazards regression. This study examines the risk of self-harm relapse over time in young adults with borderline personality disorder, with relapse as a time-to-event outcome and multiple demographic and clinical predictors. Cox proportional hazards regression is the appropriate method because it models the effect of several independent variables on the hazard (risk) of an event occurring at any point in time, while accounting for censoring. The model produces hazard ratios (HRs), which quantify how each predictor influences the risk of relapse over the follow-up period.

Q17. The statements and options are paired as follows.

1. A. Phi correlation coefficient. Both variables (adherence and relapse) are binary (yes/no). Phi correlation coefficient is a special case of Pearson's correlation, used to measure the association between two dichotomous variables in a 2×2 contingency table.
2. B. Pearson's correlation coefficient. Both variables are continuous and normally distributed. Pearson's correlation coefficient (r) measures the strength and direction of a linear relationship between two continuous variables. If caffeine intake increases, reaction time may decrease (negative correlation).
3. C. Spearman's correlation coefficient. Both variables are ordinal (ranked categories). Spearman's correlation is used for ordinal or non-normally distributed continuous data when assessing monotonic relationships. Unlike Pearson's correlation, Spearman's correlation does not assume linearity.
4. D. Poisson regression. The dependent variable (number of suicide attempts) is count data (i.e. 0, 1, 2, 3, . . .). Poisson regression is used when modelling count data and assumes that the event rates follow a Poisson distribution. Predictors (e.g. BPD severity) influence the expected number of occurrences (suicide attempts).
5. E. Linear regression. The dependent variable (PTSD score) is continuous. The independent variable (age) is also continuous. Linear regression models the relationship between a continuous predictor and a continuous outcome, assuming a linear association.
6. G. Cox proportional hazards model. Time-to-event data (time until schizophrenia diagnosis). The Cox proportional hazards model is used to estimate the risk of an event occurring over time, adjusting for covariates like trauma history. Unlike logistic regression, it considers the timing of the event rather than just whether the event occurred.
7. H. Multiple logistic regression. The dependent variable (relapse: yes/no) is binary. The are multiple independent variables (depression severity, age, medication adherence). Multiple logistic regression is used when there are multiple predictors for a binary outcome.

8. A. Phi correlation coefficient. Both variables are binary (yes/no). Phi correlation coefficient is used when assessing correlation between two dichotomous variables in a 2 × 2 table.
9. D. Poisson regression. The dependent variable (ER visits per year) is count data. Poisson regression models count data and estimates the expected number of occurrences based on independent variables.

Further Reading

Agresti A. *Categorical Data Analysis*. 3rd ed. Hoboken, NJ: Wiley; 2013.

Anderson TW, Darling DA. A test of goodness of fit. *J Am Stat Assoc*. 1954;**49**(268):765–9.

Bonferroni CE. Teoria statistica delle classi e calcolo delle probabilità. *Pubblicazioni del R Istituto Superiore di Scienze Economiche e Commerciali di Firenze*. 1936;**8**:3–62.

Cameron AC, Trivedi PK. *Regression Analysis of Count Data*. 2nd ed. Cambridge: Cambridge University Press; 2013.

Cohen J. *Statistical Power Analysis for the Behavioral Sciences*. 2nd ed. Hillsdale, NJ: Lawrence Erlbaum; 1988.

Cox DR. Regression models and life-tables. *J R Stat Soc B*. 1972;**34**(2):187–220.

D'Agostino RB. Transformation to normality of the null distribution of g_1. *Biometrika*. 1970;**57**(3):679–81.

Dunnett CW. A multiple comparison procedure for comparing several treatments with a control. *J Am Stat Assoc*. 1955;**50**(272):1096–121.

Fisher RA. On the interpretation of χ^2 from contingency tables, and the calculation of P. *J R Stat Soc*. 1922;**85**(1):87–94.

Harrell FE Jr. *Regression Modeling Strategies*. 2nd ed. Cham: Springer; 2015.

Hedges LV. Distribution theory for Glass's estimator of effect size and related estimators. *J Educ Stat*. 1981;**6**(2):107–28.

Holm S. A simple sequentially rejective multiple test procedure. *Scand J Stat*. 1979;**6**(2):65–70.

Hosmer DW, Lemeshow S, Sturdivant RX. *Applied Logistic Regression*. 3rd ed. Hoboken, NJ: Wiley; 2013.

Kaplan EL, Meier P. Nonparametric estimation from incomplete observations. *J Am Stat Assoc*. 1958;**53**(282):457–81.

Levene H. Robust tests for equality of variances. In: Olkin I, ed. *Contributions to Probability and Statistics*. Stanford, CA: Stanford University Press; 1960. pp. 278–92.

Lilliefors HW. On the Kolmogorov–Smirnov test for normality with mean and variance unknown. *J Am Stat Assoc*. 1967;**62**(318):399–402.

Mantel N. Evaluation of survival data and two new rank order statistics arising in its consideration. *Cancer Chemother Rep*. 1966;**50**(3):163–70.

McNemar Q. Note on the sampling error of the difference between correlated proportions or percentages. *Psychometrika*. 1947;**12**(2):153–7.

Scheffé H. A method for judging all contrasts in the analysis of variance. *Biometrika*. 1953;**40** (1–2):87–104.

Schoenfeld D. Partial residuals for the proportional hazards regression model. *Biometrika*. 1982;**69**(1):239–41.

Shapiro SS, Wilk MB. An analysis of variance test for normality (complete samples). *Biometrika*. 1965;**52**(3–4):591–611.

Student. The probable error of a mean. *Biometrika*. 1908;**6**(1):1–25.

Tukey JW. Comparing individual means in the analysis of variance. *Biometrics*. 1949;**5**(2):99–114.

Welch BL. The generalization of 'Student's' problem when several different population variances are involved. *Biometrika*. 1947;**34** (1–2):28–35.

Chapter 13

Economic Analysis

Introduction

Economic analysis in medicine, also known as health economics, applies economic principles to evaluate healthcare costs, resource allocation, and decision-making. The goal is to improve efficiency, effectiveness, and equity in healthcare delivery.

A key component of economic evaluation is understanding different types of healthcare costs, which are categorized as direct, indirect, intangible, and opportunity costs.

Direct Costs

Direct costs are expenses directly related to healthcare services. These can be further divided into:

- **Direct medical costs:** expenses for medical services, including:
  - hospital admissions
  - medications
  - consultations
  - investigations
  - treatment procedures.
- **Direct non-medical costs:** non-healthcare expenses incurred by patients and families, such as:
  - travel expenses
  - accommodation
  - out-of-pocket costs for care.

Examples of direct costs are those for antipsychotic medications for schizophrenia, psychotherapy fees, and hospital admissions for acute psychiatric crises.

Indirect Costs

Indirect costs represent the loss of productivity due to illness, disability, or premature death. These costs reflect the broader economic impact of health conditions. Indirect costs are usually considered from a societal perspective, as they occur outside the healthcare system. Examples include:

- reduced work productivity or job loss due to severe depression or anxiety disorders
- the financial burden on caregivers who must reduce work hours to support a relative with dementia.

Intangible Costs

Intangible costs refer to the psychological and emotional burdens experienced by patients and their families. These costs are difficult to quantify, yet they significantly impact overall wellbeing. Examples include:

- emotional distress in patients with bipolar disorder
- stress and anxiety experienced by family members of individuals with severe personality disorders.

Opportunity Cost

Opportunity cost represents the benefits lost when one healthcare intervention is chosen over another. It reflects not just financial costs, but also the alternative uses of resources. One example is allocating mental health funding to community-based therapy programmes instead of expanding inpatient services for acute psychiatric care. The opportunity cost is the potential benefits lost by not investing in inpatient care.

Table 13.1 compares the different categories of costs.

Table 13.1 Comparison table: different types of costs in economic evaluation studies

Cost type	Definition	Examples in psychiatry	Quantification
Direct costs	Costs directly associated with treatment and healthcare provision	Medication costs, therapy session fees, hospitalization expenses	Usually quantifiable in monetary terms using healthcare utilization data
Indirect costs	Costs related to loss of productivity and economic output	Loss of income due to depression, caregiver's reduced productivity	Estimated through productivity loss
Intangible costs	Non-monetary costs, including emotional and psychological impact	Anxiety in family members, reduced quality of life in patients with chronic mental illness	Difficult to quantify, often assessed through quality-of-life measures
Opportunity costs	The cost of forgoing the next best alternative when a choice is made	Allocating resources to therapy instead of inpatient services	Conceptual and comparative, not directly monetary

Discounting

Discounting is the process of adjusting the value of costs and benefits that occur in the future to reflect their present-day value.

Why Is Discounting Important?

- **Time preference:** people generally prefer benefits sooner rather than later and costs later rather than sooner.
- **Opportunity cost:** money spent today could be invested elsewhere, generating returns over time.

- **Uncertainty over time:** future costs and benefits may change due to inflation or unforeseen factors.

A 'discount rate' is used to reduce the value of future costs and benefits. A higher discount rate means that future values are reduced more significantly.

How Is Discounting Applied?

The present value of future costs or benefits is calculated using the following formula:

$$PV = \frac{FV}{(1+r)^t},$$

where PV is the present value; FV is the future value; r is the discount rate; and t is the time in years.

Health Evaluation and Health-Related Quality of Life

Health evaluation and health-related quality of life (HRQoL) studies assess individual preferences for health outcomes. Two key methods used in cost–utility analyses, where outcomes are expressed in **quality-adjusted life years (QALYs)**, are:

1. standard gamble (SG)
2. time trade-off (TTO).

Standard Gamble

The SG method is used to elicit individual preferences for different health states. It is based on the concept of a hypothetical gamble where the individual chooses between:

- Option 1: remaining in their current health state with certainty.
- Option 2: taking a gamble with:
  - a probability (p) of achieving perfect health
  - a probability ($1 - p$) of experiencing a worse health state or death.

This method is grounded in expected utility theory and is particularly useful in risk-based decision-making. For example, a patient with major depressive disorder may be asked to choose between:

- remaining in their current depressive state with certainty
- taking a gamble with new treatment where:
  - there is a 70% chance of full recovery (perfect mental health)
  - there is a 30% chance of severe deterioration (e.g. hospitalization or treatment-resistant depression).

Time Trade-Off

The TTO method measures how much time an individual is willing to sacrifice in exchange for perfect health. Participants choose between:

- Option A: living a certain number of years in their current health state.
- Option B: living a shorter time in perfect health.

This method assesses how individuals balance longevity and quality of life (QoL). For example, a patient with multiple sclerosis (MS) is asked to choose between:

- living 10 years with MS symptoms, managing relapses, and residual disabilities
- living 8 years in perfect health, free from symptoms, if a new treatment were available.

Economic Evaluation Methods

Health economists use different methods to analyse healthcare interventions by assessing inputs (costs) and outputs (benefits). While inputs are always monetary, the outputs can be either monetary or health-related outcomes.

The primary economic evaluation methods include **cost-minimization analysis** (CMA), **cost–benefit analysis** (CBA), **cost-effectiveness analysis** (CEA), **cost–utility analysis** (CUA), and **cost–consequence analysis** (CCA).

Cost-Minimization Analysis

- **Definition:** a method used to compare the costs of two or more healthcare interventions that are assumed to have equivalent outcomes.
- **Focus:** solely on input costs, as effectiveness is considered the same.
- **Best used for:** when two treatments or interventions produce identical health benefits, making cost the deciding factor.

For example, comparing paroxetine and citalopram, assuming both have the same effectiveness, but selecting the cheaper option based on cost alone.

Cost–Benefit Analysis

Cost–benefit analysis is a method used to compare the costs and benefits of a healthcare intervention or programme in monetary terms. In this approach, both inputs (costs) and outputs (benefits) are converted into monetary values and then compared to determine whether an intervention is economically justified. In practice, CBA is less commonly used in healthcare than cost-effectiveness or cost–utility analysis, because valuing health outcomes in monetary terms can be ethically and methodologically challenging. The following outlines the steps for conducting a CBA.

Define the Scope

- Clarify the objectives, timeframe, and alternatives being considered.
- Determine the perspective of the analysis (e.g. healthcare system, society, or payer).

Identify Costs and Benefits

- List all financial and non-financial impacts associated with the intervention.

Inputs (Costs)

Costs in CBA include direct, indirect, and intangible costs.

Direct Costs

Direct costs are immediate expenses related to healthcare services. These can be divided into:

- **Direct healthcare costs:** hospital stays, medications, doctor visits, diagnostic tests, therapies.

- **Direct non-healthcare costs:** transportation, home modifications, assistive devices, and special equipment.

For example, the cost of antipsychotic medications for schizophrenia or hospital admission for acute psychiatric crises.

Indirect Costs

Indirect costs arise from loss of productivity due to illness, disability, or premature death. These costs are often estimated using:

- **Human capital approach**, which values lost productivity based on wages and time lost from work.
- **Friction cost approach**, which accounts for the time taken to replace a worker due to illness.

Other indirect costs include:

- caregiver burden (lost work hours of a family caregiver)
- reduced QoL due to chronic illness.

For example, a caregiver reducing work hours to support a relative with dementia or a worker losing income due to major depressive disorder.

Intangible Costs

Intangible costs are non-monetary burdens, such as:

- pain and suffering
- emotional distress of patients and families.

These are difficult to quantify but are important for understanding the full impact of a disease. For example, the emotional distress experienced by family members of an individual with a severe personality disorder.

Assign Monetary Values to Benefits

In CBA, benefits (outputs) are converted into monetary values using different valuation methods:

- Human capital approach:
  - Values health benefits based on increased earning potential from improved health.
  - Criticism: does not fully capture QoL improvements.
- **Willingness-to-pay** (WTP) method:
  - Asks individuals how much they would pay to achieve a health improvement or avoid a health risk.
  - Uses surveys or experiments to measure preferences.
  - A preferred method as it captures personal valuation of health benefits.
- Contingent valuation (CV):
  - A specific type of WTP survey, where individuals are asked to assign a monetary value to a hypothetical health scenario.
- Revealed preference approach:
  - Estimates value by observing real-world behaviours (e.g. how much people are willing to pay for safety features in cars).

An example of assigning a monetary benefit is assessing how much individuals would be willing to pay for a new depression treatment that reduces symptoms by 50% compared to standard care.

Discount Future Costs and Benefits

Since money has a time value, future costs and benefits need to be discounted to their present value. Common discounting metrics include net present value (NPV) and present value (PV).

Net Present Value

Net present value is the difference between the present value of benefits and the present value of costs. The formula is:

$$NPV = \Sigma \frac{Bt - Ct}{(1+r)^t},$$

where B_t = benefits in year t; C_t = costs in year t; r = discount rate; and t = time period.

Present Value

Present value converts a future cost or benefit into its present value using the formula:

$$PV = \frac{FV}{(1-r)^t},$$

where PV = present value; FV = future value (amount of money to be received or paid in the future); r = discount rate; and t = time period (years into the future).

For example, a mental health programme costing £1 million today is expected to generate £5 million in economic benefits over 10 years. Discounting ensures that future benefits are adjusted for inflation and time preference.

Calculate Economic Evaluation Metrics

This is done using the benefit–cost ratio (BCR), a metric that compares the total benefits to the total costs using the formula:

$$BCR = \frac{\text{Total benefits}}{\text{Total costs}}.$$

- If BCR > 1, the intervention is economically viable.
- If BCR < 1, costs outweigh the benefits, making the intervention not cost-beneficial.
- BCR should be interpreted alongside NPV, because a high BCR can occur even when absolute net benefit is small.

For example, if a suicide prevention programme has a BCR of 3.2, it means that for every £1 spent, there is a £3.20 return in benefits (e.g. reduced hospital admissions, increased productivity).

Perform Sensitivity Analysis

- **Why?** Healthcare costs and benefits are uncertain and depend on assumptions.

- **How?** Sensitivity analysis tests how changes in key assumptions (e.g. discount rate, cost estimates) affect outcomes.
- **Example:** how does the BCR change if programme costs increase by 20% (or if the discount rate changes from 3.5% to 1.5%)?

Make Recommendations

- If the benefits outweigh the costs, the healthcare intervention is recommended.
- If costs exceed benefits, alternative strategies should be considered.

Cost-Effectiveness Analysis

Cost-effectiveness analysis is used to compare the costs and health outcomes of different interventions without converting outcomes into monetary values. Instead, outcomes are measured in natural health units, such as:

- life years gained
- cases of disease prevented
- improvements in mental health scores.

Cost-effectiveness analysis helps healthcare decision-makers allocate resources efficiently by determining which intervention provides the best health benefits for the cost incurred. The steps in conducting a CEA are as follows.

Define the Perspective

- Determine whose costs and benefits will be included in the analysis.
- Perspectives may include:
  - healthcare provider (e.g. NHS, private insurers)
  - societal perspective (including patients, families, employers, and social services).

Identify Interventions

- Clearly define the interventions being compared.
- Examples:
  - a new drug vs standard treatment for depression
  - a cancer screening programme vs no screening
  - cognitive behavioural therapy (CBT) vs medication for anxiety disorders.

Measure Inputs (Costs)

- Direct costs:
  - medical costs: staff salaries, hospital stays, medications, therapy costs
  - non-medical costs: patient transportation, caregiver expenses.
- Indirect costs:
  - productivity losses due to illness
  - time taken off work for treatment or caregiving.

Measure Outputs (Health Outcomes)

Health outcomes are measured in natural units, such as:

- lives saved
- reduction in symptoms
- cases of disease prevented
- improved QoL scores.

Unlike CBA, CEA does not convert outcomes into monetary values, but retains them in health-specific units.

Calculate the Cost-Effectiveness Ratio

The incremental cost-effectiveness ratio (ICER) compares the additional cost of an intervention per unit of health outcome gained compared to the standard intervention. The formula is:

$$\text{ICER} = \frac{C_1 - C_0}{E_1 - E_0},$$

where C_1 is the cost of the new intervention; C_0 is the cost of the standard intervention; E_1 is the effectiveness of the new intervention (e.g. cases prevented, life years gained); and E_0 is the effectiveness of the standard intervention.

For example, a study compares whether a new CBT programme for depression is more cost-effective than standard care. The cost per additional case of depression improved is calculated as follows:

- Standard care: cost = £500; cases improved = 20
- CBT programme: cost = £800; cases improved = 30
- ICER = $\frac{C_1 - C_0}{E_1 - E_0} = \frac{£800 - £500}{30 - 20}$ = £30 per additional case improved.

This means that for each additional case of depression improved, the CBT programme costs an extra £30 compared to standard care.

Interpret the Results

- Decision-makers compare the ICER to a WTP threshold per unit outcome gained.
- If ICER is below the threshold, the new intervention is considered cost-effective.

For example:

- If the WTP threshold is £50 per additional case improved, and the ICER is £30, the CBT programme would be deemed cost-effective and implemented.
- If the ICER were £100, exceeding the WTP threshold, the intervention may not be adopted due to excessive costs relative to benefits.

Cost–Utility Analysis

Cost–utility analysis is a specialized form of cost-effectiveness analysis that evaluates healthcare interventions based on both the quantity and quality of life gained. It expresses outcomes in terms of QALYs, making it particularly useful for comparing interventions across different disease areas.

Unlike CEA, which measures outcomes in natural units (e.g. lives saved, cases prevented), CUA standardizes health outcomes using QALYs, allowing comparisons between different types of interventions.

The steps in conducting a CUA are as follows.

Define the Decision Problem

- Clearly state the purpose of the analysis (e.g. comparing two or more healthcare interventions).
- Define the perspective (e.g. healthcare system, societal).
- Specify the time horizon over which costs and outcomes will be evaluated.

Identify and Measure Inputs (Costs)

Like other types of economic evaluations, CUA considers:

- Direct costs:
  - medical: treatment costs, medications, hospital stays
  - non-medical: transportation, caregiver expenses.
- Indirect costs:
  - productivity losses (e.g. work absenteeism due to illness).

Indirect costs are usually included only when the analysis takes a societal perspective; they are typically excluded in healthcare payer perspectives (e.g. NICE/NHS).

Identify and Measure Outputs (Quality-Adjusted Health Outcomes)

- **Quantity of life:** Measured in years.
- **Quality of life:** Measured using utility values from instruments such as:
  - EQ-5D (measures mobility, self-care, usual activities, pain/discomfort, anxiety/depression)
  - SF-36 (assesses multiple health domains).
- **QALY:**
  - A measure combining both length and quality of life.
  - Utility values range from 1 (full health) to 0 (death).
  - Negative values are allowed, indicating health states worse than death.

Calculate QALYs

The formula to calculate QALYs is:

$$\text{QALY} = \text{Quality of life utility score} \times \text{Years lived in that health state.}$$

For example:

- A patient lives 5 years with a quality of life utility score of 0.8.
- QALY = 0.8 × 5 = 4 QALYs.

Compute the Incremental Cost–Utility Ratio

The incremental cost–utility ratio (ICUR) calculates the additional cost required to gain one extra QALY:

$$\text{ICUR} = \frac{C_1 - C_0}{Q_1 - Q_0},$$

where C_1 is the cost of the new intervention; C_0 is the cost of the standard intervention; Q_1 is the QALYs gained from the new intervention; and Q_0 is the QALYs gained from the standard intervention.

For example, the ICUR for a new antipsychotic medication is compared to an existing standard antipsychotic for schizophrenia in Table 13.2.

Table 13.2 Inputs and total costs of new versus existing medication over a 10-year period

Inputs (costs)	New medication	Existing medication
Annual cost (£)	£1,500	£500
Time horizon (years)	10	10
Total cost (£)	£15,000	£5,000

From the information in Table 13.2, the ICUR can be calculated:

- New medication over 10 years: 0.75, 0.80, 0.85, 0.85, 0.85, 0.85, 0.85, 0.85, 0.85, 0.85 = 8.35
- Existing medication over 10 years: 0.60, 0.65, 0.70, 0.75, 0.75, 0.75, 0.75, 0.75, 0.75, 0.75 = 7.20

Therefore:

$$\text{ICUR} = \frac{C_1 - C_0}{Q_1 - Q_0} = \frac{15,000 - 5000}{8.35 - 7.2}$$

$$= \frac{10,000}{1.15} = £8,695.65 \text{ per QALY gained.}$$

Interpret Results and Conduct Sensitivity Analysis

- ICUR is compared to a WTP threshold to determine cost-effectiveness.
- Example: NICE sets a threshold of £20,000–£30,000 per QALY (higher thresholds may apply in special circumstances, such as end-of-life treatments).
  - If ICUR <£20,000, the intervention is cost-effective and recommended.
  - If ICUR >£30,000, the intervention may not be cost-effective.
  - If ICUR is between £20,000 and £30,000, other factors (e.g. severity of disease, ethical considerations) are considered.

The sensitivity analysis tests how robust the results are by varying key assumptions (e.g. costs, QALY estimates, discount rate), and determines whether cost-effectiveness conclusions hold under different scenarios. Key assumptions (e.g. costs, QALY estimates, discount rate) are used to assess how sensitive the results are to these changes.

Present and Report Findings

- Clearly summarize results using tables, graphs, and text.
- Acknowledge limitations (e.g. uncertainty in utility values, variations in cost estimates).
- Provide policy recommendations based on findings.

Cost–Consequence Analysis

Cost–consequence analysis is an economic evaluation method that presents costs and multiple health outcomes separately, without combining them into a single measure (e.g. an ICER or cost per QALY). This approach allows decision-makers to consider different aspects of an intervention independently.

Example of CCA in Mental Health

A study compares CBT and medication for depression. Instead of summarizing results in a single cost-effectiveness ratio, CCA presents findings as shown in Table 13.3.

Table 13.3 Comparison of costs and multiple outcomes for CBT and medication in depression management

Outcome	CBT	Medication
Cost per patient (£)	800	500
Reduction in depression severity score	40%	30%
Side effects	Minimal	Moderate
Patient satisfaction	High	Moderate
Work productivity improvement	25%	15%

Advantages of CCA

- **Transparency:** provides a clear breakdown of multiple outcomes.
- **Flexibility:** allows different stakeholders (clinicians, policymakers, patients) to prioritize outcomes relevant to them.
- **Comprehensive decision-making:** useful when interventions impact various domains, such as quality of life, social factors, and healthcare utilization.

Limitations

- **Complexity in decision-making:** no single measure to guide choices, requiring subjective judgement.
- **Data interpretation challenges:** requires careful comparison of multiple factors rather than a straightforward cost-effectiveness ratio.

When to Use CCA

- When multiple outcomes are important for decision-making.
- When stakeholders prioritize different factors (e.g. cost, clinical efficacy, quality of life).
- When a single summary measure (e.g. cost per QALY) is not suitable.

Chapter Summary

Economic evaluation in healthcare involves assessing different types of costs:

- Direct costs: expenses directly linked to healthcare, including medical costs (hospitalization, medications, consultations) and non-medical costs (travel, accommodation).
- Indirect costs: economic losses due to reduced productivity, job loss, or caregiver burden.

- Intangible costs: psychological and emotional burdens on patients and families, such as distress or reduced QoL.
- Opportunity cost: the benefits lost when choosing one healthcare intervention over another, such as funding community therapy instead of inpatient care.

Health-related quality of life is measured using QALYs, often assessed through:

- Standard gamble: patients choose between staying in their current health state or taking a risk for potential perfect health.
- Time trade-off: patients decide how many years of life they would trade for improved health quality.

Economic evaluation methods in healthcare help assess the costs and benefits of different interventions. The primary approaches include:

- Cost-minimization analysis: compares costs of interventions with identical outcomes, choosing the cheaper option. For example, comparing two equally effective antidepressants and selecting the less expensive one.
- Cost–benefit analysis: converts both costs and benefits into monetary terms to assess whether an intervention is economically justified. For example, calculating the financial return of a suicide prevention programme based on reduced hospital admissions and increased productivity.
- Cost-effectiveness analysis: compares costs and health outcomes measured in natural units (e.g. life years gained, cases prevented) without converting benefits into monetary terms. For example, evaluating the cost per additional case of depression improved with CBT compared to standard care.
- Cost–utility analysis: a type of CEA that incorporates both quality and quantity of life, using QALYs as the outcome measure. For example, comparing two antipsychotics by calculating the cost per QALY gained.
- Cost–consequence analysis: evaluates healthcare interventions by presenting costs and multiple health outcomes separately, allowing decision-makers to assess different factors independently. It offers transparency, flexibility, and comprehensive decision-making when multiple outcomes are important. However, it can be complex and requires careful interpretation. It is useful when a single cost-effectiveness ratio (e.g. cost per QALY) is not appropriate.

Practice Questions

Q1. A healthcare organization is evaluating a new treatment for chronic pain. The treatment is expected to improve both the length and quality of patients' lives. Which economic evaluation method is most suitable for comparing this new treatment with the current standard care?

A. Cost-minimization analysis
B. Cost–benefit analysis
C. Cost-effectiveness analysis
D. Cost–utility analysis
E. Budget impact analysis

Q2. A mental health service is comparing two interventions for managing treatment-resistant depression. Intervention A involves weekly CBT sessions at a cost of £800 per patient per year, resulting in an average improvement of 0.6 QALYs per patient per year. Intervention B involves weekly CBT sessions combined with medication management by a psychiatrist, costing £1200 per patient per year, resulting in an average improvement of 0.8 QALYs per patient per year. What is the incremental cost–utility ratio of Intervention B compared to Intervention A?

A. £500 per QALY
B. £1,000 per QALY
C. £2,000 per QALY
D. £4,000 per QALY
E. £5,000 per QALY

Q3. In health economic evaluations, which technique is used to account for the difference in value between costs or benefits received today versus those received in the future?

A. Costing
B. Sensitivity analysis
C. Discounting
D. Marginal analysis
E. Budget impact analysis

Q4. In which of the following situations is cost-effectiveness analysis the most appropriate method of economic evaluation?

A. When the goal is to determine the most cost-effective way to improve a specific health outcome, measured in natural units (e.g. symptom-free days).
B. When both the quality and quantity of life are important dimensions of the health benefits.
C. When all costs and benefits, including non-health-related benefits, need to be expressed in monetary terms.
D. When comparing interventions that are assumed to have the same effectiveness to determine the lowest-cost option.
E. When evaluating a new intervention's overall economic impact on society, including indirect costs such as productivity loss.

Q5. A 45-year-old woman with bipolar disorder is unable to work due to frequent mood episodes. She requires ongoing psychiatric care and relies on her family for daily support. What type of cost is primarily associated with her condition?

A. Direct costs
B. Indirect costs
C. Incremental costs
D. Intangible costs
E. Opportunity costs

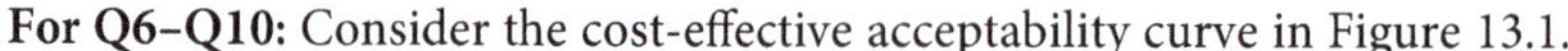

For Q6–Q10: Consider the cost-effective acceptability curve in Figure 13.1.

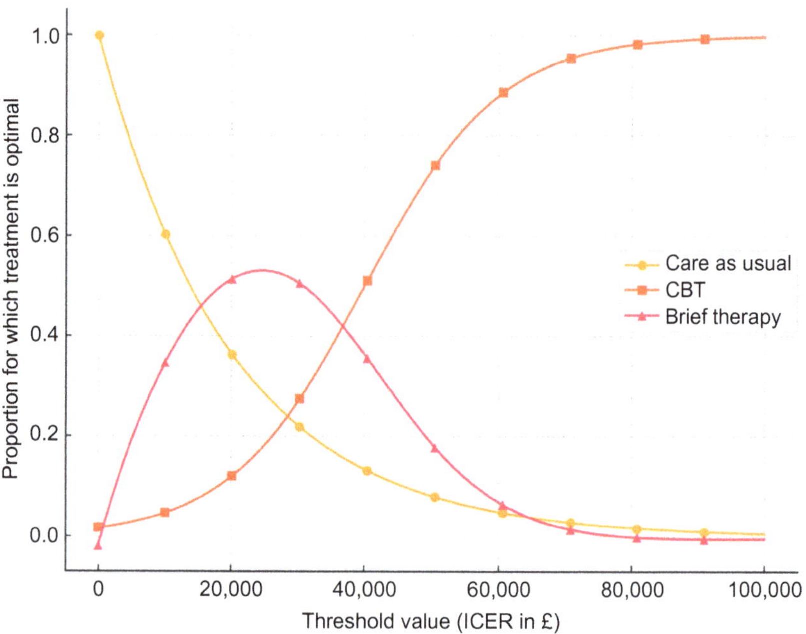

Figure 13.1 Cost-effectiveness acceptability curve comparing care as usual, CBT, and brief therapy across different willingness-to-pay thresholds (ICER in £).

Q6. At which threshold does care as usual have the highest probability of being optimal?

A. £0–£10,000
B. £10,000–£30,000
C. £30,000–£50,000
D. £50,000–£70,000
E. £70,000–£100,000

Q7. At which threshold does brief therapy reach its peak probability of being optimal?

A. £0–£10,000
B. £10,000–£30,000
C. £30,000–£50,000
D. £50,000–£70,000
E. £70,000–£100,000

Q8. NICE typically considers interventions cost-effective if they fall below a threshold of £20,000–£30,000 per QALY. At this threshold, which treatment is the most optimal?

A. Care as usual
B. CBT
C. Brief therapy

D. Equally split between CBT and brief therapy
E. No clear optimal treatment

Q9. Which of the following statements is most accurate based on the CEAC graph?
A. Care as usual remains the most optimal treatment across all threshold values.
B. CBT becomes the most cost-effective treatment after approximately £30,000 per QALY.
C. Brief therapy maintains the highest probability of being optimal even at higher ICER thresholds.
D. At ICER > £70,000, care as usual becomes the dominant option again.
E. At ICER = £50,000, all treatments have an equal probability of being optimal.

Q10. Which interpretation best describes the overall trend in the CEAC graph?
A. Care as usual is the best option regardless of willingness to pay.
B. CBT gradually becomes the dominant treatment as the ICER threshold increases.
C. Brief therapy is the most cost-effective treatment across all threshold values.
D. NICE should prioritize care as usual for cost-effectiveness.
E. At higher ICER thresholds, all treatments converge to the same probability.

Q11. Match the cost type with the correct description from the options in the two lists below.
1. A patient with schizophrenia requires long-term inpatient care. The cost of their medication, hospital stay, and psychiatrist consultations are accounted for in an economic analysis.
2. A new mental health intervention programme for PTSD is evaluated. The researchers calculate the additional cost of implementing this programme compared to standard care.
3. A healthcare provider considers using hospital beds for psychiatric patients instead of general medical patients. The economic analysis considers the value of the alternative use of these beds.
4. A study calculates the financial losses due to caregivers missing work while supporting a family member with dementia.
5. A policy change aims to improve mental health services for young adults. However, the emotional distress and stigma associated with untreated mental illness are factored into the overall burden.
6. A hospital is evaluating the cost of adding one additional bed in a psychiatric ward. The focus is on the cost of this single additional unit rather than the total programme cost.
7. An economic study examines the costs and health benefits of a new depression treatment, measuring outcomes in QALYs (quality-adjusted life years).
8. A study finds that two different SSRIs have identical effectiveness in treating depression. The analysis focuses solely on finding the cheapest option.
9. A healthcare economist analyses whether a new CBT intervention is cost-effective by comparing the additional cost per unit of health benefit (e.g. cases of depression prevented).
10. A researcher examines the long-term benefits of an early intervention psychosis programme and applies a lower weight to future costs and benefits.

A. Direct cost
B. Indirect cost
C. Intangible cost
D. Incremental cost
E. Marginal cost
F. Opportunity cost
G. Discounting
H. Cost–utility analysis
I. Cost-effectiveness analysis
J. Cost-minimization analysis

Answers

Q1. Correct answer: D. Cost-utility analysis. Uses QALYs, which combine both quantity and quality of life, making it ideal for this scenario.
Why the other options are incorrect:

A. Cost-minimization analysis is only appropriate when outcomes are equivalent, which isn't the case here.
B. Cost–benefit analysis measures outcomes in monetary terms, which might not fully capture the QoL improvements.
C. Cost-effectiveness analysis measures outcomes in natural units (e.g. life years gained), but doesn't incorporate QoL adjustments.
E. Budget impact analysis focuses on the financial impact on a budget, not the comparative effectiveness of interventions.

Q2. Correct answer: C. £2.000 per QALY. The incremental cost of Intervention B compared with Intervention A is:
Incremental cost: cost of intervention B – cost of intervention A
= £1200 – £800 = £400
Incremental QALYs: QALYs of intervention B – QALYs of intervention A
0.8 – 0.6 = 0.2 QALYs
ICUR: incremental cost / incremental QALYs
= £400 / 0.2 QALYs
= £2000 per QALYs

Q3. Correct answer: C. Discounting. This is the method used to adjust future costs and benefits to their present value.
Why the other options are incorrect:

A. Costing is the process of determining the expenses associated with a healthcare intervention.
B. Sensitivity analysis examines how results change when key assumptions or parameters are varied.
D. Marginal analysis examines the additional costs and benefits of a small change in input or output.

E. Budget impact analysis assesses the financial consequences of adopting a new intervention on a specific budget.

Q4. Correct answer: A. When the goal is to determine the most cost-effective way to improve a specific health outcome, measured in natural units (e.g. symptom-free days). Cost-effectiveness analysis is used when health benefits are measured in natural units (e.g. symptom-free days, life years gained, cases prevented) rather than monetary terms or QALYs. As CEA evaluates cost per unit of health improvement, it is ideal for assessing interventions based on natural health measures.
Why the other options are incorrect:

B. When both the quality and quantity of life are important dimensions of the health benefits. This describes cost-utility analysis, which uses QALYs.
C. When all costs and benefits, including non-health-related benefits, need to be expressed in monetary terms. This describes cost–benefit analysis, which converts all costs and benefits into monetary values.
D. When comparing interventions that are assumed to have the same effectiveness to determine the lowest-cost option. This describes cost-minimization analysis, which applies when two interventions have identical effectiveness and the goal is to find the cheaper option.
E. When evaluating a new intervention's overall economic impact on society, including indirect costs such as productivity loss. This is often used in cost–benefit analysis, which considers economic costs beyond direct healthcare expenses.

Q5. Correct answer: B. Indirect costs. Indirect costs refer to loss of productivity, lost wages, and the economic impact on caregivers due to illness. Since the patient is unable to work because of bipolar disorder, her condition results in lost income and reduced workforce participation, which are key components of indirect costs.
Why the other options are incorrect:

A. Direct costs include medical expenses such as psychiatric care, medication, and therapy. However, the question focuses on her inability to work, making indirect costs the better choice.
C. Incremental costs refer to additional costs incurred when introducing a new treatment compared to an existing one. This does not apply here.
D. Intangible costs cover pain, suffering, distress, and QoL reductions, which are relevant but not the primary focus of this question.
E. Opportunity costs involve forgone benefits from choosing one intervention over another (e.g. allocating healthcare resources differently). This question focuses on economic losses due to illness, which fall under indirect costs.

Q6. Correct answer A. £0–£10,000. Care as usual has the highest probability of being optimal at very low willingness-to-pay thresholds, because it is the least costly option. As the threshold increases, more expensive interventions (brief therapy and CBT) become more likely to be considered cost-effective, so the probability for care as usual declines.
Q7. Correct answer. B. £10,000–£30,000. Brief therapy reaches its highest probability in this range, before declining.

Q8. Correct answer: C. Brief therapy. At £20,000–£30,000, the CEAC graph shows that brief therapy has the highest probability of being the optimal treatment before CBT takes over at higher thresholds.

Q9. Correct answer: B. CBT becomes the most cost-effective treatment after approximately £30,000 per QALY. Care as usual is optimal at low ICER values; brief therapy dominates at mid-range values (~£20,000–£30,000); CBT becomes the most preferred treatment beyond £30,000 and continues to dominate as WTP increases. There is no point where all treatments are equally optimal at ICER = £50,000.

Q10. Correct answer. B. CBT gradually becomes the dominant treatment as the ICER threshold increases. Care as usual is only optimal at low ICER values; brief therapy is optimal at mid-range ICER values (~£20,000–£30,000); CBT takes over as the dominant cost-effective treatment at higher WTP thresholds.

Q11. The correct pairs are listed below:

1. A. Direct cost. Covers costs directly related to the provision of healthcare services, such as medications, hospital stays, and psychiatrist consultations.
2. D. Incremental cost. Measures the additional cost of implementing a new intervention compared to the existing standard care.
3. F. Opportunity cost. The value of the best alternative forgone – in this case, psychiatric beds could have been used for other medical patients.
4. B. Indirect cost. Indirect costs include productivity losses due to illness or caregiving responsibilities.
5. C. Intangible cost. Psychological and emotional burdens, such as stigma and distress, that are difficult to quantify financially.
6. E. Marginal cost. Refers to the additional cost of producing one more unit of service (e.g. adding one more hospital bed).
7. H. Cost–utility analysis. Measures outcomes in terms of both quantity and quality of life (e.g. QALYs).
8. J. Cost-minimization analysis. Used when interventions have equivalent outcomes, focusing only on cost differences.
9. I. Cost-effectiveness analysis. Evaluates the cost per unit of health benefit gained (e.g. cost per depression case improved).
10. G. Discounting. Applies a lower weight to future costs and benefits, as money has a time value.

Further Reading

Briggs AH, Claxton K, Sculpher MJ. *Decision Modelling for Health Economic Evaluation.* Oxford: Oxford University Press; 2006.

Dolan P. Modeling valuations for EuroQol health states. *Med Care.* 1997;**35**(11):1095–108. doi: https://doi.org/10.1097/00005650-199711000-00002.

Drummond MF, Sculpher MJ, Claxton K, Stoddart GL, Torrance GW. *Methods for the Economic Evaluation of Health Care Programmes.* 4th ed. Oxford: Oxford University Press; 2015.

EuroQol Group. EuroQol: a new facility for the measurement of health-related quality of life. *Health Policy.* 1990;**16**(3):199–208. doi: https://doi.org/10.1016/0168-8510(90)90421-9.

Fenwick E, Claxton K, Sculpher M. Representing uncertainty: the role of cost-effectiveness acceptability curves. *Health Econ.* 2001;**10**(8): 779–87. doi: https://doi.org/10.1002/hec.635.

Gold MR, Siegel JE, Russell LB, Weinstein MC, eds. *Cost-Effectiveness in Health and Medicine*. New York: Oxford University Press; 1996.

National Institute for Health and Care Excellence (NICE). *Guide to the Methods of Technology Appraisal 2013*. London: NICE; 2013. Available from: www.nice.org.uk/process/pmg9.

National Institute for Health and Care Excellence (NICE). *NICE Health Technology Evaluations: The Manual*. London: NICE; 2022. Available from: www.nice.org.uk/process/pmg36.

Neumann PJ, Ganiats TG, Russell LB, Sanders GD, Siegel JE, eds. *Cost-Effectiveness in Health and Medicine*. 2nd ed. Oxford: Oxford University Press; 2016.

Torrance GW. Measurement of health state utilities for economic appraisal: a review. *J Health Econ*. 1986;**5**(1):1–30. doi: https://doi.org/10.1016/0167-6296(86)90020-2.

Weinstein MC, Stason WB. Foundations of cost-effectiveness analysis for health and medical practices. *N Engl J Med*. 1977;**296**(13):716–21. doi: https://doi.org/10.1056/NEJM197703312961304.

Chapter 14

Qualitative Studies

Introduction

Qualitative studies play a crucial role in psychiatry by exploring the subjective experiences, perceptions, attitudes, and beliefs of patients, carers, healthcare providers, and other stakeholders. Unlike quantitative research, which focuses on numerical data and statistical analysis, qualitative research seeks to understand the 'why' and 'how' behind health-related behaviours, decisions, and outcomes. It provides in-depth insights into complex phenomena that cannot be easily quantified.

These studies involve the collection and analysis of non-numerical data (textual or visual) and typically have small sample sizes but offer high levels of detail and contextual richness. The analysis in qualitative research is interpretative and thematic rather than statistical.

Qualitative studies can be used in conjunction with quantitative research to:

- generate hypotheses and develop theories to explain psychiatric phenomena
- explore research questions at the preliminary stage of large-scale studies
- develop or refine research instruments or assessment scales
- enhance the interpretation and contextualization of findings from quantitative studies
- identify unexpected findings or anomalies in trial outcomes
- assess the coherence, acceptability, and cultural validity of quantitative research.

Sampling Techniques in Qualitative Studies

Unlike quantitative research, qualitative studies do not aim for statistical representativeness but rather focus on depth of understanding and meaning. Sampling is typically purposeful, allowing researchers to select participants who can provide rich, relevant, and diverse perspectives on the research topic.

In this section, different sampling methods used in qualitative research are discussed.

Convenience Sampling

- Participants are selected based on their availability and willingness to participate.
- This method is useful when time, resources, or access to participants are limited.
- Example: interviewing psychiatric outpatients who are available during clinic hours to explore their experiences with anxiety management.

Purposive (Judgement) Sampling

- Researchers intentionally select participants based on their specific knowledge, experience, or characteristics related to the study topic.
- This method ensures information-rich cases that provide deep insights into a phenomenon.
- Example: selecting patients who have undergone electroconvulsive therapy for severe depression.

Types of Purposive Sampling

- **Maximum variation sampling:** participants with widely differing characteristics are selected to capture diverse experiences and identify common patterns.
- **Deviant (extreme) case sampling:** selecting outliers or unusual cases to understand exceptional circumstances.
- **Critical case sampling:** choosing participants with experiences that are crucial to the study (e.g. interviewing crisis team staff about psychiatric emergency interventions).
- **Key informant sampling:** interviewing experts or individuals with specialized knowledge, such as senior psychiatrists, psychologists, or mental health advocates, to gain deeper insights into service delivery or treatment implementation challenges.

During data interpretation, researchers may also use:

- **Confirming sampling:** selecting participants who support emerging explanations or theories.
- **Disconfirming sampling:** selecting participants who challenge emerging themes, helping to test and refine interpretations.

Quota Sampling

- Researchers divide the population into subgroups and ensure that a predefined number of participants are selected from each group.
- This method ensures diversity across key demographic characteristics.
- Example: including equal numbers of male and female participants across different age groups in a study on mental illness stigma.

Criterion Sampling

- Participants are selected based on specific predefined criteria relevant to the research question.
- This method is useful for targeting specific conditions or experiences.
- Example: selecting only individuals diagnosed with post-traumatic stress disorder (PTSD) for a study on trauma-focused therapy.

Homogeneous Sampling

- Participants are selected based on shared characteristics or experiences to deeply explore a specific subgroup.
- Useful when studying a narrow and well-defined population.

- Example: interviewing adolescent females with eating disorders to explore their unique challenges in recovery.

Snowball Sampling

- Used for recruiting hard-to-reach or marginalized populations.
- Existing participants refer or recruit others with similar experiences, creating a 'snowball effect'.
- Example: recruiting sex workers or individuals with substance misuse disorders by asking current participants to suggest others.

Theoretical Sampling

- Participants are selected iteratively to refine emerging theories.
- Commonly used in **grounded theory**[1] methodology, where data collection and analysis occur simultaneously.
- Example: interviewing individuals with bipolar disorder at different stages of illness to refine a theory on coping mechanisms.

Comparison of Sampling Techniques in Qualitative Studies

Table 14.1 compares key sampling techniques used in qualitative studies, providing descriptions, applications in psychiatry, and illustrative examples.

Table 14.1 Comparison of sampling techniques in qualitative studies

Sampling technique	Description	Use in psychiatry	Example
Purposive Sampling	Selecting participants based on specific criteria or experiences	Exploring targeted experiences	Patients with experience of ECT for severe depression
Snowball sampling	Participants recruit future participants through their networks	Reaching marginalized or hard-to-access groups	Engaging individuals with substance use disorders
Convenience sampling	Choosing participants who are readily available	When resources or time are limited	Interviewing patients attending a psychiatry outpatient clinic
Theoretical sampling	Participants are selected to refine emerging theories	Developing theories through grounded theory research	Developing a theory on coping strategies in bipolar disorder
Quota sampling	Ensuring representation of specific subgroups	Balancing representation of demographics or traits	Including different age groups in a study on mental health stigma
Criterion sampling	Selecting participants who meet predefined criteria	Focusing on specific characteristics or diagnoses	Including only PTSD patients in a therapy evaluation study

[1] **Grounded theory:** An inductive qualitative method that develops theory from data through iterative coding and constant comparison. Sampling is often theoretical and continues until saturation.

Table 14.1 (cont.)

Sampling technique	Description	Use in psychiatry	Example
Maximum variation sampling	Capturing a broad range of experiences and perspectives	Understanding patterns across varied contexts	Studying schizophrenia with participants at different symptom levels
Homogeneous sampling	Selecting participants with similar characteristics	Deep exploration of specific subgroups	Focusing on adolescent females with eating disorders

Data Collection Methods in Qualitative Studies

In qualitative research, data collection methods are designed to explore deep insights, rich descriptions, and complex understandings of human experiences, behaviours, and social phenomena. These methods prioritize open-ended, non-numerical data, allowing participants to express their thoughts, feelings, and experiences in their own words. In this section, key data collection methods used in qualitative research are described.

Interviews

Interviews involve one-on-one conversations between the researcher and the participant, focusing on specific topics related to the research question. They can range from structured to unstructured, with semi-structured interviews being the most commonly used in qualitative research.

Interviews can be categorized as four different types:

- Structured interviews:
  - The researcher follows a predetermined set of questions in a fixed order for every participant.
  - Many questions are close-ended (e.g. multiple-choice, yes/no).
  - Ensures consistency across interviews and minimizes researcher bias.
  - Limitations: limited flexibility, which may restrict participants from providing in-depth responses.
  - Example: a researcher asks patients a standardized set of questions about medication adherence.

- Semi-structured interviews:
  - The researcher prepares a set of open-ended questions but allows flexibility to explore new topics that arise during the conversation.
  - Encourages a more natural and conversational flow.
  - Allows probing deeper into participants' responses.
  - Example: exploring the lived experiences of individuals with bipolar disorder and allowing the conversation to evolve naturally.

- Unstructured interviews:
  - The interviewer begins with a broad topic and lets the conversation evolve naturally.
  - The participant has greater control over the direction of the discussion.

  - Particularly useful for exploratory research where the researcher aims to gain a broad understanding of a phenomenon.
  - Example: understanding coping mechanisms used in daily life by individuals with schizophrenia.

- In-depth interviews:
  - A form of semi-structured or unstructured interview that aims to obtain detailed personal accounts of participants' experiences.
  - Conducted in a one-on-one setting, allowing for personalized exploration of the topic.
  - Requires advanced interviewer skills to build rapport and encourage participants to share openly.
  - Example: interviewing individuals who have recovered from major depressive disorder to understand their recovery journey.
  - Challenges of in-depth interviews include:

    Requirement for skilled interviewers to guide discussions effectively.

    Time-consuming data analysis due to large volumes of narrative data.

    Limited generalizability due to small sample sizes.

    Conducting and transcribing interviews is resource-intensive.

Focus Groups

Focus groups involve a small group of participants (typically 6–10) who discuss a specific topic or issue together. A moderator facilitates the discussion, ensuring that it remains focused and balanced, allowing all participants to contribute.

Key Features of Focus Groups

- Group interaction allows participants to build on each other's ideas.
- Provides insights into shared experiences and differences in perspectives.
- Useful for exploring social norms, attitudes, and collective beliefs.

Advantages of Focus Groups

Rich data: the group dynamic generates deeper discussions than individual interviews.

Diverse perspectives: brings together people with different backgrounds and experiences.

Interactive: participants feel more comfortable engaging in discussion-based research.

Cost-effective: a more efficient way to collect data from multiple participants simultaneously.

Examples of a Focus Group in Psychiatry

- **Exploring mental health stigma:** a focus group consisting of patients, caregivers, and healthcare providers discusses perceptions of stigma surrounding schizophrenia.
- **Evaluating a new therapy intervention:** a focus group of psychotherapists shares their experiences of using cognitive behavioural therapy (CBT) for PTSD.

Challenges of Focus Groups

- Dominant participants may overshadow quieter individuals, affecting data quality.
- The discussion can be steered off-topic, requiring strong moderation.
- Confidentiality concerns may limit disclosure of sensitive issues.

Observation

Observation is a key data collection method in qualitative research, where the researchers systematically examine behaviours, interactions, and contexts within real-world settings. Unlike interviews or focus groups, observations allow researchers to capture actual behaviour rather than reported behaviour.

Types of Observation

Participant Observation

- In participant observation, researchers actively engage in the environment while maintaining an analytical and reflexive stance.
- This approach provides insider perspectives and a deeper understanding of social processes but it requires careful balancing between participation and objectivity.
- Example: researchers spend several weeks on an inpatient psychiatric ward, actively engaging with patients and staff during daily activities. By participating in ward routines and observing patient–staff interactions, researchers gain insights into treatment adherence, ward culture, and interpersonal dynamics.

Non-Participant Observation

- In non-participant observation, the researchers remain detached observers, minimizing interaction with participants in order to reduce their influence on behaviour.
- This is useful in settings where observer presence could affect natural behaviour.
- Example: researchers observe interactions in outpatient psychiatry waiting area (with ethical approval and patient consent) to observe non-verbal cues such as body language, signs of anxiety, patient interactions with staff, and the impact of the clinical environment on patient engagement.

Overt Observation

- Participants are aware they are being observed. While this promotes transparency and ethical integrity, it may result in the **Hawthorne effect**,[2] where individuals alter their behaviour when they know they are being observed.
- Example: psychiatrists or researchers observe psychotherapy sessions, taking notes on therapeutic alliance, communication patterns, and patient responses with both the patients and therapists aware of the observers' role.

[2] **Hawthorne effect:** Behaviour change caused simply by awareness of being observed; typically wanes with prolonged observation or habituation.

Covert Observation

- In covert observation, researchers observe without revealing their role to participants. Although this can yield more natural behaviour, it raises significant ethical concerns regarding consent and privacy and is therefore rarely used in clinical research.
- Example: researchers analyse pre-recorded group therapy sessions, where participants had previously given consent for recordings to be used for research purposes, focusing on spontaneous interactions and emotional expression.

Methods of Data Collection in Observations

Field Notes

- Researchers systematically record observations related to the setting, behaviours, and contextual details. Field notes may include direct quotations, descriptions of non-verbal behaviour, and reflective comments to aid interpretation.

Structured Observation

- Researchers use predefined checklists or rating scales to systematically record specific behaviours. This approach increases consistency and is useful in clinical or evaluative settings.
- Example: researchers assess eye contact, speech patterns, and affect during psychiatric assessments using a structured observation schedule.

Unstructured Observation

- Researchers record detailed, free-form notes without predefined categories, allowing a holistic and flexible account of the environment and interactions. This approach is common in ethnographic research.
- Example: researchers spend time in a community mental health centre, documenting how staff and patients interact, how treatment is delivered, and how individuals engage with services.

Challenges of Observation Method

Observer Bias

- The researchers' own perceptions and expectations may influence how behaviours are interpreted.
- Mitigation strategy: use multiple observers, reflexive journaling, or structured coding frameworks.

Hawthorne Effect

- Participants may alter their behaviour when they know they are being observed.
- Mitigation strategy: prolonged observation periods allow participants to become accustomed and adjust to the researchers' presence and act more naturally.

Time-Consuming Process

- Observation requires substantial time for data collection transcription, coding, and analysis.

- Mitigation strategy: clearly define a clear research question to focus observations and limit unnecessary data collection.

Ethical Considerations in Observational Research

- **Informed consent:** participants must be aware of observation unless observing behaviour in public settings where consent is not required.
- **Privacy and confidentiality:** researchers must protect participant identities and ensure data are securely stored.
- **Minimizing harm:** observations should be non-intrusive and must not interfere with clinical care or participant wellbeing.

Role-Play

Role-play is an interactive data collection method in which participants act out specific scenarios relevant to the research topic. This approach allows researchers to observe how individuals behave and interact in different contexts, offering insights into attitudes, beliefs, and decision-making processes. Role-play is particularly useful for exploring social dynamics and power relationships within various settings, such as workplaces, families, or communities. By examining how participants portray different roles, researchers can uncover underlying perspectives and assumptions associated with those roles or situations.

In addition to understanding behaviour, role-play can be used to test interventions or training programmes by assessing how participants apply new knowledge or skills in simulated scenarios. For example, a psychiatrist can engage in role-play sessions where trained standardized patients simulate clinical consultations, such as a patient expressing reluctance to take prescribed medication due to concerns about side effects. This method provides a structured yet flexible approach to evaluating communication skills and clinical decision-making.

Diary Methods

Diary methods involve participants keeping a written record of their thoughts, feelings, experiences, and behaviours over a specified period. These diaries provide rich qualitative insights into how individuals experience the world around them. Diaries may be structured, semi-structured, or unstructured, depending on the level of guidance provided to participants.

Structured diaries contain predefined prompts or questions, ensuring consistency in data collection, whereas semi-structured and unstructured diaries allow participants more freedom to document their experiences in their own words. This method is particularly valuable for capturing longitudinal changes, providing researchers with detailed narratives that might be difficult to obtain through interviews or surveys alone.

Document Analysis

Document analysis is the systematic review and interpretation of existing documents, such as medical records, policy documents, diaries, letters, emails, meeting minutes, and historical texts. This method provides contextual insights, historical understanding, and supplementary data that support findings from other qualitative research methods.

For example, researchers may analyse therapy session notes to explore treatment progress and patient–therapist interactions. Document analysis can also be used to triangulate findings from interviews and observations, enhancing the validity of research conclusions.

Case Studies

The case study method involves an in-depth exploration of a single case or a small number of related cases to understand a phenomenon within its real-life context. Case studies provide a holistic perspective, integrating various sources of data, including interviews, observations, and document analysis.

For example, a researcher may conduct a case study of a patient with a rare psychiatric disorder to examine treatment challenges and therapeutic outcomes. This method is particularly useful for capturing complex, nuanced experiences that may not be adequately addressed through broader quantitative studies.

Narrative Inquiry

Narrative inquiry focuses on collecting and analysing personal stories, life histories, or narratives to explore how individuals make sense of their experiences. This approach emphasizes the storytelling aspect of human experience, considering both the content of the narratives and the meanings derived from them.

For instance, analysing the life stories of trauma survivors can provide insights into how individuals reconstruct their identities following adverse experiences. Narrative inquiry is particularly valuable for understanding subjective experiences and how people attribute meaning to key life events.

Ethnography

Ethnography is an immersive research approach that involves long-term engagement in a cultural or social setting to observe behaviours, interactions, and practices. This method provides contextual and cultural insights by capturing lived experiences within their natural environment.

For example, ethnographic research in a residential mental health facility may explore daily routines, support systems, and staff–patient interactions to better understand the lived experience of individuals receiving care.

A key component of ethnographic research is ethnographic interviewing, which focuses on exploring cultural, social, and experiential dimensions within a group or community. Unlike structured interviews, ethnographic interviews are open-ended and conversational, allowing for deeper exploration of participants' perspectives. They typically involve:

- open-ended questions to encourage detailed responses
- interactive dialogue to foster engagement
- probing follow-up questions and prompts to clarify or expand on key themes
- a semi-structured format, with key themes guiding the discussion while allowing for flexibility.

Ethnographic methods are particularly useful for capturing unspoken norms, rituals, and belief systems that shape behaviour within a particular context.

Table 14.2 summarizes the main qualitative data collection methods, highlighting their descriptions, strengths, and examples of application in psychiatric research.

Table 14.2 Qualitative data collection methods

Method	Description	Strengths	Example of use in psychiatry
Interviews	One-on-one conversations to explore personal experiences	In-depth insights, flexibility	Interviewing patients with bipolar disorder about treatment experiences
Focus groups	Group discussions facilitated by a moderator	Captures group dynamics, diverse perspectives	Exploring caregivers' challenges in dementia care
Observations	Watching and recording behaviours in natural settings	Provides contextual understanding and real-world insights	Observing interactions in a psychiatric ward
Document analysis	Reviewing existing documents to extract information	Useful for contextual and historical insights	Analysing therapy session notes for treatment progress
Case studies	In-depth exploration of specific cases.	Combines multiple data sources, detailed analysis	Studying a patient with a rare mental health condition
Narrative inquiry	Analysing personal stories to understand experiences	Captures personal meaning and identity processes	Collecting narratives from trauma survivors
Ethnography	Immersing in a culture to observe behaviours and practices	Provides rich cultural and contextual data	Understanding social dynamics in a mental health community setting

Iterative Approach

The iterative approach in qualitative research is a cyclical process in which data collection, analysis, and reflection occur repeatedly throughout the study. Rather than following a linear sequence, researchers continuously refine their research questions, sampling strategies, and methods based on emerging insights.

Early data analysis informs subsequent data collection, leading to modifications in interview questions, observation focus, or participant selection. This flexibility allows researchers to respond to unexpected findings and refine their theoretical framework as the study progresses, making it particularly valuable in exploratory research.

Iteration continues until new data no longer reveal significant insights, indicating that data **saturation**[3] has been reached. Methods such as grounded theory and ethnography

[3] **Saturation (data/theoretical):** Point where further data add no new codes/themes (data saturation) or no new theoretical insights to the evolving model (theoretical saturation); used to judge when to stop sampling.

heavily rely on the iterative process to develop a rich, contextual understanding of the subject matter.

Grounded Theory

Grounded theory is a systematic qualitative research methodology that focuses on generating theories directly from data rather than starting with a preconceived hypothesis. Researchers collect data and analyse it inductively, allowing patterns, themes, and theoretical concepts to emerge based on participants' perspectives.

This methodology follows an inductive approach, ensuring that theories develop from the data itself, rather than being imposed externally. A key feature of grounded theory is its iterative process, where data collection and analysis occur concurrently, with each phase informing the other in a continuous cycle.

The process of theoretical sampling guides the selection of new participants or data sources based on emerging theoretical needs, ensuring that the developing theory remains relevant and grounded in the data. Theoretical saturation is reached when no new insights or categories emerge, marking the completion of data analysis.

Methods of Data Analysis

Qualitative data analysis involves systematically examining non-numerical data such as text, audio, or video to identify patterns, themes, and meanings. Various methods exist, each with a distinct approach and focus. Below are some of the primary methods used in qualitative research.

Thematic Analysis

Thematic analysis is one of the most widely used methods for identifying, analysing, and reporting patterns (themes) within qualitative data. It involves a systematic process that typically includes:

- becoming familiar with the data
- generating initial codes
- searching for potential themes
- reviewing and refining themes
- defining, naming, and reporting themes.

This approach is highly flexible, as it can be applied across different epistemological and theoretical frameworks, making it suitable for a wide range of disciplines. It is particularly effective for exploring *commonalities*, *differences*, and *complexities* in experiences, behaviours, or opinions, while still allowing for rich, detailed descriptions of the data.

Content Analysis

Content analysis[4] is a systematic method for organizing and interpreting textual, visual, or audio data. It involves coding material into categories – which may be predefined

[4] **Content analysis:** A systematic approach to categorizing and quantifying textual or visual data to identify patterns. It may use deductive (predefined) or inductive (emergent) coding.

(deductive) or emerge from the data itself (inductive) – to identify patterns, frequencies, and relationships.

While often used to *quantify content* (e.g. how often a theme or word appears), content analysis also enables researchers to interpret meanings and contexts, bridging both quantitative and qualitative approaches.

This method is especially valuable for analysing large datasets, such as social media posts, interviews, media reports, or policy documents, where it can reveal trends, highlight dominant discourses, or uncover hidden assumptions.

Narrative Analysis

Narrative analysis focuses on the stories people tell and the ways in which these stories are structured and conveyed. It examines both the *content* (what is said) and the *form* (how it is said), exploring how individuals construct meaning and identity through storytelling. Key elements such as *plot, characters, sequencing*, and *context* are analysed to understand how experiences are framed and interpreted.

Narrative analysis is particularly valuable for research that seeks to capture personal experiences within broader cultural or social contexts. It highlights not only what happened, but also *why and how people choose to tell their stories in a particular way*. This makes it especially useful in fields such as psychology, sociology, education, and health research.

Discourse Analysis

Discourse analysis is a qualitative method that examines how language is used in texts, conversations, or other forms of communication to construct meanings, shape social realities, and reinforce or challenge power dynamics. Unlike **content analysis**, which emphasizes *what* is said, discourse analysis also explores *how* it is said, including the structure of language, tone, context, and the social or political functions of speech.

Researchers using discourse analysis often focus on:

- **Word choice and framing:** how certain terms (e.g. 'immigrant' vs 'migrant') carry different social or political connotations.
- **Context and setting:** how meaning shifts depending on who is speaking, to whom, and in what situation.
- **Power and ideology:** how language reflects or reproduces power relations, authority, or social norms.

Example: analysing media coverage of mental health might reveal whether language frames individuals as 'patients in need of care' versus 'risks to society', highlighting how discourse can shape public attitudes and policy.

Phenomenological Analysis

Phenomenological analysis seeks to explore and describe the *lived experiences* of individuals, with the goal of capturing the *essence* of a phenomenon as it is perceived by those who have experienced it. This method emphasizes understanding *subjective meaning* rather than producing objective explanations.

Researchers typically:

- engage in **bracketing,**[5] setting aside their own assumptions to minimize bias
- collect detailed personal accounts, often through in-depth interviews
- identify recurring themes that reflect shared aspects of experience
- focus on how participants interpret and make sense of their world.

This approach is widely used in health, psychology, and social sciences, where insight into personal and subjective perspectives is essential.

Framework Analysis

Framework analysis employs a *matrix-based approach* to organize and interpret qualitative data systematically. Data are charted into a framework of *key themes* and *sub-themes,* which enables researchers to make structured comparisons across participants, cases, or groups. Key steps usually include:

- familiarization with the data
- identifying a thematic framework, often informed by research objectives or questions
- indexing or coding the data against the framework
- charting, where data are summarized and entered into a matrix
- mapping and interpretation, allowing researchers to identify patterns, relationships, and explanations.

This method is particularly useful in *applied policy research* or studies with predefined objectives, where both depth and systematic organization of data are required. Unlike purely inductive approaches, framework analysis accommodates both *pre-set aims* and *emergent themes.*

Grounded Theory Analysis

Grounded theory is an inductive approach designed to generate theory that emerges directly from the data rather than testing pre-existing hypotheses. Researchers move iteratively between data collection and analysis to refine emerging concepts. The method typically involves:

- **Open coding:** breaking down data into discrete parts and identifying initial concepts.
- **Axial coding:** linking concepts into categories and exploring relationships between them.
- **Selective coding:** integrating categories around a central theme to build a coherent theoretical framework.

A hallmark of grounded theory is the use of *constant comparison* – each piece of data is continually compared with others to refine categories and test emerging ideas.

Grounded theory is especially well-suited for exploratory research, where the goal is to build new theoretical insights into social processes, behaviours, or experiences. It is widely applied in sociology, psychology, health research, and organizational studies.

[5] **Bracketing:** Temporarily setting aside the researcher's preconceptions (epoché) to minimize their influence during data collection and analysis; common in phenomenology and supported by reflexive memos.

Interpretative Phenomenological Analysis

Interpretative phenomenological analysis (IPA) is a qualitative approach that explores how individuals perceive, interpret, and make sense of their personal and social experiences. It goes beyond describing lived experience to examine the *subjective meaning-making process*, recognizing that both participant and researcher play a role in interpreting the data (a '**double hermeneutic**').[6]

Interpretative phenomenological analysis provides rich, detailed accounts of individual experiences and is particularly suited for exploring significant life events – such as illness, trauma, or identity changes – where understanding personal meaning is central. It is most widely applied in psychological and health research, but its use has expanded into education and social sciences.

Constant Comparative Method

The constant comparative method is an iterative process of continuously comparing data segments – such as incidents, events, or statements – to refine codes, develop categories, and identify emerging patterns. While it is a core component of grounded theory, it can also be applied independently in thematic or content analysis to strengthen rigour.

Through repeated comparison, researchers ensure that categories evolve directly from the data and remain sensitive to new insights. For example, if multiple interviewees express a sense of 'feeling overwhelmed', these instances may be grouped and refined into a broader category of stress or emotional burden.

By cycling between new data and existing categories, the constant comparative method produces findings that are both systematic and grounded in the dataset as a whole, ensuring depth, consistency, and credibility.

Table 14.3 provides a summary of major qualitative data analysis methods, outlining their descriptions, key features, and typical applications.

Table 14.3 Qualitative data analysis methods

Method	Description	Key features	Usage/ applications
Thematic analysis	Identification and analysis of patterns or themes within qualitative data	Coding data and grouping codes into broader themes	Exploring common experiences, behaviours, or opinions in various fields
Content analysis	Systematic categorization and quantification of textual information	Coding text into predetermined or emergent categories; frequency counts	Analysing large volumes of text (e.g. media, policy documents, social media)

[6] **Double hermeneutic (IPA):** Two-stage meaning-making: participants interpret their experiences, and the researcher interprets those interpretations; acknowledges co-construction of findings.

Table 14.3 (cont.)

Method	Description	Key features	Usage/ applications
Narrative analysis	Focus on the stories people tell and the structure of these narratives	Examining plot, characters, and context within personal narratives	Studying personal experiences, life histories, and storytelling in various contexts
Discourse analysis	Examination of language use and communication to understand social realities and power dynamics	Analysing language structure, context, and the implications of communication	Media studies, political communication, and research on social interactions
Grounded theory analysis	Developing theory inductively from the data itself	Iterative coding (open, axial, selective), constant comparative analysis, and theoretical sampling	Exploratory research to generate new theoretical insights across disciplines
Phenomenological analysis	Exploration of lived experiences to capture the essence of a phenomenon	Deep, reflective analysis of personal narratives to understand core experiences	Health, psychology, and studies focusing on personal experiences
Framework analysis	Systematic, matrix-based method for organizing and analysing qualitative data	Charting data into matrices for comparison across cases and themes	Applied policy research and studies with predefined research questions
Interpretative phenomenological analysis (IPA)	Focus on how individuals make sense of their personal and social experiences	Detailed, interpretative examination of personal meaning-making processes (double hermeneutic)	Psychological and health research exploring individual perceptions and experiences
Constant comparative method	Continuous comparison of data segments to refine categories and identify patterns	Iterative comparison of data to ensure emerging categories are robust and comprehensive	Integral to grounded theory; used to enhance thematic or content analysis

Strategies to Enhance the Trustworthiness and Rigour of Qualitative Research

Ensuring trustworthiness and rigour in qualitative research is essential for producing credible and meaningful findings. The following strategies enhance the credibility, dependability, confirmability, and transparency of qualitative research.

Reflexivity

Reflexivity is the process by which researchers continuously examine and acknowledge their own assumptions, values, and potential biases throughout the research process. It emphasizes self-awareness, recognizing that the researcher is not a neutral, detached observer but an active participant whose background, beliefs, and interactions can shape the study.

Common reflexive practices include:

- keeping reflective journals to document thoughts, reactions, and potential biases

- explicitly stating positionality (e.g. cultural, social, or professional background)[7]
- documenting methodological and analytical decision-making.

By making these influences transparent, reflexivity not only deepens the researcher's understanding of the process, but also enhances the credibility and trustworthiness of the findings, enabling readers to judge how interpretations may have been shaped.

Bracketing

Bracketing is a specific technique, most often associated with phenomenological research, in which researchers deliberately attempt to set aside or 'suspend' their preconceptions, assumptions, and prior knowledge while engaging with participants' data. The goal is to minimize the intrusion of the researcher's worldview and focus instead on how participants themselves experience and describe a phenomenon.

Bracketing typically involves consciously identifying personal assumptions before data collection and consciously striving not to allow these assumptions to influence interviews, coding, or interpretation. While reflexivity acknowledges and documents the researcher's influence, bracketing seeks to temporarily reduce or neutralize that influence during analysis.

Table 14.4 highlights the distinctions between reflexivity and bracketing across definition, purpose, process, application, and outcomes.

Table 14.4 Distinction between reflexivity and bracketing in qualitative research

Aspect	Reflexivity	Bracketing
Definition	Ongoing self-examination by the researcher regarding their own assumptions, values, and potential biases throughout the research process	The deliberate process of setting aside or 'putting in brackets' the researcher's preconceptions to view data as objectively as possible
Purpose	To acknowledge, document, and account for the influence of the researcher's perspective on the study	To minimize the influence of the researcher's pre-existing beliefs and biases during data collection and analysis
Process	A continuous, reflective practice integrated throughout all stages of research (design, data collection, analysis, and interpretation)	A specific, often initial step – particularly in phenomenological research – aimed at suspending judgements and assumptions
Application	Employed continuously, with researchers regularly revisiting and questioning their influence on the study	Applied mainly during the early stages of data collection and analysis to ensure an open, unbiased engagement with the data
Outcome	Greater transparency in how personal views may shape the research, contributing to the study's credibility	A more focused and neutral analysis, as researchers aim to 'bracket' their prior understanding to better capture participants' perspectives

[7] **Positionality:** The researcher's social/professional location (e.g. gender, culture, role) and standpoint; making it explicit helps readers judge potential influence on data collection/interpretation (links to reflexivity).

Triangulation

Triangulation enhances the credibility and trustworthiness of qualitative research by using multiple sources, methods, or perspectives to validate findings. By examining a phenomenon from different angles, triangulation reduces bias and increases validity.

The main types of triangulation include:

- **Data triangulation:** using multiple sources of data, such as interviews, observations, and documents, to gain a comprehensive understanding.
- **Method triangulation:** employing different research methods, such as interviews and focus groups, to explore the same phenomenon.
- **Investigator triangulation:** involving multiple researchers in the data collection and analysis process to introduce diverse perspectives.
- **Theory triangulation:** applying multiple theoretical frameworks to interpret the data.

For example, researchers studying workplace culture might use data triangulation by collecting data through employee interviews, workplace observations, and analysis of company policies.

Member Checking

Member checking (also called participant validation) is a technique used to enhance the credibility and validity of qualitative research findings by involving participants directly in the process of analysis and interpretation. In simple terms, it allows participants to 'check back' with the researcher to confirm whether their views, experiences, and meanings have been accurately captured.

This process can involve reviewing interview transcripts, summaries, codes, or preliminary findings. Participants then provide feedback on their accuracy and resonance.

The benefits include:

- Validates findings by confirming their accuracy.
- Reduces misinterpretations that may result from researcher bias or assumptions.
- Strengthens participant involvement, giving them a sense of ownership in how their narratives are represented.

The limitations include:

- Participants may feel pressured to agree with the researcher's interpretation.
- Practical constraints arise if participants have limited time, interest, or availability.
- Some argue it may not always guarantee validity, since participants' views may evolve over time.

Peer Debriefing

Peer debriefing is a strategy used to enhance the credibility and trustworthiness of qualitative research by involving colleagues or experts who are not directly involved in the research. Unlike member checking, which involves participants, peer debriefing draws on external peers to provide external critical perspective of the researcher's methods, analysis, and interpretations.

Through open discussion, peers can:

- challenge assumptions and highlight potential blind spots
- question the consistency of coding and thematic development
- suggest alternative interpretations that the researcher may not have considered
- help identify areas where personal bias or over-interpretation may have influenced analysis.

Auditing

Auditing is a quality assurance process involving the systematic and independent examination of the research process and outputs to assess their trustworthiness and rigour. An audit is typically conducted by an independent reviewer, to ensure transparency and methodological coherence.

The auditing process may involve reviewing:

- raw data (e.g. interview transcripts, field notes)
- analytical decisions (e.g. coding frameworks, thematic development)
- final interpretations to verify that they are grounded in the data.

Constant Comparison

Constant comparison is an iterative analytical technique, most commonly used in grounded theory, to develop and refine interpretations and theories directly from the data. It involves systematically comparing different segments of data – such as codes, categories, or themes – throughout the research process.

By continuously comparing data, researchers can:

- identify patterns, similarities, and differences
- refine emerging categories
- develop robust theoretical constructs that are firmly grounded in the data.

Neutral and Indirect Questioning Techniques

Neutral and indirect questioning techniques are strategies used in qualitative interviews to encourage participants to share their views openly while minimizing the risk of bias or discomfort.

- **Neutral questioning** involves phrasing questions in a balanced, non-leading way so participants are not steered toward a particular answer. Example: instead of asking, 'Did you find the service helpful?', a neutral version would be, 'How did you find the service?'
- **Indirect questioning** uses open-ended, scenario-based, or third-person prompts to explore sensitive issues more safely. Example: asking, 'Some people in your situation feel anxious – how do you think others might cope?' allows participants to reflect without feeling personally exposed.

These techniques reduce social desirability bias and help capture more authentic, nuanced accounts, especially when discussing sensitive or complex topics.

Table 14.5 outlines key techniques for reducing bias in qualitative research, with their definitions and intended outcomes.

Table 14.5 Techniques to reduce bias in qualitative research

Technique	Definition	Purpose/outcome
Reflexivity	Ongoing self-examination by the researcher of personal assumptions, values, and biases throughout the study	Acknowledge and document researcher influence, enhancing transparency and reducing subjective distortions
Bracketing	The deliberate process of setting aside preconceptions during data collection and analysis	Minimize the impact of prior beliefs, ensuring a more neutral engagement with participants' data
Triangulation	Using multiple data sources or methods (e.g. interviews, observations, document analysis) to cross-check findings	Enhance credibility by reducing reliance on a single data source and counterbalancing individual biases
Member checking	Involving participants in reviewing and confirming data interpretations	Validate that interpretations accurately reflect participants' intended meanings, reducing bias
Peer debriefing	Engaging colleagues or external experts to review the research process and findings	Provide external checks, challenge assumptions, and refine interpretations to mitigate bias
Neutral and indirect questioning	Using non-leading, open-ended, and hypothetical or projective questions during interviews	Reduce pressure for socially desirable responses, encouraging more authentic and honest disclosures
Confidentiality and anonymity assurances	Clearly communicating that participants' responses will remain confidential or anonymous	Alleviate concerns about judgement, fostering an environment where participants feel safe to share openly
Documentation and **audit trails**[8]	Maintaining detailed records of every research step, including data collection, coding, and analysis decisions	Ensure transparency and enable external review, confirming that conclusions are data-driven and unbiased
Constant comparison	An iterative analytical process (often used in grounded theory) that involves continuously comparing and contrasting data segments	Enhance consistency and rigour in data analysis by systematically identifying emerging patterns and reducing interpretative bias

Quantifying Qualitative Data Using Scaling Techniques

Although qualitative research is primarily exploratory and interpretative, scaling techniques can be used to systematically quantify aspects of qualitative data, allowing researchers to measure attitudes, experiences, and perceptions in a structured manner. These techniques help bridge the gap between qualitative richness and quantitative measurement, particularly in mixed-methods research designs.

[8] **Audit trail:** Transparent record of decisions, materials and analytic steps (e.g. protocols, memos, codebooks) enabling external review of rigour and dependability.

Thurstone Scale

The Thurstone scale is designed to measure attitudes or beliefs by developing a set of statements that represent varying degrees of a particular viewpoint. A panel of judges rates these statements based on their perceived intensity or favourability. Statements with known scale values are then selected and presented to respondents, who indicate which statements they agree with. A median or mean scale value is calculated to quantify respondents' positions.

This method is useful in psychological and social research where attitudes need to be ranked along a continuum. For example, a Thurstone scale could be used to measure the severity of stigma experienced by individuals with a mental health condition.

Likert Scale

The Likert scale is one of the most widely used scaling methods in survey-based qualitative and mixed-methods research. Participants rate their level of agreement with a series of statements on a numerical scale (e.g. 1–5 or 1–7), typically ranging from 'strongly disagree' to 'strongly agree'.

This approach enables researchers to quantify subjective attitudes, beliefs, or opinions, allowing for descriptive and inferential statistical analysis. Likert scales are commonly used in surveys, questionnaires, and psychological assessments, making them particularly useful for capturing structured feedback on topics such as treatment satisfaction, perceived stress, or workplace experience.

Guttman Scale

The Guttman scale presents a series of statements that are progressively more extreme in relation to the construct being measured. It is based on the assumption of cumulativeness, whereby agreement with a given item implies agreement with all preceding, less extreme items.

This scale is useful for measuring cumulative attitudes or behaviours. Higher scores reflect stronger endorsement or more severe manifestations of the concept being measured. For example, a Guttman scale could be used to assess the severity of anxiety symptoms, where mild symptoms are listed first, followed by progressively more severe symptoms.

Visual Analogue Scale

The visual analogue scale (VAS) is a continuous measurement tool that presents a horizontal or vertical line (usually 100 mm long) with anchors at each end representing the extreme limits of a subjective experience. Participants mark a point on the line to indicate their perceived state, which is then measured numerically.

VAS is particularly useful for measuring subjective experiences such as pain, fatigue, stress, or quality of life. It allows for a more nuanced measurement of intensity or severity. For example, a VAS could be used in clinical psychology or pain research to assess perceived distress in individuals with chronic illness (Figure 14.1).

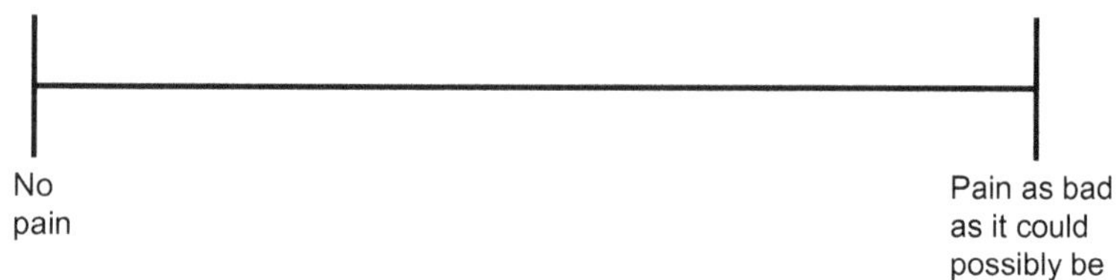

Figure 14.1 Visual analogue scale for pain measurement.

Chapter Summary

Sampling Techniques in Qualitative Research

- Convenience sampling: participants are selected based on availability and willingness to participate, making it a time-efficient method. Example: interviewing psychiatric outpatients during clinic hours to explore anxiety management.
- Purposive sampling: researchers intentionally select participants based on their knowledge, experience, or characteristics related to the study. Example: studying patients who have undergone electroconvulsive therapy for severe depression.
- Types of purposive sampling include:
  - maximum variation sampling (capturing diverse experiences)
  - deviant case sampling (studying outliers or exceptional cases)
  - critical case sampling (focusing on participants with crucial experiences)
  - key informant sampling (interviewing experts in the field).
- Quota sampling: researchers ensure diverse representation by selecting a predetermined number of participants from specific subgroups. Example: including equal numbers of male and female participants in a study on mental illness stigma.
- Criterion sampling: participants must meet predefined criteria relevant to the research question. Example: selecting individuals diagnosed with PTSD for a study on trauma-focused therapy.
- Homogeneous sampling: participants share common characteristics or experiences, allowing for an in-depth exploration of a specific subgroup. Example: studying adolescent females with eating disorders to understand their unique recovery challenges.
- Snowball sampling: used to recruit hard-to-reach or marginalized populations by relying on existing participants to refer others. Example: recruiting individuals with substance misuse disorders through participant referrals.
- Theoretical sampling: participants are selected iteratively to refine emerging theories, commonly used in grounded theory. Example: interviewing individuals with bipolar disorder at different illness stages to refine a theory on coping mechanisms.

Data Collection Methods in Qualitative Research

- Interviews: one-on-one conversations where participants share their experiences. They can be structured (fixed questions), semi-structured (flexible but guided), unstructured (free-flowing), or in-depth (detailed exploration of personal experiences). Example: interviewing individuals with bipolar disorder about their lived experiences.

- Focus groups: small groups (typically 6–10 participants) discussing a topic, facilitated by a moderator. This method captures group dynamics, shared experiences, and diverse perspectives. Example: a focus group of caregivers discussing challenges in dementia care.
- Observations: researchers observe and record behaviours in real-world settings to capture natural interactions and context. Observations can be participant (researcher engages in the environment) or non-participant (researcher remains a detached observer). Example: observing interactions in a psychiatric ward.
- Role-play: participants act out scenarios related to the research topic, helping researchers study decision-making, attitudes, and social dynamics in a controlled but realistic setting. Example: psychiatrists engaging in role-play sessions to assess patient communication skills.
- Diary methods: participants keep a written record of their thoughts, feelings, and experiences over a period of time. Diaries may be structured (with prompts), semi-structured, or unstructured. Example: patients documenting their daily mood and coping strategies in a mental health study.
- Document analysis: reviewing existing documents such as medical records, policy documents, letters, and emails to extract insights and historical context. Example: analysing therapy session notes to study treatment progress.
- Case studies: in-depth exploration of one or a few cases within their real-life context. This method integrates multiple sources of data, including interviews, observations, and document analysis. Example: studying a patient with a rare psychiatric disorder to examine treatment challenges.
- Narrative inquiry: collecting and analysing personal stories to understand how individuals make sense of their experiences. Example: analysing life stories of trauma survivors to explore identity reconstruction.
- Ethnography: an immersive approach where researchers engage in a cultural or social setting for an extended period to understand interactions and behaviours. Example: studying support systems in a residential mental health facility.
- Iterative approach: data collection and analysis occur simultaneously in cycles, allowing for refinement of research questions and sampling based on emerging insights. Example: ethnographic studies where researchers adjust their focus based on ongoing observations.
- Grounded theory: a systematic approach where data collection and analysis occur iteratively, allowing patterns and theories to emerge from the data itself rather than being pre-imposed. Example: interviewing individuals with bipolar disorder at different illness stages to develop a theory on coping mechanisms.

Methods of Data Analysis

- Content analysis: a systematic approach to categorizing data to identify trends.
- Narrative analysis: focuses on storytelling and analysing narrative content.
- Discourse analysis: examines language, interactions, and power dynamics.
- Grounded theory analysis: iterative coding method to develop theories.
- Phenomenological analysis: captures participants' lived experiences.
- Framework analysis: links data to research questions using a matrix.

- IPA: explores how individuals make sense of their world.
- Constant comparative method: iterative coding to identify patterns.

Scaling Techniques for Quantifying Qualitative Data

- Thurstone scale: measures attitudes by having a panel of judges rank statements based on their intensity. Respondents indicate agreement, and a median score is calculated. This method is useful in ranking attitudes, such as measuring mental health stigma.
- Likert scale: one of the most commonly used scaling techniques, where participants rate their level of agreement on a numerical scale (e.g. 1–5). It is widely used in surveys and psychological assessments to measure opinions, treatment satisfaction, or stress levels.
- Guttman scale: presents a hierarchical series of statements, where agreeing to a more extreme statement implies agreement with all preceding ones. It is effective for measuring cumulative attitudes or behaviours, such as assessing anxiety severity from mild to severe symptoms.
- Visual analogue scale: a continuous scale where participants mark a point on a line representing the extremes of a concept (e.g. no pain to extreme pain). It is useful for measuring subjective experiences such as pain, fatigue, or distress in clinical and psychological research.

Practice Questions

Q1. Which qualitative research strategy involves seeking feedback from participants to verify the accuracy and credibility of the researcher's interpretations?

A. Theoretical sampling
B. Data saturation
C. Member checking
D. Reflexivity
E. Triangulation

Q2. When should a researcher stop data collection in a qualitative study?

A. When the researcher has interviewed an equal number of participants from each demographic group.
B. When additional interviews begin to confirm existing findings rather than introduce new insights.
C. When the sample size reaches 100 participants, ensuring statistical significance.
D. When the research findings align with the initial hypothesis.
E. When the study duration reaches a predetermined time limit.

Q3. A researcher plans to analyse television advertisements to examine how mental health issues are portrayed in mainstream media. The researcher systematically identifies recurring themes, classifies visual and verbal elements, and quantifies the frequency of certain portrayals. Which qualitative research method would be the most appropriate approach?

A. Content analysis
B. Discourse analysis
C. Thematic analysis

D. Conversation analysis
E. Narrative analysis

Q4. A researcher wants to study how psychiatric nurses in forensic mental health units perceive their role in managing violent patients. The study aims to explore their experiences, coping strategies, and the impact of workplace violence on their mental well-being. Which research approach is most appropriate?

A. A randomized controlled trial comparing two de-escalation techniques used in forensic psychiatry
B. A national survey measuring nurses' attitudes toward violence in forensic settings using a structured questionnaire
C. A statistical analysis of incident reports on violent behaviour in psychiatric hospitals over a five-year period
D. A qualitative study using semi-structured interviews with forensic psychiatric nurses about their experiences and coping strategies
E. A cohort study tracking long-term stress-related outcomes in psychiatric nurses exposed to violent incidents

Q5. Which of the following techniques is most appropriate for converting these qualitative perceptions into quantitative data?

A. Chi-square test
B. Thematic analysis
C. Visual analogue scale
D. Phenomenological analysis
E. Spearman's rank correlation

Q6. A researcher conducting a qualitative study on coping mechanisms in schizophrenia continuously compares new interview data with previously collected and analysed data. This process helps to refine emerging themes and develop new conceptual insights based on patterns identified in the data. What is this process called?

A. Theoretical sampling
B. Grounded theory coding
C. Constant comparison
D. Inductive reasoning
E. Content analysis

Q7. A researcher conducts a study exploring how individuals diagnosed with schizophrenia experience and make sense of their illness. The study focuses on their lived experiences, emotions, and the meaning they attribute to their condition. Which qualitative research method is most appropriate for this study?

A. Grounded theory
B. Ethnographic analysis
C. Narrative analysis
D. Phenomenological analysis
E. Thematic analysis

Q8. A researcher conducting a study on patient experiences with psychiatric hospitalization collects interview data, codes the data for emerging themes, and then uses these themes to guide further data collection and refine the analysis. This process is repeated until a well-supported theoretical framework emerges. What is this research approach called?

A. Thematic analysis
B. Inductive coding
C. Grounded theory
D. Ethnographic analysis
E. Case study method

Q9. Match the sampling type that would be most appropriate for the studies listed from the options in the two lists below.

A. Convenience sampling
B. Maximum variation sampling
C. Purposive sampling
D. Snowball sampling
E. Systematic sampling
F. Theoretical sampling

1. What are the lived experiences of transgender individuals in rural communities regarding mental health stigma?
2. What are the challenges faced by refugees when accessing mental health support in the UK?
3. How do patients with schizophrenia experience medication adherence in community care?
4. What are the cultural beliefs of South Asian communities regarding depression and help-seeking behaviours?

Q10. Match the most appropriate data collection method with the research topic from the options in the two lists below.

A. Semi-structured interviews
B. Focus groups
C. Participant observation
D. Document analysis
E. Narrative inquiry
F. Diary method

1. How do individuals with bipolar disorder describe their journey from diagnosis to recovery?
2. What are the interactions between psychiatric nurses and patients in an inpatient mental health facility?
3. How do caregivers of dementia patients collectively perceive the challenges of providing long-term care?
4. What are the key themes in historical policy documents regarding mental health service provision?
5. What are the daily emotional experiences of adolescents diagnosed with anxiety disorders?

Answers

Q1. Correct answer: C. Member checking. Member checking is a qualitative research strategy where participants review and verify the accuracy of the researcher's interpretations of their data. This process enhances the credibility and validity of the findings by ensuring that the participant's intended meaning has been accurately captured.
Why the other options are incorrect:

A. Theoretical sampling involves selecting new participants based on emerging theoretical needs, commonly used in grounded theory research.
B. Data saturation occurs when no new themes or insights emerge from further data collection, indicating sufficient data has been gathered.
D. Reflexivity refers to the researcher's self-examination of biases, assumptions, and influence on the research process.
E. Triangulation involves using multiple sources, methods, or researchers to validate findings.

Q2. Correct answer: B. When additional interviews begin to confirm existing findings rather than introduce new insights. Qualitative research follows an iterative and exploratory approach, meaning data collection continues until data saturation is reached. Saturation occurs when new interviews or observations no longer yield new themes or insights, indicating that further data collection would be redundant. This ensures that the study has achieved depth and richness in understanding the research question.
Why the other options are incorrect:

A. Interviewing an equal number of participants from each demographic group: qualitative research focuses on depth, not balancing numerical representation.
C. Sample size reaching 100 participants for statistical significance: statistical significance is a quantitative concept; qualitative research does not require a fixed sample size.
D. Aligning with the initial hypothesis: qualitative studies are exploratory, and findings are not judged based on pre-existing hypotheses.
E. Reaching a predetermined time limit: stopping based on time constraints may lead to incomplete findings, rather than achieving data saturation.

Q3. Correct answer: A. Content analysis. The researcher is systematically coding and categorizing media messages based on recurring themes and representations. Content analysis is commonly used to study media representations, advertisements, and written or visual content by classifying elements into meaningful categories for analysis. It allows for both qualitative interpretation and quantification of media portrayals.
Why the other options are incorrect:

B. Discourse analysis focuses on how language constructs meaning and power within communication, rather than systematically coding specific portrayals in media.
C. Thematic analysis is used to identify themes in interview transcripts or participant narratives, not structured media content.
D. Conversation analysis studies spoken interactions, such as doctor–patient conversations, not media content.

E. Narrative analysis focuses on how individuals construct stories about their experiences, rather than analysing media portrayals at a broad level.

Q4. Correct answer: D. A qualitative study using semi-structured interviews with forensic psychiatric nurses about their experiences and coping strategies. The study focuses on understanding subjective experiences, which is best explored using qualitative methods such as interviews, focus groups, or thematic analysis. Qualitative research is ideal for capturing personal narratives, emotions, and complex social dynamics that cannot be quantified through surveys or statistical analysis.
Why the other options are incorrect:

A. A randomized controlled trial is not suitable because the research question is exploratory rather than testing an intervention.
B. A national survey using structured questionnaires would provide quantitative data on attitudes but would not capture in-depth personal experiences.
C. Statistical analysis of incident reports would measure frequency and patterns of violence, but not how nurses perceive and cope with it.
E. A cohort study tracking long-term stress-related outcomes focuses on long-term effects but does not explore subjective experiences in depth.

Q5. Correct answer: C. Visual analogue scale. The VAS is a quantitative method used to convert subjective qualitative perceptions into numerical data. It allows participants to indicate their feelings, experiences, or attitudes by marking a point along a continuous line, typically from 0 to 100 mm.
Why the other options are incorrect:

A. Chi-square test: a statistical test used to compare categorical data, but does not convert qualitative perceptions into numerical form.
B. Thematic analysis: a purely qualitative method used to identify themes in textual data, without numerical transformation.
D. Phenomenological analysis: a qualitative approach focused on understanding lived experiences but does not provide numerical conversion.
E. Spearman's rank correlation: a statistical method that measures associations between ranked data, rather than converting qualitative perceptions into a measurable scale.

Q6. Correct answer: C. Constant comparison. Constant comparison is a technique used in qualitative research, particularly in grounded theory, where newly collected data is continuously compared with existing data to refine categories and concepts. This process enhances theoretical development by ensuring that themes are well supported and consistently grounded in the data.
Why the other options are incorrect:

A. Theoretical sampling: a sampling strategy in grounded theory where data collection is guided by emerging concepts rather than a pre-set sample.
B. Grounded theory coding: refers to the stages of coding (open, axial, selective) used to analyse data but does not describe the iterative comparison process.

D. Inductive reasoning: a broad reasoning approach in qualitative research but does not specifically involve comparing data iteratively.
E. Content analysis: a method used for categorizing and quantifying text data, but it does not involve systematic comparison of new and old data.

Q7. Correct answer: D. Phenomenological analysis. Phenomenological analysis is a qualitative research approach that explores how individuals experience a particular phenomenon and the meaning they assign to it. This method focuses on personal lived experiences, making it ideal for studying subjective experiences of mental health, illness, trauma, or personal transformation.

Why the other options are incorrect:

A. Grounded theory: used to develop new theories from data, rather than solely exploring lived experiences.
B. Ethnographic analysis: focuses on studying cultures and social interactions, not individual subjective experiences.
C. Narrative analysis: examines how individuals construct and tell their life stories, rather than focusing on the essence of an experience.
E. Thematic analysis: identifies patterns across multiple participants' responses, but does not deeply explore individual meaning-making as phenomenology does.

Q8. Correct answer: C. Grounded theory. Grounded theory is a systematic qualitative research method that involves iterative cycles of data collection, coding, and analysis to develop theory directly from the data rather than starting with a preconceived hypothesis. The core principle of grounded theory is that theoretical development emerges from continuous comparison and refinement of data.

Why the other options are incorrect:

A. Thematic analysis focuses on identifying themes in qualitative data, but it does not necessarily involve the iterative cycles leading to theory development.
B. Inductive coding refers to coding without pre-existing categories, but does not describe the full process of developing a grounded theory.
D. Ethnographic analysis involves long-term immersion in a cultural or social setting, but is not designed primarily for theory generation.
E. Case study method focuses on detailed analysis of a single case or small set of cases, rather than developing theory from iterative data collection and coding.

Q9. The answers are paired as below.

1. D. Snowball sampling. Transgender individuals in rural communities may be a hard-to-reach population, so referrals from participants would be useful.
2. D. Snowball sampling. Refugees may be difficult to access, and snowball sampling allows for recruitment through social networks.
3. F. Theoretical sampling. If the study aims to refine emerging theories on medication adherence, theoretical sampling is appropriate.
4. C. Purposive sampling. A study on cultural beliefs requires selecting individuals with relevant ethnic backgrounds, making purposive sampling the best fit.

Q10. The answers are paired as below.

1. E. Narrative inquiry. The focus on personal life stories makes narrative inquiry the best approach.
2. C. Participant observation. Directly observing interactions allows for rich, contextual data on patient–nurse engagement.
3. B. Focus groups. A group setting encourages discussion on shared caregiving experiences.
4. D. Document analysis. Reviewing policy documents helps uncover historical trends in mental health services.
5. F. Diary method. Capturing daily emotional experiences is best achieved through personal diary entries.

Further Reading

Braun V, Clarke V. Using thematic analysis in psychology. *Qual Res Psychol.* 2006;**3**(2):77–101. doi: https://doi.org/10.1191/1478088706qp063oa.

Carcary M. The research audit trail: enhancing trustworthiness in qualitative inquiry. *Electron J Bus Res Methods.* 2009;7(1):11–24.

Charmaz K. *Constructing Grounded Theory.* London: Sage; 2006.

Denzin NK. *The Research Act: A Theoretical Introduction to Sociological Methods.* 2nd ed. New York: McGraw-Hill; 1978.

Fairclough N. *Discourse and Social Change.* Cambridge: Polity Press; 1992.

Finlay L. 'Outing' the researcher: the provenance, process, and practice of reflexivity. *Qual Health Res.* 2002;**12**(4):531–45.

Gale NK, Heath G, Cameron E, Rashid S, Redwood S. Using the framework method for the analysis of qualitative data in multi-disciplinary health research. *BMC Med Res Methodol.* 2013;**13**:117. doi: https://doi.org/10.1186/1471-2288-13-117.

Giorgi A. *The Descriptive Phenomenological Method in Psychology.* Pittsburgh, PA: Duquesne University Press; 2009.

Glaser BG, Strauss AL. *The Discovery of Grounded Theory: Strategies for Qualitative Research.* Chicago, IL: Aldine; 1967.

Guttman L. A basis for scaling qualitative data. *Am Sociol Rev.* 1944;**9**(2):139–50.

Hammersley M, Atkinson P. *Ethnography: Principles in Practice.* 3rd ed. London: Routledge; 2007.

Huskisson EC. Measurement of pain. *Lancet.* 1974;**304**(7889):1127–31.

Krippendorff K. *Content Analysis: An Introduction to Its Methodology.* 3rd ed. Thousand Oaks, CA: Sage; 2013.

Likert R. A technique for the measurement of attitudes. *Arch Psychol.* 1932;**140**:1–55.

Lincoln YS, Guba EG. *Naturalistic Inquiry.* Newbury Park, CA: Sage; 1985.

Riessman CK. *Narrative Methods for the Human Sciences.* Thousand Oaks, CA: Sage; 2008.

Ritchie J, Spencer L. Qualitative data analysis for applied policy research. In: Bryman A, Burgess RG, eds. *Analysing Qualitative Data.* London: Routledge; 1994. pp. 173–94.

Smith JA, Flowers P, Larkin M. *Interpretative Phenomenological Analysis: Theory, Method and Research.* London: Sage; 2009.

Thurstone LL. Attitudes can be measured. *Am J Sociol.* 1928;**33**(4):529–54.

Tufford L, Newman P. Bracketing in qualitative research. *Qual Soc Work.* 2012;**11**(1):80–96. doi: https://doi.org/10.1177/1473325010368316.

Chapter 15

Audit and Quality Improvement

Clinical Audit

Introduction

Clinical audit is a quality improvement process that systematically reviews clinical care against explicit criteria to ensure it meets established standards and identifies areas for improvement. It is a cyclical process that involves comparing actual practice against predefined standards, identifying gaps, implementing changes to improve patient care, and reassessing to ensure the effectiveness of these improvements.

Unlike research, which aims to generate new knowledge applicable to broader populations to establish what constitutes best practice, clinical audit focuses on assessing whether current practice meets existing standards. Therefore, a key difference from research is that audit results are typically only relevant within the specific setting, whereas research findings can be generalized beyond the immediate population. Unlike research, clinical audits do not usually require research ethics committee (REC) approval, as they evaluate existing services rather than testing new interventions.

Methodology

1. **Standards:** audits use existing guidelines, best practices, or national standards as benchmarks.
2. **Data collection:** data is gathered on current practices, often through patient records, surveys, or observations.
3. **Analysis:** the collected data is compared against standards to identify gaps or areas where practice deviates from the ideal.
4. **Action plan:** based on the findings, an action plan is developed to implement changes and improve the quality of care.
5. **Re-audit:** after a sufficient period, a re-audit is conducted to assess the effectiveness of the implemented changes.

Figure 15.1 shows the clinical audit cycle.

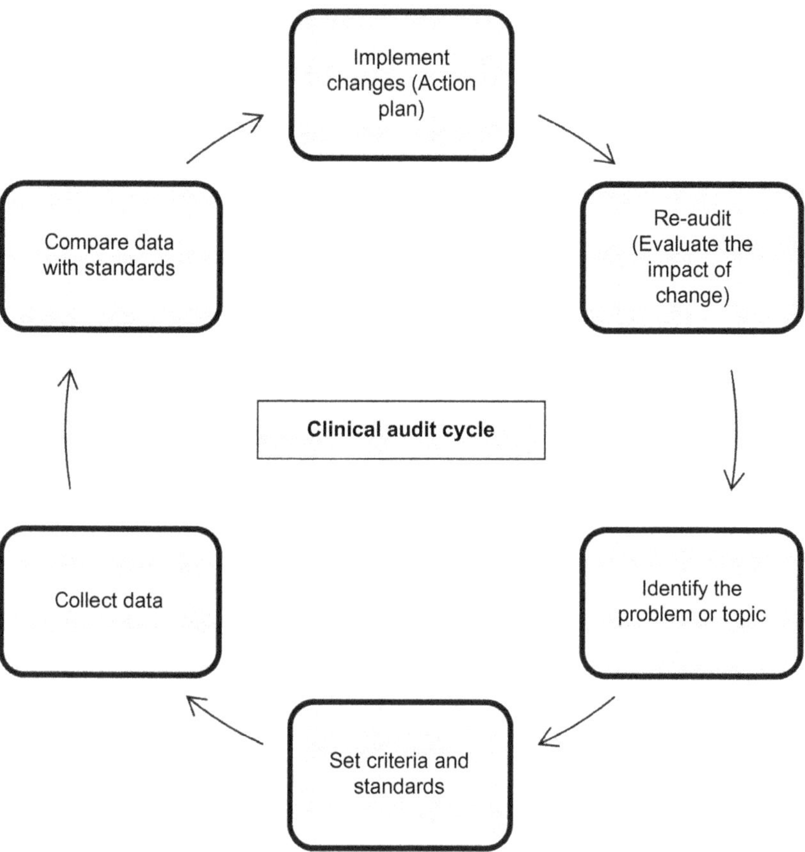

Figure 15.1 The clinical audit cycle.

Clinical Audit vs Research

Clinical audit and research serve different purposes in healthcare improvement. Clinical audit ensures adherence to best practices and drives quality improvement within a specific setting, while research seeks to generate new knowledge applicable across broader populations.

Table 15.1 outlines the key differences between clinical audit and research across their goals, focus, data sources, methods, and outcomes.

Table 15.1 Key differences between clinical audit and research

Feature	Clinical audit	Research
Primary goal	Evaluate and improve current practice	Generate new knowledge
Focus	Current service quality	New treatments, diagnoses, or understanding
Standards	Existing guidelines, protocols, standards	Aims to develop new knowledge/standards

Table 15.1 (cont.)

Feature	Clinical audit	Research
Data source	Existing patient records, observations, etc.	May involve experiments, surveys, new data collection
Methodology	Comparison against standards, gap analysis	Study design, data analysis, hypothesis testing
Generalizability	Local/specific to the audited area	Aims for broader applicability
Ethical review	Often less stringent, focuses on service improvement	More rigorous, especially for interventions
Outcome	Action plan for local improvement	Publication, new knowledge, potential change in practice
Purpose	Quality assurance, improvement	Knowledge generation, advancement of the field
Timescale	Usually shorter-term	Can be short- or long-term

Quality Improvement

Quality improvement (QI) is a continuous and systematic process aimed at enhancing the quality of healthcare services and patient outcomes. It involves using various methods and tools to identify areas for improvement, implement changes, and monitor their effectiveness.

Key Principles of Quality Improvement

- **Patient-centredness:** QI focuses on meeting the needs and preferences of patients and ensuring their experience is positive.
- **Safety:** QI aims to minimize risks and prevent harm to patients during healthcare delivery.
- **Effectiveness:** QI promotes the use of evidence-based practices and ensures that treatments and interventions are effective.
- **Efficiency:** QI seeks to optimize resource utilization and reduce waste in healthcare processes.
- **Timeliness:** QI strives to provide timely access to care and reduce unnecessary delays.
- **Equity:** QI aims to address disparities in healthcare access and outcomes and ensure equitable care for all populations.

Methodology of Quality Improvement

Quality improvement initiatives typically follow a structured approach, often involving the following steps:

1. Identify an area for improvement: this could be based on patient feedback, clinical audit findings, or performance data.
2. Form a QI team: a team of healthcare professionals involved in the area of focus is formed to lead the improvement effort.
3. Analyse the current situation: the team gathers data to understand the current processes, identify bottlenecks, and pinpoint areas for improvement.
4. Develop and test interventions: the team brainstorms potential solutions and designs interventions to address the identified issues.

5. Implement changes: the interventions are implemented in a controlled setting, often using a pilot approach.
6. Monitor and evaluate: the team collects data to assess the impact of the changes and determine if they have led to measurable improvements.
7. Sustain improvements: if the interventions are successful, the team works to embed them into routine practice and ensure long-term sustainability and prevent a return to old habits.

Common QI Methodologies

Plan–Do–Study–Act Cycle

The Plan–Do–Study–Act (**PDSA**) cycle[1] is a structured, cyclical framework for continuous quality improvement. It involves planning a change, testing it on a small scale, studying the results, and acting on what is learned. The process is iterative, allowing refinements over multiple cycles.

Plan

- Define the objective by clearly specifying the problem and the desired improvement.
- Develop a detailed plan, outlining:
  - *who* will be involved
  - *what* changes will be implemented
  - *where* and *when* the test will take place
  - *how* impact will be measured.
- Predict the expected outcome to provide a benchmark for evaluation.

Do

- Implement the planned change on a small scale.
- Document observations systematically.
- Collect data to monitor both expected and unexpected effects.

Study

- Analyse the collected data to assess whether the change produced improvement.
- Compare actual outcomes with predicted outcomes.
- Summarize findings, noting lessons learned and any unintended consequences.

Act

- Decide whether to adopt the change (make it standard practice), adapt it (refine and retest), or abandon it (if ineffective).
- Plan the next PDSA cycle, building on what has been learned.

Example

In a mental health clinic, a PDSA cycle was used to reduce missed appointments. Text message reminders were introduced as the intervention. Data analysis showed a measurable

[1] **PDSA:** A structured, iterative method for testing and refining changes in practice through four stages: Plan, Do, Study, and Act. Start with small, rapid cycles; track outcomes, process and balancing measures.

reduction in the *did not attend* (DNA) rate, so the change was adopted and integrated into routine practice.

Lean

A systematic approach to improving processes by eliminating waste and increasing efficiency, originally derived from the Toyota Production System. In a healthcare context, this often focuses on improving patient flow.

Six Sigma

Six Sigma[2] is a data-driven methodology focused on minimizing variability and defects in processes. Key concepts include:

- **Customer focus:** quality is defined by customer needs.
- **Data-driven approach:** uses statistical tools to guide decisions.
- **Process improvement:** reduces variation to achieve consistent results.
- **DMAIC cycle:** define, measure, analyse, improve, and control.

Institute for Healthcare Improvement (IHI) Model for Improvement (Nolan Model)

The **IHI Model for Improvement**[3] is a widely used quality improvement (QI) framework developed by Associates in Process Improvement and promoted by the IHI. It provides a structured approach to improving healthcare services through two distinct parts:

1. Three key questions:

- What are we trying to accomplish? (Aim)
- How will we know that a change is an improvement? (Measures)
- What changes can we make that will result in improvement? (Changes)

2. The PDSA cycle, which serves as the core mechanism for testing and refining changes iteratively. By using the Model for Improvement alongside the PDSA cycle, healthcare teams can ensure that improvements are goal-driven, measurable, and sustainable.

This model is used alongside the PDSA and other QI methodologies to ensure measurable, goal-driven improvements in healthcare settings.

Tools and Techniques Used in QI

- **Process mapping:**[4] a visual representation of a workflow that shows each step in a process, helping to identify inefficiencies, redundancies, or bottlenecks.
- **Data analysis:** the systematic use of quantitative and qualitative data to measure performance, monitor change, and assess the impact of improvement initiatives.

---

[2] **Six Sigma (DMAIC):** Structured reduction of variation: define–measure–analyse–improve–control. Emphasizes good measurement, cause-and-effect, and sustaining gains; $6\sigma \approx 3.4$ defects per million opportunities on critical-to-quality metrics.

[3] **Model for improvement (Nolan/IHI):** Three questions (aim, measures, changes), plus PDSA cycles; track outcome, process and balancing measures to detect trade-offs.

[4] **Process mapping:** Visual depiction of steps/hand-offs (flowchart); swim-lanes add roles; value-stream maps add times, waits, and waste; baseline before testing changes.

- **Root cause analysis (RCA):**[5] a structured method for identifying the fundamental underlying causes of a problem, rather than just addressing immediate symptoms.
- **Fishbone diagram (Ishikawa diagram):**[6] a visual brainstorming tool shaped like a fish skeleton, used to categorize and display potential causes of a problem across domains such as people, processes, environment, and equipment.
- **Run charts:**[7] line graphs that display data points plotted over time, enabling detection of trends, shifts, or cycles in performance.
- **Control charts:**[8] an advanced form of run chart that adds statistically calculated upper and lower control limits, helping to distinguish between **common cause** (natural) variation and **special cause**[9] (abnormal) variation.

Benefits of Quality Improvement

- **Improved patient outcomes:** enhances clinical care and patient experience.
- **Enhanced safety:** reduces errors and harm.
- **Increased efficiency:** streamlines processes and reduces waste.
- **Better staff morale:** empowers staff to contribute to improvements.
- **Cost savings:** reduces unnecessary expenditure through optimized processes.

Table 15.2 highlights the key differences between clinical audit and QI, illustrating how each contributes to improving healthcare delivery.

Table 15.2 Comparison of clinical audit and quality improvement

Feature	Clinical audit	Quality improvement
Primary goal	Evaluate current practice against standards	Continuously improve processes and outcomes
Focus	Compliance with standards, identifying gaps	Enhancing efficiency, effectiveness, and patient experience
Methodology	Set standards – collect data – compare performance to standards – implement changes – re-audit	Identify areas for improvement – analyse processes – develop and test interventions – implement and monitor changes

[5] **Root cause analysis (RCA):** Structured investigation of what, how, and why an incident occurred to prevent recurrence. Use the Five Whys and fishbone; assign actions, owners and deadlines.

[6] **Fishbone diagram (Ishikawa diagram):** A cause-and-effect tool that organizes possible causes of a problem into categories (e.g. methods, materials, equipment, people, environment, measurement). It supports structured brainstorming and root cause analysis. Branches should be populated with evidence rather than assumptions.

[7] **Run chart:** A time series plot with a median used to detect non-random variation. Rules identify shifts, trends, too few/many runs, or astronomical data points. The median should be recalculated if a sustained shift occurs.

[8] **Control charts (SPC):** A time series graph with a centreline and statistically derived control limits to distinguish common cause from special cause variation. It supports real-time quality monitoring.

[9] **Common vs special cause:** Common cause is a routine system variation (fix the process); special cause is an unusual, assignable variation (investigate the event). Treating common cause as special (or vice versa) wastes effort or misses systemic fixes.

Table 15.2 (cont.)

Feature	Clinical audit	Quality improvement
Scope	Often focused on a specific clinical area or process	Can be broader, addressing system-level issues
Data	Primarily retrospective, using existing records	May involve real-time data collection and analysis
Timescale	Typically shorter cycles with defined start and end points	Ongoing, iterative process
Change	Often focused on correcting deviations from standards	May involve more innovative and transformative changes
Measures	Primarily quantitative, measuring compliance	Can include both quantitative and qualitative measures
Patient involvement	May involve patient feedback but often focuses on clinical data	Actively seeks patient input and engagement
Example	Auditing adherence to guidelines for prescribing antipsychotic medication.	Enhancing communication between healthcare providers

Chapter Summary

Clinical Audit

A clinical audit is a structured quality improvement process that evaluates current clinical practice against predefined standards (e.g. hospital guidelines, NICE recommendations). It is a cyclical process that includes:

1. setting standards based on best practices
2. collecting data on current clinical practice
3. comparing data with established standards
4. developing an action plan for improvement
5. conducting a re-audit to assess whether improvements have been achieved.

Unlike research, which generates new knowledge and aims to establish what 'best practice' is, clinical audit is focused on improving local healthcare practices and evaluates if 'best practice' is being followed.

Quality Improvement

Quality improvement is a systematic and continuous approach to enhancing healthcare services and patient outcomes. It focuses on process improvements rather than just compliance with standards.

Key Principles of QI

- Patient-centredness: focuses on patient needs and experiences.
- Safety: minimizes risks and prevents harm.
- Effectiveness: ensures use of evidence-based practices.
- Efficiency: reduces waste and optimizes resources.
- Timeliness: improves access and reduces waiting times.
- Equity: ensures fair and equal healthcare access.

QI Methodologies

- PDSA cycle: a step-by-step iterative approach to testing and refining changes.
- Lean: focuses on eliminating waste and increasing efficiency.
- Six Sigma: a data-driven methodology to reduce variability and improve quality.
- Institute for Healthcare Improvement (IHI) model: developed by Associates in Process Improvement (Nolan *et al.*), it uses three fundamental questions and the PDSA cycle for systematic improvement.

Benefits of QI

- Better patient outcomes and safety
- increased efficiency and reduced waste
- improved staff morale through engagement in change
- cost savings by optimizing processes.

Practice Questions

Q1. Which of the following is *not* a formal step in the clinical audit cycle?

A. Setting standards and criteria for best practice
B. Collecting data on current practice
C. Implementing changes based on audit findings
D. Evaluating the impact of changes through re-audit
E. Applying statistical tests to see if the results can be generalized to other populations

Q2. What is the primary source of clinical audit standards?

A. Expert opinions published in medical textbooks
B. Findings from a single case report
C. Conclusions drawn from qualitative research interviews
D. The opinion of a senior clinician in the department
E. Established guidelines

Q3. Which of the following is an example of a clinical audit?

A. Conducting interviews with patients to explore their experiences of psychiatric care
B. Evaluating whether a new cognitive behavioural therapy (CBT) programme improves patient outcomes
C. Comparing the percentage of patients with schizophrenia who received clozapine as per NICE guidelines
D. Collecting data on the number of patients with a history of childhood trauma who developed depression in adulthood
E. Investigating whether a new electronic prescribing system reduces medication errors

Q4. Which tool is commonly used in QI to identify potential causes of a problem?
  A. Fishbone diagram
  B. Randomized controlled trial
  C. Systematic review
  D. Cohort study
  E. Financial audit

Q5. What is a primary goal of using run charts and control charts in QI?
  A. To visualize performance trends over time
  B. To generate new medical theories
  C. To test pharmaceutical efficacy in clinical trials
  D. To assess only qualitative feedback from patients
  E. To replace electronic medical records

Q6. Which of the following is one of the three key questions in the Nolan model for improvement?
  A. What resources are required to implement change?
  B. What are the potential financial risks of the project?
  C. How will the improvement impact staffing levels?
  D. What are we trying to accomplish?
  E. How long should we observe changes before deciding on further action?

Q7. Which of the following steps is categorized as the 'Act' phase of the PDSA cycle in quality improvement?
  A. Implementing the intervention on a small scale
  B. Identifying areas for improvement and setting objectives
  C. Analysing collected data and comparing results to predictions
  D. Developing a strategy to sustain successful changes or modify unsuccessful ones
  E. Documenting observations and collecting feedback during implementation

Q8. A psychiatry trainee notices that patients with depression admitted to an inpatient unit are not consistently receiving a structured suicide risk assessment upon admission. They decide to conduct a QI project using the PDSA cycle. What should be the next step?
  A. Collecting and analysing data on how often suicide risk assessments are completed upon admission
  B. Implementing a new standardized suicide risk assessment tool immediately
  C. Reporting the issue to the hospital board for further investigation
  D. Presenting the problem at a national psychiatry conference
  E. Discontinuing all current risk assessments and replacing them with a new approach

Answers

Q1. Correct answer: E. Applying statistical tests to see if the results can be generalized to other populations. A clinical audit is a QI process that involves comparing current practice against established standards, implementing improvements, and reassessing through re-audit. Clinical audit focuses on improving local practice against established standards. It's about checking and improving local service delivery. Generalizing results to other populations is more aligned with research methodology, not the core purpose of clinical audit.

Q2. Correct answer: E. Established guidelines. A clinical audit evaluates current practice against predefined standards, which are derived from authoritative clinical guidelines, such as NICE guidelines, Royal College of Psychiatrists guidelines, and local hospital protocols and policies.
Why the other options are incorrect:

A. Expert opinions published in medical textbooks: while informative, textbooks do not provide up-to-date, evidence-based clinical standards.
B. Findings from a single case report: case reports describe individual cases, not general standards of care.
C. Conclusions drawn from qualitative research interviews: qualitative studies provide insights but do not define clinical benchmarks.
D. The opinion of a senior clinician in the department: individual opinions may vary and are not sufficient to define objective audit standards.

Q3. Correct answer: C. Comparing the percentage of patients with schizophrenia who received clozapine as per NICE guidelines. A clinical audit involves measuring current practice against an established gold standard, such as NICE guidelines, to ensure adherence and identify areas for improvement. Comparing clozapine prescriptions for schizophrenia against NICE recommendations is a classic audit approach.
Why the other options are incorrect:

A. Conducting interviews with patients to explore their experiences of psychiatric care. This is qualitative research, focusing on patient experiences rather than comparing practice with a standard.
B. Evaluating whether a new CBT programme improves patient outcomes. This is a QI or research project, assessing effectiveness rather than adherence to guidelines.
D. Collecting data on patients with childhood trauma who developed depression. This is observational research, exploring associations rather than auditing practice.
E. Investigating whether a new electronic prescribing system reduces medication errors. This is service evaluation or QI, as it assesses the impact of a change rather than auditing current practice against a guideline.

Q4. Correct answer: A. Fishbone diagram. A fishbone (Ishikawa) diagram helps teams visually identify and categorize root causes of a problem.

Q5. Correct answer: A. To visualize performance trends over time. These charts are used to monitor variations in process performance over time, helping teams identify improvements or deviations.

Q6. Correct answer: D. What are we trying to accomplish? This is one of the three fundamental questions in the Nolan model for improvement, which helps guide QI projects. The model ensures teams define clear goals, measure outcomes effectively, and implement meaningful changes. The other options focus on operational or financial concerns, which are important but not part of the core Nolan framework.

Q7. Correct answer: D. Developing a strategy to sustain successful changes or modify unsuccessful ones. The 'Act' phase of the PDSA cycle focuses on deciding the next steps based on the findings from the 'Study' phase. It involves:

- adopting the change if it worked well
- adapting the change if modifications are needed
- abandoning the change if it did not lead to improvement.

Why the other options are incorrect:

A. `Implementing the intervention on a small scale: this occurs in the 'Do' phase.
B. Identifying areas for improvement and setting objectives: this is part of the 'Plan' phase.
C. Analysing collected data and comparing results to predictions: this is done in the 'Study' phase.
E. Documenting observations and collecting feedback during implementation: this is also part of the 'Do' phase.

Q8. Correct answer: A. Collecting and analysing data on how often suicide risk assessments are completed upon admission. The next step in the PDSA cycle after identifying a problem is the 'Plan' phase, which involves gathering baseline data, understanding the existing process, and identifying gaps before implementing a solution.
Why the other options are incorrect:

B. Implementing a new standardized suicide risk assessment tool immediately: this would fall under the 'Do' phase, which comes after planning and data collection.
C. Reporting the issue to the hospital board for further investigation: while stakeholder engagement is important, it is not a required step in the PDSA framework at this stage.
D. Presenting the problem at a national psychiatry conference: dissemination of findings happens much later, after the QI project has been tested and evaluated.
E. Discontinuing all current risk assessments and replacing them with a new approach: a QI project typically improves processes rather than abruptly stopping them without an alternative plan.

Further Reading

Benneyan JC, Lloyd RC, Plsek PE. Statistical process control as a tool for research and healthcare improvement. *Qual Saf Health Care.* 2003;**12**(6):458–64.

Deming WE. *Out of the Crisis.* Cambridge, MA: MIT Press; 1986.

Institute for Healthcare Improvement. *Science of Improvement: How to Improve.* Boston, MA: IHI; 2009.

Ishikawa K. *Guide to Quality Control.* Rev. ed. Tokyo: Asian Productivity Organization; 1986.

Langley GJ, Moen R, Nolan KM, et al. *The Improvement Guide: A Practical Approach to Enhancing Organizational Performance.* 2nd ed. San Francisco, CA: Jossey-Bass; 2009.

Lloyd RC. *Quality Health Care: A Guide to Developing and Using Indicators.* 2nd ed. Burlington, MA: Jones & Bartlett; 2017.

Montgomery DC. *Introduction to Statistical Quality Control.* 8th ed. Hoboken, NJ: Wiley; 2019.

National Institute for Health and Care Excellence (NICE). *Clinical Audit: A Guide for*

NHS Boards and Partners. London: NICE; 2002.

Ohno T. *Toyota Production System: Beyond Large-Scale Production*. Portland, OR: Productivity Press; 1988.

Perla RJ, Provost LP, Murray SK. The run chart: a simple analytical tool for learning from variation in healthcare processes. *BMJ Qual Saf*. 2011;**20**(1):46–51.

The Health Foundation. *Quality Improvement Made Simple*. 2nd ed. London: The Health Foundation; 2013.

Womack JP, Jones DT. *Lean Thinking*. New York: Simon & Schuster; 1996.

Chapter 16 Research Ethics, Ethical Approval, and Reporting Standards in Research Studies

Research Ethics and the Ethical Approval Process in the UK

Introduction

Research ethics refers to the principles, standards, and guidelines that ensure research involving human participants, personal data, or biological samples is conducted in an ethical, safe, and responsible manner.

It aims to protect participants' rights, dignity, and wellbeing while maintaining scientific integrity.

Key Principles of Research Ethics

Research ethics in the UK are based on international guidelines (e.g. the Helsinki Declaration) and national frameworks (e.g. UK Policy Framework for Health and Social Care Research). The key principles include:

1. Respect for autonomy:
   - Participants must give informed consent before taking part.
   - They should have the right to withdraw at any time.
2. Beneficence maximizing benefit:
   - Research should maximize benefits while minimizing risks.
   - Participants should not be exposed to unnecessary harm.
3. Non-maleficence (do no harm):
   - Researchers must identify and mitigate risks (e.g. psychological distress, confidentiality breaches).
   - Risks should be justified by potential benefits.
4. Justice (fairness and equity):
   - Research should be inclusive and non-discriminatory.
   - The benefits and burdens of research should be fairly distributed.

5. Confidentiality and data protection
   - Personal data must be stored securely and comply with **UK General Data Protection Regulation (UK GDPR) and the Data Protection Act 2018.**[1]
   - Identifiable data should be anonymized or pseudonymized where possible.
6. Scientific integrity:
   - Research must be honest, transparent, and reproducible.
   - Plagiarism, data fabrication, or misconduct is strictly prohibited.

Who Regulates Research Ethics in the UK?

Research ethics in the UK are overseen by various bodies, depending on the research context.

Health and Social Care Research (NHS, Clinical Research)

- **Health Research Authority (HRA):** oversees ethical approval for research involving NHS patients, staff, or facilities.
- **National Health Service Research Ethics Committees (NHS REC):** reviews research proposals involving human participants, tissue, or personal data.
- **Medicines and Healthcare Products Regulatory Agency (MHRA):** regulates clinical trials of medicinal products and medical devices.

HRA approval vs NHS REC: HRA and HCRW approval is the governance approval required for NHS research in England and Wales. This process may incorporate Research Ethics Committee (REC) review, rather than requiring a separate sequential application. For clinical trials of investigational medicinal products (CTIMPs), a Combined Review process is used via IRAS, in which MHRA and REC review are coordinated within a single application.

MHRA vs REC: For CTIMPs (clinical trial of an investigational medicinal product (drug trials)) and many device studies you need *MHRA authorization* (regulatory) *in addition to* an NHS REC opinion (ethical).

Academic and Non-NHS Research

- **University Research Ethics Committees (URECs):** handle ethics approval for social sciences, humanities, and non-NHS medical research.
- **UK Research Integrity Office (UKRIO):** provides ethical guidance for universities and independent researchers.

Social Care and Sensitive Research

- **Social Care Research Ethics Committee** (SCREC):[2] reviews research involving social care services and vulnerable populations.

---

[1] **UK GDPR and Data Protection Act 2018:** UK legislation governing lawful, fair, and transparent processing of personal data, including research uses. It mandates minimization, security, and rights for data subjects.

[2] **SCREC (Social Care REC):** National REC for research in social care and with vulnerable groups in those settings; routes through IRAS where applicable.

- **Confidentiality Advisory Group (CAG):** grants permission for researchers to access confidential patient data without consent in limited cases. The CAG can permit use of confidential patient information without consent in specific circumstances (public interest, impracticable consent) via the Health Service (Control of Patient Information) Regs 2002 (often called 's251').

Ethical Approval Process in the UK

Before conducting research involving human participants, ethical approval must be obtained. The process involves the following.

Determining If Approval Is Required

Ethical approval is needed if research involves:

- human participants (interviews, experiments)
- personal or sensitive data
- biological samples (e.g. blood, tissue)
- NHS staff, patients, or social care users.

Identifying the Right Ethics Committee

- **NHS REC via HRA:** if research involves NHS patients, staff, or facilities.
- **University REC:** if research is academic and does not involve the NHS.
- **SCREC:** if the study involves social care users.

Submitting an Application

- **NHS studies:** apply via the Integrated Research Application System (**IRAS**).[3]
- **University research**: apply via institutional ethics review portals.
- Applications must include a research protocol, consent forms, risk assessments, and data protection plan.

Ethics Review and Approval

- Timelines vary depending on the review pathway, the completeness of the application, and whether further information is requested
- Possible outcomes: approved, conditional approval (requiring changes), or rejected.

Research Misconduct and Ethics Violations

Ethical breaches in research can lead to severe consequences, including *legal action*, *loss of funding*, and *professional misconduct investigations*. Common violations include:

- **Plagiarism:** using others' work without proper citation.
- **Data fabrication:** making up research data or results.
- **Data falsification:** manipulating data to support desired conclusions.
- **Breach of confidentiality:** exposing participants' personal data.
- **Failure to obtain ethical approval:** conducting research without prior ethics approval.

---

[3] **IRAS (Integrated Research Application System):** Single online system to prepare and submit one application for all required UK health/social care approvals (e.g. REC, HRA, R&D, MHRA); generates a project IRASID.

Special Considerations in Research Ethics

Some research topics require additional safeguards.

Research with Vulnerable Populations

- Includes children, prisoners, elderly, and people lacking mental capacity.
- Requires extra informed consent procedures and safeguarding measures.

Research Using Personal Data

- Must comply with UK GDPR and Data Protection Act 2018.
- Anonymization should be used where possible.
- Some projects require Confidentiality Advisory Group approval to use patient-identifiable data without consent.
- Anonymization vs pseudonymization: *Anonymized* data are not identifiable by anyone; *pseudonymized* data can be relinked by a key holder, and remain personal data. Ethics and UK GDPR treat these differently.

Research Involving Deception

- Some psychological and social research uses deception (e.g. placebo studies).
- This requires justification and post-study debriefing for participants.

Deception and debrief: deception must be *justified, minimally intrusive*, and followed by timely *debriefing* that explains the purpose and offers withdrawal of data where appropriate.

Key Legislation and Guidelines

- **UK Policy Framework for Health and Social Care Research (HRA):** sets out the principles, standards, and responsibilities for the design, management, and conduct of health and social care research in the UK, ensuring that research is ethical, scientifically robust, and compliant with legal and governance requirements.
- **Declaration of Helsinki**: international guidelines for medical research ethics.
- **UK General Data Protection Regulation (UK GDPR):** data protection for research participants.
- Mental Capacity Act 2005:[4] guidelines for research involving individuals who lack capacity.
- Human Tissue Act 2004:[5] regulations for research using human tissue samples.

Summary of Research Ethics in the UK

The following list provides a summary of the core aspects of research ethics in the UK, including principles, regulating bodies, approval processes, potential misconduct risks, and special considerations:

- **core principles:** Respect, beneficence, non-maleficence, justice, confidentiality, scientific integrity

---

[4] **Mental Capacity Act 2005:** When capacity is lacking, a consultee advises on likely wishes; the researcher decides with safeguards. Extra protections apply for minimal burden and assent.

[5] **Human Tissue Act 2004 (HTA):** UK consent-centred framework; storage of relevant material for research is licensable (unless exempt). Institutions need HTA licenses and governance.

- **regulating bodies:** HRA, NHS REC, MHRA, UKRIO, SCREC, URECs
- **approval process:** identify need → choose ethics committee → submit IRAS/university application → review → approval
- **misconduct risks:** plagiarism, data fraud, privacy violations, lack of consent
- **special considerations:** vulnerable populations, personal data, deception in research.

Reporting Standards and Guidelines for Research Studies

CONSORT

CONSORT (Consolidated Standards of Reporting Trials) provides guidelines designed to improve the quality of reporting for randomized controlled trials (RCTs), which are considered the highest level of evidence. Key aspects include:

- a 25-item checklist covering various aspects of the trial, from the title and abstract to the discussion of results
- a flow diagram representing the progress of participants through the trial.

PRISMA

PRISMA (Preferred Reporting Items for Systematic Reviews and Meta-Analyses) is a set of evidence-based minimum recommendations for reporting systematic reviews and meta-analyses, which synthesize data from multiple studies to provide strong evidence. PRISMA consists of:

- a 27-item checklist addressing various aspects of the review, including the title, abstract, introduction, methods, results, and discussion
- a flow diagram that visually represents the flow of information through the different phases of a systematic review, including identification, screening, eligibility, and inclusion of studies.

QUOROM

QUOROM (Quality of Reporting of Meta-Analyses) was a reporting guideline developed to improve the quality of reporting in meta-analyses of RCTs. It has since been superseded by the PRISMA statement.

PROSPERO

PROSPERO (the International Prospective Register of Systematic Reviews)[6] is an online database where researchers register their protocols for systematic reviews. PROSPERO registers protocols for systematic reviews with a health-related outcome. Its key purposes include:

- increasing transparency in systematic reviews
- reducing duplication of reviews
- minimizing reporting bias.

---

[6] **PROSPERO:** An international database for registering systematic review protocols. Registration improves transparency and reduces duplication.

ISRCTN

ISRCTN (International Standard Randomised Controlled Trial Number)[7] is a unique identification number assigned to clinical trials. The ISRCTN Registry provides a publicly accessible database of registered clinical trials.

STARD

STARD (Standards for Reporting Diagnostic Accuracy Studies) is a guideline designed to improve the completeness and transparency of reporting in studies evaluating the accuracy of diagnostic tests. It aims to ensure diagnostic accuracy studies are reported in a way that allows readers to assess their potential for bias and applicability. STARD includes:

- a 30-item checklist covering study design, patient selection, index test, reference standard, statistical methods, and results
- emphasis on clear and detailed reporting of how a diagnostic test was evaluated.

STROBE

STROBE (Strengthening the Reporting of Observational Studies in Epidemiology) provides recommendations to improve the quality of reporting for observational studies in epidemiology. It applies to cohort, case–control, and cross-sectional studies. The purpose of STROBE is to:

- ensure studies are reported in a way that allows readers to critically appraise their validity and generalizability
- promote reliable and transparent epidemiological research.

AGREE

AGREE (Appraisal of Guidelines for Research and Evaluation) is a tool used to assess the quality and reporting of clinical practice guidelines. It provides a systematic and standardized approach to evaluating the methodological rigour and transparency of these guidelines. The AGREE instrument consists of six domains:

1. scope and purpose
2. stakeholder involvement
3. rigour of development
4. clarity of presentation
5. applicability
6. editorial independence

Each item in AGREE is scored on a seven-point scale, allowing for a quantitative assessment of guideline quality.

SRQR

SRQR (Standards for Reporting Qualitative Research) is designed to improve the transparency and quality of reporting in qualitative research studies. It provides a framework for

[7] **ISRCTN:** A registry that issues International Standard Randomized Controlled Trial Numbers for unique trial identification. It supports transparency and tracking.

researchers to report their studies comprehensively and clearly. SRQR consists of a 21-item checklist covering:

- study design
- methods
- data analysis
- findings.

COREQ

COREQ (Consolidated Criteria for Reporting Qualitative Research) is a 32 item checklist developed to ensure comprehensive reporting of qualitative studies, particularly those using interviews and focus groups. It helps researchers provide thorough and transparent reports of qualitative research.

Chapter Summary

Research Ethics and Ethical Approval Process in the UK

Research ethics ensure that studies involving human participants, personal data, or biological samples are conducted safely and responsibly. Ethical principles such as *autonomy*, *beneficence*, *non-maleficence*, *justice*, *confidentiality*, and *scientific integrity* guide research practices.

In the UK, ethical approval is regulated by bodies such as the Health Research Authority (HRA), NHS Research Ethics Committees (REC), Medicines and Healthcare Products Regulatory Agency (MHRA), university RECs, and the UK Research Integrity Office (UKRIO).

The ethical approval process involves determining whether approval is required, identifying the appropriate ethics committee, submitting an application, and undergoing review. Research misconduct, including *plagiarism*, *data fabrication*, and *failure to obtain ethical approval*, can have serious consequences.

Reporting Standards and Guidelines for Research Studies

To improve transparency, accuracy, and reproducibility in research, various reporting guidelines exist:

- **CONSORT** (for RCTs)
- **PRISMA** (for Systematic Reviews and Meta-Analyses)
- **QUOROM** (previously used for meta-analyses, now replaced by PRISMA)
- **PROSPERO** (for registering systematic review protocols)
- **ISRCTN** (for trial identification)
- **STARD** (for diagnostic accuracy studies)
- **STROBE** (for observational studies)
- **AGREE** (for evaluating clinical practice guidelines)
- **SRQR** (for qualitative research)
- **COREQ** (for detailed qualitative research reporting).

Practice Questions

Q1. Which principle focuses on maximizing benefits for participants in a study?

A. Confidentiality
B. Non-maleficence
C. Beneficence
D. Justice
E. Scientific integrity

Q2. Which UK organization is responsible for overseeing ethical approval for research involving NHS patients, staff, or facilities?

A. UK Research Integrity Office (UKRIO)
B. Health Research Authority (HRA)
C. Social Care Research Ethics Committee (SCREC)
D. Confidentiality Advisory Group (CAG)
E. University Research Ethics Committees (UREC)

Q3. Which organization regulates clinical trials of medicinal products and medical devices in the UK?

A. NHS REC
B. Health Research Authority (HRA)
C. Medicines and Healthcare Products Regulatory Agency (MHRA)
D. Social Care Research Ethics Committee (SCREC)
E. University Research Ethics Committees (UREC)

Q4. Which of the following research studies would *not* require ethical approval?

A. A study involving anonymized interviews from previous research with existing ethical approval.
B. A study collecting anonymized personal data.
C. A study using publicly available, anonymized data.
D. A study involving non-clinical NHS staff.
E. A study using biological samples like blood and tissue.

Q5. Which reporting guideline applies specifically to RCTs?

A. PRISMA
B. CONSORT
C. STARD
D. COREQ
E. AGREE

Q6. Which guideline has replaced QUOROM for systematic reviews and meta-analyses?

A. STROBE
B. PRISMA
C. AGREE

D. COREQ
E. PROSPERO

Q7. What is the purpose of PROSPERO in research?
A. To register protocols for systematic reviews.
B. To evaluate diagnostic test accuracy studies.
C. To assess the quality of observational studies.
D. To regulate clinical trials.
E. To provide ethics approval for social care research.

Q8. Which guideline focuses on improving the transparency of qualitative research reporting?
A. CONSORT
B. PRISMA
C. STARD
D. COREQ
E. STROBE

Answers

Q1. Correct answer: C. Beneficence. Beneficence requires that researchers ensure the benefits of a study outweigh the risks and that harm to participants is minimized.

Q2. Correct answer: B. Health Research Authority (HRA). The HRA oversees governance and coordination of ethical review for NHS-related research, while NHS Research Ethics Committees provide the ethical opinion.

Q3. Correct answer: C. Medicines and Healthcare Products Regulatory Agency (MHRA). The MHRA regulates clinical trials, medicinal products, and medical devices to ensure safety and compliance.

Q4. Correct answer: C. A study using publicly available, anonymized data.
Research using publicly available, anonymized data does not require ethical approval because it does not pose risks to participants.
The other options are incorrect because they all involve one of:

direct interaction with human participants (interviews, NHS staff) the use of personal data biological samples (which are directly taken from individuals).

Q5. Correct answer: B. CONSORT. The CONSORT guideline is specifically designed for RCTs.

Q6. Correct answer: B. PRISMA. PRISMA has replaced QUOROM as the standard for reporting systematic reviews and meta-analyses.

Q7. Correct answer: A. To register protocols for systematic reviews. PROSPERO is an online registry where researchers register their systematic review protocols to improve transparency.

Q8. Correct answer: D. COREQ. COREQ (Consolidated Criteria for Reporting Qualitative Research) ensures comprehensive reporting of qualitative research.

Further Reading

AGREE Research Trust. AGREE II Instrument (user manual). 2017. Available from: www.agreetrust.org/wp-content/uploads/2017/12/AGREE-II-Users-Manual-and-23-item-Instrument-2009-Update-2017.pdf

Bossuyt PM, Reitsma JB, Bruns DE, et al. STARD 2015. *BMJ*. 2015;**351**:h5527.

GOV.UK/MHRA. Clinical trials for medicines: apply for authorisation in the UK. Available from: www.gov.uk/guidance/clinical-trials-for-medicines-apply-for-authorisation-in-the-uk

Health Research Authority. Clinical trials of investigational medicinal products (CTIMPs): currently applicable legislation. Available from: www.hra.nhs.uk/planning-and-improving-research/policies-standards-legislation/clinical-trials-investigational-medicinal-products-ctimps.

Health Research Authority. Confidential patient information and the regulations (Section 251); guidance for CAG applicants. Available from: www.hra.nhs.uk/about-us/committees-and-services/confidentiality-advisory-group/guidance-cag-applicants/

Health Research Authority. Integrated Research Application System (IRAS). Available from: myresearchproject.org.uk.

Health Research Authority. Mental Capacity Act. Available from: www.hra.nhs.uk/planning-and-improving-research/policies-standards-legislation/mental-capacity-act/

Health Research Authority. UK Policy Framework for Health and Social Care Research. 2017–2025 update. Available from: www.hra.nhs.uk/planning-and-improving-research/policies-standards-legislation/uk-policy-framework-health-social-care-research/uk-policy-framework-health-and-social-care-research/

Human Tissue Authority. The Human Tissue Act 2004: legislation, consent and licensing. Available from: www.hta.gov.uk/guidance-professionals/licences-inspections-and-fees/licensing/hta-legislation-powers-consent-and

Information Commissioner's Office. The UK GDPR and UK GDPR guidance and resources. Available from: ico.org.uk.

ISRCTN Registry. About/why register. Available from: isrctn.com.

Moher D, Schulz KF, Altman DG ; CONSORT Group. CONSORT 2010 statement. *BMJ*. 2010;**340**:c869.

O'Brien BC, Harris IB, Beckman TJ, et al. SRQR. *Acad Med*. 2014;**89**(9):1245–51.

Page MJ, McKenzie JE, Bossuyt PM, et al. PRISMA 2020 statement. *BMJ*. 2021; **372**:n71.

Tong A, Sainsbury P, Craig J. COREQ. *Int J Qual Health Care*. 2007;**19**(6):349–57.

UK Parliament. Data Protection Act 2018. Available from: www.legislation.gov.uk/ukpga/2018/12/contents

University of York, CRD. PROSPERO: international prospective register of systematic reviews. Available from: crd.york.ac.uk/prospero.

von Elm E, Altman DG, Egger M, et al. STROBE statement. *PLoS Med*. 2007;**4**(10):e296–7.

World Medical Association. Declaration of Helsinki: ethical principles for medical research involving human subjects. Available from: www.wma.net/policies-post/wma-declaration-of-helsinki/

Glossary

A

Absolute benefit increase (ABI)/risk difference The difference in benefit between treatment and control groups.

Absolute risk The probability that an event (e.g. disease onset) will occur in a defined population over a specified time period. Unlike relative risk, it conveys the actual likelihood of occurrence and is useful for patient-facing communication.

Absolute risk difference (ARD) Also known as *attributable risk*, this is the numerical difference between the risk of an outcome in an exposed group compared to an unexposed group. It measures the actual change in risk – such as the number of additional cases of a disease – that can be directly attributed to a specific exposure. It is calculated as ARD = risk exposed – risk unexposed.

Absolute risk reduction (ARR)/risk difference The difference in risk between control and treatment groups.

Accuracy of a test The overall ability of a diagnostic test to correctly classify individuals as diseased or not diseased relative to a reference standard. It is the proportion of all correct results (true positives + true negatives) among all tested: (TP + TN) / (TP + TN + FP + FN). However, accuracy depends strongly on disease prevalence and can be misleading when the condition is rare, so it should be interpreted alongside sensitivity, specificity, and predictive values.

Adaptive randomization A method that adjusts treatment allocation probabilities during a trial based on interim results.

Adjusted (standardized) rate A rate modified to remove the effects of population differences (e.g. age, sex) to allow fair comparisons. Direct and indirect standardization are common approaches.

Age-specific death rate Deaths within a defined age band / population of that age band (×100,000). Use for fair comparisons across ages and as inputs to age standardization.

AGREE (Appraisal of Guidelines for Research and Evaluation) A tool to evaluate the quality, transparency, and applicability of clinical practice guidelines. It assesses domains such as scope, stakeholder involvement, rigour, clarity, and editorial independence.

Allocation concealment Prevents foreknowledge of the next assignment at enrolment (e.g. central randomization, sequentially numbered opaque sealed envelopes); distinct from blinding. Without concealment, clinicians can steer high-risk patients to a favoured arm.

Alpha (α) The prespecified probability of a type I error (false positive) in hypothesis testing. Commonly set at 0.05 in biomedical research.

Alternative hypothesis (H_1) The research proposition that there is a genuine effect or association. It contrasts with the null hypothesis, which posits no difference or association.

Amispective cohort study A hybrid cohort design with both retrospective and prospective components. Past records establish baseline exposures and outcomes, after which participants are followed forward for new outcomes. It measures incidence and can estimate risk ratios, but is vulnerable to loss to follow-up and time-varying confounding.

Analogy Causal consideration asking whether a similar exposure is known to produce a similar effect; such parallels add plausibility but are the weakest of Bradford Hill's considerations and cannot establish causation on their own.

Anonymization vs pseudonymization Anonymized data are no longer identifiable by anyone; pseudonymized data can be relinked by a key holder and remain personal data. Ethics and UK GDPR treat these differently.

ANOVA (analysis of variance) A family of tests comparing means across three or more groups by partitioning variance into between- and within-group components. Significant results typically require post-hoc tests to identify which groups differ.

Antagonism When two risk factors act together to produce a combined effect that is smaller than expected based on their individual effects.

Area under the curve (AUC) A measure summarizing the overall diagnostic accuracy of a test based on the receiver operating characteristic (ROC) curve. Values range from 0.5 (no discrimination) to 1.0 (perfect discrimination). AUC is threshold-independent but ignores clinical thresholds; pair with sensitivity/specificity at decision-relevant cut-points.

Assay sensitivity (trials) The ability of a trial to distinguish an effective treatment from a less effective or ineffective one. It is crucial in non-inferiority and equivalence designs.

As-treated analysis A method of analysing clinical trial data in which participants are analysed according to the treatment they actually received, regardless of their randomization.

Attrition (lost to follow-up) The loss of participants during a study, which can bias results if those lost differ systematically from those who remain.

Audit Systematic comparison of current practice against explicit standards to identify gaps and implement improvement; evaluates care already being provided (not designed to generate generalizable knowledge). See also *Audit cycle*.

Audit cycle Set standards → measure current practice → implement change → re-audit to confirm and sustain improvement.

Audit trail (electronic data/GCP) Metadata log recording creation/modification/deletion events with user IDs and timestamps to ensure data integrity and compliance.

Audit trail (qualitative research) Transparent record of decisions, materials and analytic steps (e.g. protocols, memos, codebooks) enabling external review of rigour and dependability.

B

Bar chart A chart using rectangular bars to represent categorical data, with bar lengths proportional to frequencies or values.

Bayes' Theorem A rule for updating the probability of a hypothesis in the light of new evidence: Posterior ∝ prior × likelihood. In diagnostics, it converts pre-test probability to post-test probability using likelihood ratios.

Bayesian analysis A framework that combines prior information with observed data to produce posterior distributions for parameters or hypotheses. It yields probabilities about effects rather than binary accept/reject decisions.

Bayesian hypothesis testing An approach that compares models or hypotheses using quantities like Bayes factors. It quantifies relative evidence rather than relying solely on p-values.

Begg's test A rank correlation test for publication bias in meta-analysis. It assesses whether study effect sizes correlate with their variances or standard errors.

Benefit–cost ratio (BCR) Monetized benefits / costs; BCR > 1 suggests net benefit. Interpret alongside net present value (NPV) because high ratios on tiny projects can mislead.

Between-subjects design A design in which different participants receive different conditions or treatments. It avoids carryover effects but generally requires larger samples than within-subjects designs.

Betweenness centrality A centrality measure reflecting how often a node lies on the shortest paths between other nodes. Nodes with high betweenness can control or mediate information flow in the network. See *Centrality*.

Bias (systematic error) A systematic deviation from the truth arising from design, conduct, or analysis flaws. Common forms include selection bias, information bias, and confounding.

Binary (dichotomous) data Variables with two categories (e.g. yes/no; event/no event). Analyses often use proportions, odds, or logistic models.

Biological gradient (dose–response relationship) A causal criterion stating that increasing exposure levels are associated with increasing (or decreasing) risk of disease.

Birth cohort Individuals born in the same period who are followed to study how early-life exposures influence later outcomes. Birth cohorts support life course epidemiology.

Bland–Altman plot A graphical method to assess agreement between two quantitative measurements by plotting their mean against their difference. Limits of agreement help identify systematic bias and outliers.

Blinding (masking) Keeps participants/clinicians/outcome assessors unaware of allocation to reduce performance/detection bias. Consider level (single-/double-/assessor-blind) and risk of unblinding.

Block randomization A method that allocates participants in small blocks to maintain balance in group sizes over time. Blocks may be fixed or randomly varied to preserve allocation concealment.

Bonferroni correction A conservative adjustment for multiple comparisons that divides α by the number of tests. It reduces type I errors but may decrease statistical power.

Boolean operators Use *AND*/*OR*/*NOT*, quotation marks (' ') for phrases, truncation (e.g. therap*), and database-specific proximity operators to tune sensitivity/specificity.

Bootstrap (resampling) A computational method that estimates sampling variability by repeatedly resampling the observed data with replacement. It is useful for non-parametric standard errors and confidence intervals.

Bootstrapped CI (BCa) Bias corrected and accelerated interval that adjusts for bias and skewness in the bootstrap distribution; typically more accurate than basic/percentile intervals, uses a large number of resamples (often thousands).

Box plot (whisker plot) A graphical display of a dataset showing the median, quartiles, and potential outliers. The 'whiskers' extend to indicate variability outside the quartiles.

Bracketing Temporarily setting aside the researcher's preconceptions (epoché) to minimize their influence during data collection and analysis; common in phenomenology and supported by reflexive memos.

Bradford Hill criteria Nine considerations proposed by Austin Bradford Hill (1965) to assess causality in epidemiological associations: strength, consistency, specificity, temporality, biological gradient, plausibility, coherence, experiment, and analogy.

Bridge node A node that connects otherwise separate parts of the network; its removal can fragment the network and disrupt information flow.

Budget impact analysis (BIA) Payer-perspective cash flow estimate (often 1–5 years) of adopting an intervention. Answers 'Can we afford it now?', complementing cost-effectiveness analysis.

C

CAG (Section 251) support UK route to use confidential patient information without consent for specific public-interest research where consent is impracticable; requires safeguards and review.

Case fatality rate (CFR) The proportion of individuals with a condition who die from it during a specified period. It indicates disease severity and effectiveness of care.

Case study (qualitative) In-depth examination of a bounded 'case' (person, team, service, event) using multiple sources (interviews, observation, documents) to illuminate processes and context. Can be single- or multiple-case; targets analytic generalization, not population estimates.

Case–control study An observational study design comparing individuals with a disease (cases) to those without (controls) to assess prior exposures. Efficient for rare diseases but prone to recall and selection bias.

Causal web A framework emphasizing how multiple interconnected factors contribute jointly to disease.

Central limit theorem (CLT) A theorem stating that the distribution of sample means approaches normality as sample size grows, regardless of the population distribution. It underpins many inferential procedures.

Centrality plot A visual comparison of centrality values across nodes to highlight the most influential elements.

Centrality A family of measures that quantify the relative importance of a node in a network. Key types include degree, betweenness, closeness, and eigenvector centrality.

Chi-square test A statistical test assessing whether observed frequencies differ from expected frequencies in categorical data. Requires adequate expected cell counts; use Fisher's exact test when cells are small.

CINAHL Nursing and allied-health literature – broadens beyond core biomedical databases.

CINeMA Confidence in NMA via domains aligned to GRADE (within-study bias, reporting bias, indirectness, imprecision, heterogeneity, incoherence); yields transparent, domain-level judgements.

Clinical audit cycle The cyclical process of planning, implementing, measuring, and reviewing changes to improve healthcare quality.

Clinical trial phases Conventional pathway: preclinical → phase I → phase II → phase III → phase IV. Modern programmes may use adaptive/seamless designs (e.g. phase I/II or II/III) with prespecified decision rules. See also: *preclinical (non-clinical) studies, phase I–IV.*

ClinicalTrials.gov Trial registry/results database – helps find ongoing/unpublished studies and assess selective reporting.

Closeness centrality A measure of how close a node is to all others in terms of path length; nodes with high closeness can quickly reach or influence other nodes. See *Centrality.*

Cluster randomized trial A trial design in which groups (e.g. schools, hospitals, general practices) rather than individuals are randomized to intervention or control arms. Analysis must account for intra-cluster correlation, since outcomes within clusters tend to be correlated.

Clustering coefficient Proportion of a node's neighbour pairs that are also connected (local transitivity); the network average reflects overall 'cliquishness'.

Cochran's Q test A chi-square statistic used in meta-analysis to test for heterogeneity across studies. A significant Q indicates variability greater than expected by chance alone, but power is limited when the number of studies is small.

Cochrane library Includes CDSR (systematic reviews) and CENTRAL (trial registry of registries); core sources for trial identification. It is a key source for high-quality syntheses.

Cochrane Risk of Bias Tool A structured tool for assessing bias in randomized trials. The original version (RoB 1) covered domains such as selection, performance, detection, attrition, and reporting bias. The revised 2019 version (RoB 2) evaluates bias across five domains: randomization process, deviations from intended interventions, missing outcome data, measurement of the outcome, and selection of the reported result.

Cohen's *d* An effect size expressing the mean difference between two groups in standard deviation units. Values of 0.2, 0.5, and 0.8 are often interpreted as small, medium, and large.

Coherence A causal criterion where an observed association should not conflict with existing biological knowledge.

Cohort study An observational study in which individuals are classified by exposure status and followed over time to assess disease incidence. Measures incidence and can estimate risk ratios; vulnerable to loss to follow-up and time-varying confounding.

Common vs special cause Common cause is a routine system variation (fix the process); special cause is an unusual, assignable variation (investigate the event). Treating common cause as special (or vice versa) wastes effort or misses systemic fixes.

Comorbidity network A network where nodes represent disorders and edges represent their co-occurrence within individuals or populations.

Component cause A factor that contributes to disease but is neither necessary nor sufficient alone. Multiple component causes often form a sufficient cause.

Confidence interval (CI) A range of plausible values for a parameter given the observed data and model assumptions (e.g. 95% CI). Narrower intervals indicate more precise estimates.

Confidentiality Advisory Group (CAG) A UK body that can authorize use of confidential patient information without consent under strict safeguards. It balances research value with privacy.

Confounding Distortion of an exposure–outcome association caused by a third variable related to both. Design (randomization, restriction, matching) and analysis (stratification, regression) can address it.

Consistency (NMA context) The agreement between direct and indirect comparisons in network meta-analysis.

CONSORT flow diagram A standard visual showing the passage of participants through enrolment, allocation, follow-up, and analysis. It clarifies attrition and exclusions.

CONSORT Reporting guidelines for randomized controlled trials that improve transparency and reproducibility. The checklist and flow diagram are widely used by journals.

Constant comparative method Iterative grounded-theory technique in which data segments ('incidents') are continually compared within and across sources to refine codes and group them into categories. Using analytic memos and ongoing sampling, categories are elaborated and integrated until *theoretical saturation* is reached.

Content analysis A systematic approach to categorizing and quantifying textual or visual data to identify patterns. It may use deductive (predefined) or inductive (emergent) coding.

Contingent valuation (CV) Survey method that elicits individuals' willingness to pay (or willingness to accept) for a specified health gain or risk reduction under a hypothetical scenario, to monetize benefits for cost–benefit analysis.

Continuous quality improvement (CQI) An ongoing process of identifying, describing, and analysing strengths and problems, then testing, implementing, and monitoring interventions to improve outcomes.

Control chart (SPC) A time series graph with a centreline and statistically derived control limits to distinguish common cause from special cause variation. It supports real-time quality monitoring.

Control event rate (CER) The proportion of participants with the outcome in the control group.

Control group A comparator group receiving standard care or placebo. It provides a baseline to attribute changes to the intervention.
Convenience sampling Non-probability sampling that recruits readily available participants (e.g. volunteers, consecutive attendees) rather than from a defined sampling frame. Fast and low-cost but prone to selection bias and limited generalizability; report the recruitment source and time window.
COREQ Consolidated criteria for reporting qualitative research (interviews/focus groups).
Correlation analysis A statistical method assessing the strength and direction of association between two continuous variables. Remember correlation does not imply causation; check scatterplots for non-linearity and outliers.
Correlation coefficient A statistic (e.g. Pearson's r, Spearman's ρ) quantifying strength and direction of association between two variables. Values range from -1 (perfect negative) to $+1$ (perfect positive).
Cost–benefit analysis (CBA) Compares costs and benefits, both expressed in monetary terms.
Cost–consequence analysis (CCA) Lists costs alongside multiple outcomes without combining them into a single ratio.
Cost-effectiveness acceptability curve (CEAC) A graphical representation showing the probability of an intervention being cost-effective across a range of willingness-to-pay thresholds.
Cost-effectiveness analysis (CEA) Compares costs to a natural health outcome (e.g. life years gained).
Cost-minimization analysis (CMA) Identifies the least costly option among equally effective interventions.
Cost–utility analysis (CUA) An evaluation comparing costs with utility-based outcomes such as QALYs. It facilitates comparison across diverse interventions.
Cox proportional hazards model A semi-parametric regression for time to event data estimating hazard ratios. It assumes proportional hazards over time.
Criterion sampling Purposive strategy that selects all cases meeting a prespecified criterion (e.g. diagnosis, exposure level, or event). Ensures relevance and comparability; state the criterion and rationale, noting it is not intended for statistical generalization.
Criterion vs standard (audit) A criterion states what should happen; a standard sets the compliance target (e.g. ≥95% within 48 h). Both should be measurable and time bound.
Critical case sampling Purposive strategy that selects cases with strategic importance (where the phenomenon is most/least likely to occur) so findings have strong logical leverage – for example, 'if it works here, it will work anywhere', or the converse. Suited to testing propositions and illuminating mechanisms in depth; not for statistical generalization.
Crossover trial A trial where participants receive treatments sequentially, serving as their own control.
Cross-sectional study An observational study design measuring exposure and outcome at the same time point, providing a snapshot of associations.
Crude death rate The total number of deaths in a population during a period divided by the population size (e.g. per 1,000). It does not adjust for age or other factors.
Cytoscape Open source environment widely used in bioinformatics/neuroscience for complex biological network visualization and plugin-based analysis.

D

DALY (disability-adjusted life year) A measure of overall disease burden combining years of life lost due to premature mortality and years lived with disability. It supports cross-disease comparisons in health economics.
Data analysis Using data systematically to track performance, monitor change, and evaluate outcomes.
Data saturation (qualitative) The point in data collection when no new themes or insights emerge. It guides sample size decisions in qualitative studies.
Data triangulation Using multiple data sources to corroborate findings. Together with method and investigator triangulation, it strengthens credibility.
Deception and debrief Any deception must be necessary, proportionate, and followed by timely debrief with the option to withdraw data. Record rationale and mitigate distress.
Decision tree (economic modelling) A diagram that maps clinical pathways, probabilities, costs, and outcomes over short horizons. Complex or recurrent processes often require Markov models instead.
Declaration of Helsinki An international statement of ethical principles for human research, covering consent, risk–benefit, and

transparency. It underpins many national regulations and ethics reviews.

Deductive reasoning A form of reasoning in which conclusions about specific cases are derived from general principles or established rules. In clinical and scientific contexts, deductive reasoning involves applying known laws, definitions, or formulas (such as dosage calculations or diagnostic criteria) to individual situations.

Degree centrality The simplest centrality measure, counting the number of direct connections a node has. Nodes with high degree centrality are immediately influential. See *Centrality*.

Degrees of freedom (df) The number of independent pieces of information available to estimate a parameter. Many test statistics (t, χ^2, F) depend on df for significance.

Density plot (KDE) A smoothed estimate of the distribution formed by summing kernels (often Gaussian) placed at each data point; the bandwidth controls smoothness. The curve integrates to 1 and approximates the probability density.

Dependent variable (outcome) The variable measured to assess the effect of the exposure or intervention. It is also called the response or outcome variable.

Descriptive statistics Methods that summarize data (e.g. mean, median, standard deviation, range, IQR). They provide essential context before inferential analysis.

Deterministic causation A cause that, if present, is sufficient to produce the effect in a given context (no randomness once conditions are fixed).

Deviant (extreme) case sampling Purposive selection of unusually successful/unsuccessful or otherwise outlier cases to make underlying processes most visible and test boundary conditions. Useful for mechanism-finding and hypothesis generation; not for statistical generalization. State the criteria for 'extreme' and the selection rationale.

Diagnostic gold standard The best available method against which new tests are measured.

Diary methods Prospective self-recording of behaviours, symptoms, experiences or exposures by participants at scheduled intervals (time-based) or when events occur (event-based). Can use paper/e-diaries or ecological momentary assessment via mobile prompts. Reduces recall bias and captures within-day variation; report mode, prompting schedule, compliance/missingness handling, timestamping and reminders.

Direct age standardization Applies age-specific rates to a standard population to remove age-structure differences, enabling fair comparisons across places/times.

Direct costs Resources directly used to deliver healthcare (e.g. consultations, investigations, procedures, bed-days, medicines, devices); may also include direct non-medical costs such as patient travel or formal social care, depending on perspective.

Discounting (economic evaluation) Adjusting future costs and health outcomes to present value using a discount rate. It reflects time preference in cost-effectiveness analyses.

Discourse analysis A qualitative method examining how language constructs meaning, identities, and power relations. It considers context, form, and function of language use.

Document analysis Systematic examination of existing texts and artefacts (e.g. medical records, policies, minutes, emails, media) to address a research question using content/thematic or discourse approaches.

Dose–response relationship (biological gradient) A principle of causality: increasing exposure should increase disease risk (or decrease risk in protective factors).

Dot plot Displays each observation (or stacked duplicates) on a number line, preserving exact values without binning useful for small to moderate sample sizes and for comparing groups side-by-side.

Double hermeneutic Two-stage meaning-making: participants interpret their experiences, and the researcher interprets those interpretations; acknowledges co-construction of findings.

Double-blind trial Participants and investigators are both unaware of group allocations.

Dunnett's test A post-hoc comparison of multiple treatments against a single control following ANOVA. It controls for type I error while focusing on treatment vs control contrasts.

E

Ecological fallacy Mistakenly inferring individual-level effects from group-level associations; guard against with individual-level data or multilevel models.

Ecological study Uses group-level exposures/outcomes (e.g. countries/regions). Efficient for hypothesis generation, but cannot ascribe effects to individuals.

Effect modification When the effect of an exposure on an outcome differs across levels of a third variable (an effect modifier). Reporting stratum-specific estimates clarifies the interaction.

Effect size A quantitative index of the magnitude of an effect (e.g. Cohen's *d*, OR, RR, η^2). Unlike *p*-values, effect sizes reflect practical importance.

Egger's test Regression test for funnel-plot asymmetry (small study effects) in meta-analysis: regress the standard normal deviate (effect size / SE) on study precision (1 / SE); a non-zero intercept suggests asymmetry (e.g. publication or reporting bias).

Eigenvector centrality A measure of node importance that gives higher scores to nodes connected to other highly connected nodes, capturing influence within the wider network.

Elastic net regression A penalized regression that blends L1 (lasso) and L2 (ridge) penalties. It handles correlated predictors and performs variable selection and shrinkage.

Embase Emtree-indexed biomedical/pharma database with strong conference abstract coverage. Use alongside MEDLINE to reduce retrieval bias; de-duplicate carefully.

Epidemiology The study of the distribution and determinants of health-related states in populations. It informs prevention, policy, and clinical decision-making.

Equivalence trial A trial designed to show that two treatments do not differ by more than a prespecified margin. It contrasts with noninferiority and superiority trials.

Eta squared (η^2) An ANOVA effect size expressing the proportion of total variance attributable to a factor. Partial η^2 is commonly reported in multifactor designs.

Ethical approval Formal permission from an ethics committee to conduct research involving humans, data, or tissue. It ensures risk–benefit balance, consent, and data protection.

Ethnography Field-based qualitative approach to understand how a group functions in its natural setting. Involves prolonged engagement, participant observation, reflexive fieldnotes and iterative interviewing/analysis to produce a 'thick description' of culture and practice.

Evidence synthesis Combining findings from multiple studies (e.g. systematic review, meta-analysis). It increases precision and supports generalizable conclusions.

Excess risk (attributable risk) The difference in incidence between exposed and unexposed groups, reflecting the disease burden due to exposure.

Experimental event rate (EER) The proportion of participants with the outcome in the intervention group.

Explanatory trial Randomized study designed to test efficacy under optimal, tightly controlled conditions (strict eligibility, protocolized interventions, intensive follow-up, high adherence), maximizing internal validity; contrasts with pragmatic trials of real-world effectiveness.

Exposed cohort A group of individuals with a specified exposure, followed for outcomes. Measures incidence and can estimate risk ratios; vulnerable to loss to follow-up.

Exposure (risk) window: Prespecified period after (or around) an exposure during which the risk of an outcome may change. The window should be defined a priori (start and duration) to support valid causal interpretation and to avoid bias such as reverse causation.

Eyeballing funnel plot Informal visual inspection of a funnel plot to judge whether studies are symmetrically distributed, potentially indicating publication bias.

F

***F* statistic** A ratio of between-group to within-group variance used in ANOVA and related models. Larger values relative to df indicate greater evidence against equal means.

Fagan nomogram Graph converts pre-test probability and likelihood ratio into post-test probability; helpful without a calculator.

Fail-safe *N* An estimate of how many missing 'null' studies would be needed to reduce a statistically significant meta-analysis result to non-significance. It provides a rough indication of robustness to publication bias. However, fail-safe *N* is an older and limited metric and may give false reassurance, as it does not account for the plausibility or impact of missing studies; it should be interpreted alongside other methods such as funnel plots and trim-and-fill.

Falsification theory Popper's view that scientific claims must be testable and open to refutation. Surviving severe tests strengthens confidence in a theory.

Field trial Epidemiological studies conducted in real-world community or population settings, typically to evaluate preventive interventions (e.g. vaccines, public health measures) before large-scale implementation. They focus on how an intervention works 'in the field' rather than under tightly controlled experimental conditions.

Fishbone diagram (Ishikawa diagram) A cause-and-effect tool that organizes possible causes of a problem into categories (e.g. methods, materials, equipment, people, environment, measurement). It supports structured brainstorming and root cause analysis. Branches should be populated with evidence rather than assumptions.

Fisher's exact test An exact test of association in small contingency tables. It is appropriate when expected cell counts are low.

Fisher's LSD A relatively liberal post hoc procedure following ANOVA for pairwise comparisons. It offers more power at the cost of higher type I error risk.

Fixed-effect model Assumes that all studies included in a meta-analysis estimate the same underlying true effect size, and that observed differences between study results are due solely to chance (sampling error). This contrasts with the random-effects model, which allows for genuine variation in effect sizes between studies.

Flow diagram (PRISMA/CONSORT) A structured figure depicting identification, screening, eligibility, and inclusion (PRISMA) or trial participant progress (CONSORT). It enhances transparency.

Focus group Moderated group discussion (typically 6–8 participants with shared characteristics) that explores beliefs, experiences, and norms through interaction. Uses a topic guide and probing to surface consensus/divergence; data are the dialogue and dynamics.

Forest plot A graphical display of individual study results and pooled effect estimates in a meta-analysis, showing effect size and confidence intervals.

Framework analysis Matrix-based approach for applied qualitative research. Typical stages: familiarization → identify a thematic framework → index/code → chart into a case-by-theme matrix → map and interpret. Suited to policy/practice questions and team-based, transparent analysis.

Frequency density (histogram) With unequal bins, height = frequency / bin width, so area = counts. With equal bins it reduces to the familiar frequency histogram.

Friction cost approach Values productivity loss only over the friction period (time to replace staff and restore output). Typically yields smaller, labour-market-realistic estimates than human capital.

Funnel plot A scatter plot of study size or precision against effect size, used to assess publication bias and small-study effects.

G

Galbraith (radial) plot A meta-analytic scatter plot of standardized effects versus precision that highlights heterogeneity and outliers. It aids sensitivity analyses.

Gaussian (normal) distribution A bell-shaped, symmetric distribution defined by mean and variance. Many parametric tests rely on normality assumptions.

GCP (Good Clinical Practice) An international ethical and scientific quality standard for designing, conducting, and reporting trials involving human subjects.

Gephi Open-source, interactive platform for large-graph layout, filtering, and clustering (e.g. ForceAtlas, Louvain) used for exploratory visualization.

Gini coefficient (inequality) A measure of inequality (0 = perfect equality, 1 = maximal inequality). In health economics it can summarize income or health disparities.

GRADE framework Rates certainty of evidence (high → very low) across risk of bias, inconsistency, indirectness, imprecision, and publication bias; keeps certainty distinct from recommendation strength.

Grey literature Research not formally published in books or peer-reviewed journals, such as theses, reports, conference proceedings, or regulatory documents.

Grounded theory An inductive qualitative method that develops theory from data through iterative coding and constant comparison. Sampling is often theoretical and continues until saturation.

H

Hawthorne effect Behaviour change caused simply by awareness of being observed; typically wanes with prolonged observation or habituation.

Hazard ratio (HR) A relative measure from survival analysis comparing hazard rates between groups. HR > 1 suggests higher instantaneous risk in the exposed group.

Health Research Authority (HRA) The UK body overseeing research ethics review and study approvals in the NHS. It promotes safe, ethical, and transparent research.

Heterogeneity (meta-analysis) Variation in study effects beyond chance, arising from clinical or methodological differences. It is assessed with Cochran's Q, I^2, and τ^2.

Histogram A bar-like plot displaying the distribution of continuous data by bins. It helps assess shape, spread, and potential outliers.

HMIC Health Management Information Consortium; a good source for health policy, management, and service-delivery evidence.

Homophily/assortativity (networks) The tendency for similar nodes to connect (e.g. by attributes or degree). Positive assortativity can impact diffusion and resilience.

HRA approval vs NHS REC HRA approval checks governance/organizational compliance; an NHS REC provides the ethical opinion. Many NHS studies require both.

Human capital approach Productivity loss = wage × time lost (illness/premature death); tends to yield larger indirect-cost estimates than friction cost.

Human Tissue Act 2004 (HTA) UK consent-centred framework; storage of relevant material for research is licensable (unless exempt). Institutions need HTA licences and governance.

I

I^2 Statistic The percentage of total variability in a meta-analysis due to heterogeneity rather than chance. Values around 25%, 50%, and 75% are often labelled low, moderate, and high.

ICER (incremental cost-effectiveness ratio) The ratio of the difference in costs to the difference in effects between two options (ΔCost / ΔEffect). It is compared against willingness-to-pay thresholds.

ICTRP (WHO) Aggregates national/regional trial registries, improving global ascertainment beyond US/EU; useful for non-English and LMIC trial capture.

Inception cohort A cohort recruited at a common early stage in disease or exposure to allow unbiased follow-up. Measures incidence and can estimate risk ratios; vulnerable to loss to follow-up and time-varying confounding.

Incidence rate (person-time) Events / accumulated person-time at risk; captures speed of occurrence vs risk (probability) over a fixed interval.

Incidence rate ratio (IRR) Relative rate = exposed period event rate / unexposed period rate (often from Poisson/NB models); interprets as multiplicative change in rate.

Incremental cost The difference in total costs between two alternatives (e.g. intervention A minus intervention B) for a stated perspective and time horizon. Used with the incremental health effect to compute the ICER; distinct from marginal cost (cost of one extra unit) and average cost (total cost divided by units).

Incremental cost-effectiveness ratio (ICER) The ratio of the difference in costs to the difference in effectiveness between two interventions.

Incremental cost-utility ratio (ICUR) Similar to ICER but outcomes are measured in utility terms (e.g. QALYs).

Independent *t*-test (unpaired *t*-test) A parametric statistical test used to compare the means of a continuous outcome variable between two independent groups (e.g. treatment vs control). It assumes approximately normal distribution of the outcome in each group, independence of observations, and homogeneity of variances (or uses a variance-adjusted version if this assumption is violated).

Independent variable A variable manipulated or classified to observe its effect on a dependent (outcome) variable.

In-depth interviews (qualitative) One-to-one, open-ended qualitative interviews that use a topic guide and probing to explore participants' experiences, beliefs, and context in depth. Well suited to complex or sensitive topics; not for statistical generalization. State the sampling approach, mode (face-to-face/phone/video), setting, and whether semi-structured or unstructured.

Indirect costs Productivity losses or other non-medical costs resulting from illness.

Inductive reasoning (qualitative) Bottom-up inference where codes, categories, and themes are derived from the data rather than imposed a priori; patterns are refined iteratively (e.g. constant comparison) until saturation.

Inferential statistics Statistical tests to make inferences about a population from a sample.

Information bias Systematic error arising from inaccurate measurement or misclassification of exposure, outcome, or covariates. State the expected direction (towards/away from null) and describe the design/analysis strategies to mitigate it.

Intangible costs Non-monetary burdens (e.g. pain, psychological distress, stigma, reduced quality of life) that do not involve direct resource use. Typically not priced in cost or cost-minimization analyses; in cost–utility analysis they are reflected via health-state utilities/QALYs, and in cost–benefit analysis they may be monetized using willingness-to-pay methods.

Intention-to-treat analysis Analysis of all trial participants in the groups to which they were originally randomized, regardless of adherence, preserving the benefits of randomization.

Interpretative phenomenological analysis (IPA) Qualitative, idiographic approach exploring how individuals make sense of significant experiences ('double hermeneutic': participants interpret events; researchers interpret participants' accounts).

Interval data Numerical data with equal intervals between values but no true zero (e.g. temperature in Celsius).

Inverse probability weighting (IPW) A statistical method that assigns weights to individuals based on the inverse probability of receiving a particular treatment or exposure (and/or remaining uncensored), given measured covariates. IPW is commonly used to adjust for confounding in observational studies and to account for informative censoring, creating a weighted pseudo-population in which groups are more comparable.

Inverse variance method A meta-analysis weighting approach where larger, more precise studies contribute more to the pooled estimate.

Inverse variance weighting Study weight $w_i = 1 / \mathrm{Var}(\theta^i)$; more precise studies contribute more. Consider REML/DL estimators and Hartung–Knapp CIs when heterogeneity is substantial.

IQR (interquartile range) The spread of the middle 50% of observations (Q3 – Q1). It is robust to skewness and outliers.

IRAS Single online system to prepare and submit one application for all required UK health/social care approvals (e.g. REC, HRA, R&D, MHRA); generates a project IRAS ID.

ISRCTN A registry that issues International Standard Randomized Controlled Trial Numbers for unique trial identification. It supports transparency and tracking.

Iterative approach Cyclical refinement of design, data collection, and analysis in repeated rounds informed by emerging findings and feedback. Common in qualitative research and quality improvement (e.g. PDSA cycles); document each change and its rationale to maintain transparency and rigour.

J

JAGS Just Another Gibbs Sampler. Open-source Bayesian MCMC engine similar to BUGS; integrates tightly with R, widely used for hierarchical and network models.

Judgement bias (risk of bias) Subjective decisions that can influence study selection, data extraction, or analysis. Preregistration and protocols help mitigate it.

K

Kaplan–Meier estimator A non-parametric estimator of the survival function accounting for censoring. It produces stepwise survival curves with confidence intervals.

Kendall's tau (τ) A rank-based correlation coefficient less sensitive to ties than Spearman's ρ. It reflects the proportion of concordant minus discordant pairs.

Kernel density (density plot) Smooth distribution estimate from kernels at each observation; bandwidth controls smoothness and the curve integrates to 1.

Key informant sampling Purposive strategy that recruits individuals with specialized knowledge or positional insight (e.g. service leads, community representatives, subject-matter experts) to illuminate processes, contexts, and networks. Useful for scoping and triangulation; not for prevalence estimate. State the selection criteria and reflect on potential gatekeeper/positionality bias.

Koch's postulates Classical microbiological criteria linking a specific pathogen to a disease: the organism is present in cases, can be isolated and cultured, reproduces disease in a susceptible host, and can be re-isolated. Useful historically; modern limits include asymptomatic carriage, uncultivable or polymicrobial diseases, and genomic ('molecular postulates') updates.

Kruskal–Wallis test A non-parametric alternative to one-way ANOVA for comparing medians across three or more groups. Post hoc pairwise tests may follow if significant.

L

Lasso regression (L1) A penalized regression that shrinks some coefficients to zero for variable selection. It is useful when predictors are numerous or correlated.

Last observation carried forward (LOCF) A missing-data method where the last available observation is used to replace missing values.

League tables Matrices listing all pairwise treatment comparisons (relative effects with CIs) and often rankings; aid cross-treatment interpretation at a glance.

Lean (7+1 wastes) Transport, inventory, motion, waiting, over-production, over-processing, defects, and (+1) unused skills. Map the value stream to expose queues/rework and remove non-value steps.

Leptokurtic A distribution with heavier tails and a sharper peak than normal (excess kurtosis > 0). It implies more extreme values than Gaussian.

Levene's test (homogeneity of variance) Test for equal variances across groups; robust to non-normality (uses absolute deviations from group medians/means); commonly checked before *t*-tests/ANOVA.

Likelihood ratio (LR+, LR–) Ratios indicating how much a test result changes the probability of disease. Use with pre-test odds to get post-test odds (Fagan nomogram); LR+ > 10 or LR– < 0.1 provide strong shifts in probability.

Likelihood ratio negative (LR–) Ratio of the probability of a negative test result in diseased individuals to the probability in non-diseased individuals. Values < 0.1 strongly decrease likelihood of disease. Use with pre-test odds to get post-test odds (Fagan nomogram); LR+ >10 or LR– <0.1 provide strong shifts in probability.

Likelihood ratio positive (LR+) Ratio of the probability of a positive test result in diseased individuals to the probability in non-diseased individuals. Values > 10 strongly increase likelihood of disease. Use with pre-test odds to get post-test odds (Fagan nomogram); LR+ >10 or LR– <0.1 provide strong shifts in probability.

Likert scale Ordered categorical response format (typically 1–5 or 1–7 points from 'strongly disagree' to 'strongly agree') for attitude or opinion items. Analyse single items as ordinal; summed/averaged multi-item scores are often treated as approximately interval. Report number of points, anchors, direction, and check internal consistency.

Logistic regression Models log-odds of a binary outcome as a linear function of predictors; coefficients exponentiate to odds ratios. Check linearity-in-the-logit for continuous predictors.

Lost to follow-up See *Attrition.*

Louvain algorithm Fast, greedy heuristic that optimizes modularity via node moves and community aggregation; scalable but non-deterministic across runs.

M

Mann–Whitney U test A non-parametric test comparing the distributions (often medians) of two independent groups. It is used when normality assumptions are questionable.

Marginal cost The additional cost of producing one more unit of output (e.g. one extra treatment/visit), holding other outputs fixed. In the short run it mainly reflects variable costs; distinct from average cost and from incremental cost (difference between two complete alternatives).

Markov chain Monte Carlo (MCMC) Posterior simulation (e.g. Gibbs/Metropolis). Check convergence (trace plots, $R \approx 1$, effective sample size), allow burn-in, and use posterior-predictive checks before inference.

Markov model A state transition model for chronic or recurrent processes in economic evaluation. It captures movement between health states over cycles and accumulates costs and utilities.

Maximum variation sampling Purposive approach that deliberately selects cases spanning the widest plausible range on key characteristics (e.g. age, severity, setting) to capture heterogeneity. Useful for identifying patterns that cut across diversity and edge cases; state the dimensions used and selection rationale (qualitative insight, not statistical generalizability).

Mean difference (MD) Difference between group means on the same scale (e.g. mmHg, points); typically pooled with inverse-variance methods and shown with a 95% CI. Use SMD instead if studies use different scales.

Mean The arithmetic average sensitive to extreme values. In skewed data, the median may better represent central tendency.

Mean/median imputation Replacing missing values with the mean or median of observed data.

Median The 50th percentile that splits ordered data in half. It is robust to skewness and outliers.

Mediating factor A variable that lies on the causal pathway between exposure and outcome.

Medicines and Healthcare Products Regulatory Agency (MHRA) Regulates clinical trials of medicines and medical devices in the UK.
Member checking Returning data or interpretations to participants for confirmation or clarification to enhance credibility; note that disagreement can be informative and reflects diverse perspectives.
Mental Capacity Act 2005 When capacity is lacking, a consultee advises on likely wishes; the researcher decides with safeguards. Extra protections apply for minimal burden and assent.
Meta-analysis A statistical synthesis combining results from multiple studies to obtain a pooled effect. Models may be fixed effect or random effects, depending on heterogeneity.
Meta-regression A regression across study level characteristics to explain heterogeneity in meta-analysis. It is observational and subject to ecological bias.
MHRA authorization UK regulatory authorization for CTIMPs and many device studies, in addition to an NHS REC opinion; required before starting.
Minimization (randomization) An adaptive allocation method balancing groups on prognostic factors. It improves comparability in small samples but requires allocation concealment.
Mode The most frequent value in a dataset. Some distributions are multimodal, indicating subpopulations.
Model for improvement (Nolan/IHI) Three questions (aim, measures, changes), plus PDSA cycles; track outcome, process and balancing measures to detect trade-offs.
Modularity (Q) A community-structure metric comparing within-community edge density to what would be expected by chance. Higher modularity (Q) indicates clearer community separation (dense within communities, sparse between). Note: modularity optimization can have a resolution limit (may miss small communities in large graphs).
Mosaic plot Tiles encode contingency table frequencies; tile area = cell count/percentage; useful for spotting associations.
Multiple imputation (MI) Handles missing data by creating several (m) complete datasets using an imputation model that reflects uncertainty, analysing each, then pooling estimates and standard errors using Rubin's rules. Typically assumes data are missing at random (MAR) given variables in the imputation model; include predictors of missingness and the outcome, respect variable types (e.g. logistic for binary), and align imputation with the analysis model.
Multivariable analysis Statistical modelling of a single outcome with two or more predictors to adjust for confounding (e.g. multiple linear or logistic regression); reports adjusted effects.
Multivariate analysis Modelling of two or more correlated outcomes jointly (e.g. MANOVA, multivariate regression, canonical correlation), accounting for their covariance; distinct from multivariable analysis.
mvmeta (Stata) A Stata command for multivariate and random-effects meta-analysis, widely used in frequentist network meta-analysis workflows. Companion routines allow network diagrams, treatment comparisons, and ranking of interventions.

N

Narrative analysis Qualitative analytic approach that examines the content, structure, and performance of stories to understand how participants make sense of experience. Variants include thematic (what is told), structural (how it is told), and dialogic/performance (to whom and with what effect); often used alongside transcripts, fieldnotes, and documents.
Narrative inquiry Qualitative methodology that studies experience as story over time and place, using field texts (interviews, observations, documents) co-constructed with participants. Typically idiographic and often longitudinal; emphasizes reflexivity and ethics, aiming for analytic (not statistical) generalization.
Narrative synthesis Structured, textual integration when pooling isn't appropriate: group studies, summarize effect directions and certainty, and explain heterogeneity (consider logic models/harvest plots).
Necessary cause A factor that must be present for a disease to occur. It may not be sufficient on its own to produce disease.
Negative binomial regression Generalized linear model for count outcomes (typically with a log link) that handles overdispersion by adding a dispersion parameter (e.g. $\mathrm{Var}(Y) = \mu + \kappa\mu^2$). Use when a Poisson model shows overdispersion; coefficients exponentiate to incidence rate ratios, and an offset term can account for varying exposure time.
Negative predictive value (NPV) The probability that individuals with a negative test truly do not have the disease. Predictive values

depend on disease prevalence; consider reporting across plausible prevalence ranges.

Nested case–control study A case–control study conducted within a defined cohort, efficient for rare outcomes, with exposures often measured prospectively, reducing recall bias; analysed using odds ratios.

Net present value Present value of benefits minus costs after discounting; complements BCR by reflecting scale as well as efficiency.

Network density Observed edges / possible edges (0–1), describing overall connectedness; high density often shortens path lengths.

NetworkX (Python) Python library for constructing and analysing networks (paths, centrality, communities) in computational/statistical workflows; integrates with NumPy/Pandas.

Neutral and indirect questioning (qualitative) Use of open, non-leading prompts and indirect phrasing in interviews/focus groups to reduce social desirability and demand characteristics.

Newcastle–Ottawa scale Quality appraisal for non-randomized studies using stars across selection, comparability, and outcome/exposure; provides a quick risk-of-bias signal, not a meta-analytic weight.

NHS REC (ethical opinion) NHS Research Ethics Committee that issues the ethical opinion (separate from HRA approval). Most NHS studies need both.

NHS Research Ethics Committees (NHS REC) Committees reviewing NHS-related research proposals involving participants, data, or tissue.

NICE Evidence UK portal aggregating NICE guidance and curated evidence summaries; useful for policy and implementation contexts.

***N*-of-1 trial** Prospective, multiple-crossover experiment in a single patient comparing two (or more) treatments in randomized, usually blinded periods separated by washouts. Outcomes are measured repeatedly and analysed within-person to estimate that patient's treatment effect; suited to stable chronic conditions and can be aggregated across patients for group summaries.

Nominal data Categorical variables with mutually exclusive, unordered categories (e.g. blood group, yes/no). Analyse with counts/proportions and tests like chi-square or Fisher's exact; encode as indicator (dummy) variables in regression.

Non-inferiority trial A design testing whether a new treatment is not worse than an active control by more than a specified margin. It often supports alternatives with safety or cost advantages.

Number needed to harm (NNH) Number of patients who, if treated, would lead to one additional adverse event over a stated time horizon. NNH = 1 / |RD| when RD > 0 (harm). Report the specific adverse outcome, timeframe, baseline risk, and a 95% CI; round to a whole person.

Number needed to treat (NNT) Number of patients who must be treated to prevent one additional event over a stated time horizon. NNT = 1 / |RD| where RD = EER − CER (negative for benefit). Report the timeframe, baseline risk, and a 95% CI; round to a whole person (commonly rounded up).

O

Odds The ratio of the probability of an event to the probability of it not occurring. It differs from probability and is the basis for logistic regression.

Odds ratio (OR) A measure comparing the odds of an outcome between two groups. It approximates the relative risk when outcomes are rare.

One-tailed vs two-tailed test A one-tailed test evaluates an effect in a specified direction; a two-tailed test evaluates either direction. Choice should be prespecified to avoid bias.

OpenGrey Database of grey literature (e.g. reports, theses, conference proceedings) not published in traditional journals.

Opportunity cost The value of the next best alternative forgone when a resource is used.

Ordinal data Categorical data with a natural order but unequal intervals (e.g. Likert scales). Analyses often use non-parametric or ordinal models.

Outlier An observation markedly distant from the bulk of the data. In box plots, points beyond 1.5 × IQR below Q1 or above Q3 are flagged. Outliers may reflect valid extreme values or data issues and should be interpreted in context.

Overdispersion (counts) Variance > mean (violates Poisson). Consider negative binomial, quasi-Poisson, or robust SEs; examine residuals/dispersion.

Overfitting When a model captures noise instead of signal, harming generalizability. Cross-validation and regularization help prevent it.

P

Pair plot (scatter plot matrix) Grid of scatterplots for all variable pairs; diagonals show univariate distributions; reveals linearity, clusters, and outliers.

Paired *t*-test A parametric test comparing means of two related measurements (e.g. before–after). Assumes approximately normal differences.

Pearson correlation (r) A measure of linear association between two continuous variables (−1 to +1). It is sensitive to outliers and nonlinearity.

Peer debriefing Engaging colleagues or experts to critically review data and interpretations, reducing bias.

Percentile The value at or below which a stated percentage of observations lie (e.g. 90th percentile is exceeded by 10%). For small samples it may be interpolated; the 50th percentile is the median.

Per-protocol (PP) analysis A trial analysis including only participants who adhered to the protocol (e.g. completed assigned treatment without major deviations). It can overestimate efficacy compared with intention-to-treat analysis, since non-adherent participants are excluded.

Phase 0 (microdosing studies) Early studies in humans using microdoses to study pharmacokinetics without therapeutic intent.

Phase 1 First-in-human safety/tolerability with dose escalation; characterizes PK/PD and identifies a recommended dose for phase II (often healthy volunteers or small patient cohorts). See also *Clinical trial phases.*

Phase 2 Proof-of-concept efficacy and safety in patients; refines dose/regimen (phase IIa/b), usually randomized/controlled. See also *Clinical trial phases.*

Phase 3 Confirmatory large, comparative trials testing efficacy and safety versus standard care/placebo to support marketing authorization. See also *Clinical trial phases.*

Phase 4 Post-authorization effectiveness/safety, pharmacovigilance, and rare/long-term adverse effects in routine practice; may include registries and pragmatic studies. See also *Clinical trial phases.*

Phenomenological analysis A qualitative approach describing the essence of lived experience. It involves careful reflection to bracket preconceptions (bracketing).

PICO framework Structure questions and eligibility: population/problem, intervention/exposure, comparator, outcome; often extended to PICOS (adds study design) or PICOT (adds time).

Pie chart A circular chart divided into slices to represent proportions of a whole.

Placebo effect Clinical improvement arising from expectations rather than active treatment components. It underscores the role of context and perception.

Placebo An inert intervention used as a comparator in trials. It helps isolate the specific effect of an active treatment from expectancy effects.

Plan–Do–Study–Act (PDSA) cycle A structured, iterative method for testing and refining changes in practice through four stages: Plan, Do, Study, and Act. Start with small, rapid cycles; track outcomes, process, and balancing measures.

Plausibility A causal criterion where the proposed relationship is biologically reasonable.

Poisson distribution A count distribution where the mean equals the variance, often modelling rare events per time/space. Overdispersion suggests using negative binomial models.

Poisson regression A loglinear model for count outcomes assuming a Poisson distribution. Offsets allow modelling of rates (events per person time).

Polynomial regression A regression that models non-linear relationships by including polynomial terms. It risks overfitting at high degrees.

Positionality The researcher's social/professional location (e.g. gender, culture, role) and standpoint; making it explicit helps readers judge potential influence on data collection/interpretation (links to reflexivity).

Positive predictive value (PPV) The proportion of positive test results that are true positives. PPV increases with prevalence and test specificity.

Posterior probability In Bayesian analysis, the probability assigned to a parameter or hypothesis after updating prior beliefs with observed data. It represents the updated belief given the evidence.

Post-hoc tests (multiple comparisons) Procedures (e.g. Tukey HSD, Bonferroni, Scheffé) used after a significant omnibus test to locate group differences. They control type I error inflation.

Post-test odds Odds after a test result: post-test odds = pre-test odds × likelihood ratio; convert to probability via p = odds / (1 + odds).

Post-test probability In diagnostic testing, the probability of disease after a test result, derived from the pre-test probability and the test's likelihood ratio (via Bayes' theorem or a Fagan nomogram).

Power ($1 - \beta$) of a test The probability of detecting a true effect of a specified size. It increases with larger samples, lower variability, and higher α.

Pragmatic clinical trial (PCT) Controlled clinical trials, usually randomized, designed to evaluate the effectiveness of interventions in routine healthcare practice. Unlike explanatory trials (which test efficacy under ideal conditions), pragmatic trials assess outcomes in diverse, everyday settings to inform real-world clinical and policy decision-making.

Pre-clinical (non-clinical) studies Laboratory and animal research conducted before human trials to characterize pharmacology (PK/PD), dose–response, and safety/toxicology (e.g. dose–range finding, safety pharmacology, genotoxicity, reproductive, and carcinogenicity studies) under GLP where applicable. Findings inform first-in-human dosing and support regulatory submissions; not designed to test clinical efficacy in humans.

Present value (PV) The current worth of a future sum of money, discounted at a specific rate.

Pre-test odds Odds form of pre-test probability: odds = $p/(1 - p)$; useful because LRs multiply odds linearly.

Pre-test probability The estimated likelihood of disease before testing, based on prevalence and clinical judgement. It is the starting point for Bayes-based interpretation.

Prevalence The proportion of a population with a condition at a specific time point or over a period. It informs service planning and screening policies.

PRISMA Reporting guidelines for systematic reviews and meta-analyses. The flow diagram documents study identification, screening, eligibility, and inclusion.

Probabilistic causation A cause changes the probability of an outcome rather than guaranteeing it; typical for multifactorial, population-level health outcomes.

Probability The likelihood of an event occurring (0–1 or 0–100%). Always report the time horizon and baseline risk; derive NNT/NNH = 1 / |RD| (round NNT up).

Process mapping Visual depiction of steps/hand-offs (flowchart); swim-lanes add roles; value-stream maps add times, waits, and waste; baseline before testing changes.

Propensity score methods Techniques (matching, weighting, stratification) that balance measured confounders in observational studies. They emulate some features of randomization.

Proportion The fraction of observations in a category: $p = x / n$, where x is the count in the category and n is the total. Example: for 40 smokers out of 100 patients, $p = 40/100 = 0.40$ (40%). Often reported with a 95% binomial CI (e.g. Wilson).

Proportional hazards assumption The assumption in Cox models that hazard ratios are constant over time. Violations suggest time-varying effects or alternative models.

Prospective cohort study A cohort study where exposure is measured at baseline and participants are followed forward. Measures incidence and can estimate risk ratios; vulnerable to loss to follow-up and time-varying confounding.

PROSPERO An international database for registering systematic review protocols. Registration improves transparency and reduces duplication.

PubMed NLM database with MEDLINE indexing and MeSH terms; use MeSH explosion and field tags to balance sensitivity/specificity.

Purposive (judgement) sampling Non-probability sampling that deliberately selects information-rich cases relevant to the question. Common variants include maximum variation, typical/critical case, extreme, and criterion; justify selection criteria and sample size (e.g. saturation).

***p*-Value** The probability of observing data as or more extreme than those observed, assuming the null hypothesis is true. It is not the probability the null is true and should be interpreted with effect sizes and CIs.

Q

QALY (quality-adjusted life year) A composite measure combining quantity and quality of life (utility) into a single metric. Cost utility analyses often report cost per QALY gained.

qgraph (R) R package for estimating and visualizing psychometric/symptom networks;

supports partial-correlation/graphical models, centrality plots, and bootstrapping.

Quadratic term (regression) A predictor squared (e.g. X^2) added to a regression model to capture curvature or non-linear relationships. Centring the original predictor before squaring can reduce multicollinearity with the linear term.

Qualitative research An approach focusing on meanings, experiences, and social processes using methods like interviews and observation. Rigour is enhanced via reflexivity, triangulation, and member checking.

Quality improvement (QI) Systematic, data-driven efforts to improve processes and outcomes, often using PDSA cycles, SPC charts, and root cause analysis. It differs from research by its local, iterative focus.

Quality-adjusted life year (QALY) A measure combining quantity and quality of life, used in cost–utility analysis.

QUOROM Quality of Reporting of Meta-analyses (1999) guideline for reporting meta-analyses of randomized trials; superseded by PRISMA (2009; updated 2020) for systematic reviews and meta-analyses. See also *PRISMA*.

Quota sampling Non-probability sampling in which recruiters fill prespecified quotas for key strata (e.g. age, sex, site) to mirror target proportions. Fast and practical but prone to selection bias within quotas, and lacks a calculable sampling error; report the quota variables/targets and the within-quota selection method.

R

R `(gemtc, netmeta)` `gemtc` performs Bayesian NMA via MCMC (commonly with JAGS/BUGS); netmeta implements frequentist graph-theoretic NMA with fixed/random-effects options and inconsistency checks.

Random allocation Assigning participants to study arms by chance after enrolment using a prespecified random sequence (e.g. computer-generated; possibly stratified/blocked). Purpose: balance prognostic factors on average and support causal inference. Requires allocation concealment to prevent selection bias; distinct from random selection (sampling).

Random effects model (meta-analysis) Assumes that true effect sizes vary across studies, incorporating both within-study error and between-study variance (τ^2) into the weighting. Produces wider confidence intervals when heterogeneity is present.

Random error Unpredictable variability arising from chance that widens confidence intervals but does not systematically bias results. Larger samples reduce its impact.

Random selection Choosing individuals from a defined sampling frame so each eligible member has a known, non-zero probability of inclusion (e.g. simple random, stratified, cluster, multistage). Improves representativeness/external validity; distinct from random allocation within a trial.

Randomization Assignment of participants to groups by chance to balance confounders and prevent selection bias. Allocation concealment and blinding further protect validity.

Rate Frequency of an event in a population over time.

Ratio data Interval data with a true zero, allowing ratios to be meaningful (e.g. weight, height).

Recall bias Differential accuracy/completeness of remembered exposures between groups; minimize with objective records and standardized questionnaires.

Receiver operating characteristic (ROC) curve A plot of sensitivity versus (1 – specificity) across thresholds that visualizes discrimination. The area under the curve (AUC) summarizes overall test accuracy.

Reference ('gold') standard Best available method to classify disease status against which an index test is compared; imperfections can still bias accuracy estimates.

Reflexivity Ongoing critical reflection on how the researcher's identity, assumptions, and relationships shape data collection, analysis, and interpretation. Maintain a reflexive journal.

Regression analysis A statistical technique to estimate relationships between dependent and independent variables. Check model assumptions (linearity, homoscedasticity, normality of residuals) and consider transformations or robust SEs.

Regression to the mean The tendency for extreme observations to move closer to the average on remeasurement. It can confound before–after designs without controls.

Relative benefit increase (RBI) The proportional increase in benefit in treatment vs control groups.

Relative risk (RR) The ratio of risk in the exposed group to that in the unexposed group. Values above 1 indicate increased risk; below 1 indicate protection.

Relative risk reduction (RRR) The proportional reduction in risk in treatment vs control groups. Always report the time horizon and baseline risk; derive NNT/NNH = 1 / |RD| (round NNT up).

Reliability (internal consistency) The extent to which items in a scale measure the same construct; Cronbach's alpha > 0.7 is often considered acceptable. Split-half reliability is another internal check.

Research ethics Principles ensuring human research is conducted responsibly, respecting participants' rights and wellbeing.

Residuals (regression) Differences between observed and model predicted values. Their patterns help diagnose assumption violations and model fit.

Revealed preference approach Values health or safety benefits by analysing actual choices people make in related markets (e.g. wage–risk trade-offs for hazardous jobs, hedonic pricing of housing near pollution sources, travel–cost methods for healthcare access). Infers implicit willingness to pay from behaviour rather than surveys; sensitive to market imperfections, information gaps, and equity concerns.

Reverse causality An apparent association arises because the outcome (or its early symptoms) influences the exposure, rather than the exposure causing the outcome. Most problematic in cross-sectional/retrospective designs; mitigate by establishing temporality (prospective cohorts), lagging exposures, excluding early cases, or using designs/analyses such as instrumental variables, Mendelian randomization, or self-controlled methods.

RevMan Cochrane's Review Manager for building reviews and pairwise meta-analyses (data entry, forest plots, RoB/ROBINS-I workflows); NMA generally run in R/Stata and is then reported in RevMan outputs.

Risk (exposure) window Prespecified period after/around an exposure when risk may change; define start/length a priori; SCCS may include pre-risk windows.

Risk difference (RD) Absolute risk in exposed – risk in comparator (EER – CER). RD may be positive or negative depending on outcome coding. Also referred to as absolute risk reduction (ARR) when treatment lowers risk, or absolute risk increase (ARI) when treatment raises risk.

Role-play (qualitative research) Facilitated enactment of realistic scenarios to explore decision-making, communication, and behaviour in context; data include dialogue, actions, and post-task reflections. Use alone or alongside interviews/observation; report scenario design and role instructions, analysis approach (e.g. thematic or conversation analysis), and safeguards (briefing, consent, debrief, managing potential distress).

Root cause analysis (RCA) Structured investigation of what, how, and why an incident occurred to prevent recurrence. Use the five whys and fishbone; assign actions, owners, and deadlines.

Rothman's causal pies model A model of sufficient causes as 'pies' composed of multiple component causes.

Run chart A time series plot with a median used to detect non-random variation. Rules identify shifts, trends, too few/many runs, or astronomical data points. The median should be recalculated if a sustained shift occurs.

S

Sample size calculation A priori estimation of the number of participants needed to detect a clinically meaningful effect with specified α and power. Inputs include effect size, variability, and design.

Saturation (data/theoretical) Point where further data add no new codes/themes (data saturation) or no new theoretical insights to the evolving model (theoretical saturation); used to judge when to stop sampling.

Scatter plot A graph of paired values used to visualize relationships and spot nonlinearity or outliers. Adding trend lines aids interpretation.

SCREC (Social Care REC) National REC for research in social care and with vulnerable groups in those settings; routes through IRAS where applicable.

Selection bias Systematic differences between those included and the target population (or between comparison groups); arises at sampling, recruitment, or retention.

Self-controlled case series (SCCS) Case-only design comparing event rates during exposed vs unexposed periods within individuals; controls fixed confounders by design.

Sensitivity analysis (systematic reviews/meta-analysis) Tests how results change when varying key assumptions inclusion criteria, or analytic decisions. It is used to assess the robustness and stability of conclusions (e.g. excluding high-risk-of-bias studies or comparing fixed vs random effects models).

Sensitivity (diagnostic testing) The proportion of true positives correctly identified by a test. High sensitivity is useful for ruling out disease when a test result is negative.

Shortest-path length Minimum number of edges (or weighted cost) between two nodes; network average is the characteristic path length; short paths aid fast diffusion.

Six Sigma (DMAIC) Structured reduction of variation: define–measure–analyse–improve–control. Emphasizes good measurement, cause-and-effect, and sustaining gains; $6\sigma \approx 3.4$ defects per million opportunities on critical-to-quality metrics.

Snowball sampling Non-probability chain-referral recruitment where initial 'seeds' nominate further participants, useful for hidden or hard-to-reach groups. Practical but prone to network/selection bias and duplication; not suitable for prevalence estimates. Report seed selection, number of waves, stopping rule, and any safeguards (e.g. anonymity). A weighted variant is respondent-driven sampling.

Social Care Research Ethics Committee (SCREC) Reviews research involving social care users and vulnerable groups.

Sole cause A single factor that can independently cause a disease.

Spearman's rank correlation A non-parametric correlation assessing monotonic relationships between ranked variables. It is robust to outliers and nonnormality.

Specificity The proportion of true negatives correctly identified. High specificity helps rule in disease.

Spectrum bias Diagnostic accuracy varies with case mix/severity; non-representative spectra mislead estimates; sample across the full clinical spectrum.

SRQR A 21-item reporting guideline for qualitative research outlining what to report on problem formulation, context, researcher reflexivity, sampling, ethics, data collection/analysis, techniques to enhance trustworthiness, and presentation of findings.

Standard deviation (SD) A measure of dispersion around the mean reflecting average distance of observations. In normal data, ~95% lie within ±1.96 SD of the mean.

Standard error (SE) The standard deviation of a sampling distribution (e.g. of the mean or proportion). It quantifies precision; smaller SE yields narrower CIs.

Standard error of a proportion An estimate of precision for a sample proportion: $SE = \sqrt{[p(1 - p)/n]}$. It supports binomial confidence intervals.

Standard error of the mean (SEM) Standard deviation of the sampling distribution of the mean; estimated as $SE = s / \sqrt{n}$ (or $\sigma / \sqrt{n}$ if the population SD is known).

Standard gamble (SG) Utility elicitation method: a respondent chooses between living in health state H with certainty versus a gamble between full health (probability p) and immediate death ($1 - p$). The indifference probability p is taken as the utility of H (anchored at 1 = full health, 0 = death).

Standardized mean difference (SMD) An effect size expressing mean differences in SD units, enabling pooling across different scales. Hedges' g corrects small sample bias.

Standardized mortality ratio (SMR) Ratio of observed to expected deaths (based on standard population rates), usually expressed ×100. A value >100 indicates higher-than-expected mortality; <100 indicates lower-than-expected mortality.

Standardized rate A summary rate adjusted to a common population structure (typically age) to enable fair comparisons across populations or time. Methods include direct standardization (apply study-specific rates to a standard population to get an age-standardized rate) and indirect standardization (compare observed vs expected events; yields ratios such as the SMR).

STARD Reporting guidelines for diagnostic accuracy studies that improve completeness and transparency. Items cover patient selection, index tests, reference standards, and flow.

Stata (mvmeta) mvmeta fits multivariate meta-analytic models and underpins frequentist NMA workflows (with companion commands for network plots, inconsistency, and ranking).

Stem-and-leaf plot A textual histogram that preserves the original numbers (stems = leading digits, leaves = trailing digits); quickly shows shape and outliers and can be 'back-to-back' for two groups.

Stratified analysis An approach that examines associations within levels of a potential confounder or effect modifier. It helps identify Simpson's paradox and interaction.

Stratified randomization Randomization performed separately within prespecified strata (e.g. site, sex, disease stage) to balance key prognostic factors across arms; typically uses permuted blocks within each stratum. Use a small number of important strata, maintain allocation concealment, and consider minimization if many factors need balancing.

Strength of association A causal criterion where stronger associations are more likely to be causal.

STROBE Reporting guidelines for observational studies (cohort, case–control, cross-sectional). They encourage clear reporting of design, analysis, and bias handling.

SUCRA 'Surface under the cumulative ranking' (0–100%): summarizes how often a treatment ranks near 'best' in a network meta-analysis. Interpret with effect sizes, uncertainty (CIs/predictive intervals), and checks for heterogeneity/incoherence.

Sufficient cause A set of component causes that together inevitably produce disease. Different sufficient causes may exist for the same outcome.

Survey See *Cross-sectional study.*

Survival analysis Methods for time to event data accounting for censoring (e.g. Kaplan–Meier, Cox model). Outcomes include hazard ratios and median survival.

Susser's causal web model Conceptual framework portraying disease causation as a network of interacting proximal and distal causes across biological, behavioural, social, and environmental levels. Emphasizes pathways, interactions, and feedbacks rather than single necessary causes, helping identify multiple points for prevention (upstream and downstream).

Synergism When two risk factors together produce a greater effect than the sum of their separate effects.

Systematic error Directional deviation of an estimate from the truth caused by flaws in design, conduct, measurement, or analysis (e.g. selection bias, confounding, misclassification). Not reduced by larger sample size; mitigate through design (randomization, blinding, standardized measurement) and appropriate analysis. See also: *Error*; *Random error.*

T

Tau² (τ^2) The estimated between study variance in random effects meta-analysis. Larger τ^2 indicates more heterogeneity beyond sampling error.

Temporal precedence The requirement that exposure occurs before outcome to infer causality. Cohort and trial designs establish temporality more clearly than cross-sectional studies.

Temporality A causal criterion where exposure must occur before the outcome.

Thematic analysis A flexible qualitative method for identifying and reporting patterns (themes) across data. Phases include familiarization, coding, theme development, and refinement.

Theoretical sampling In grounded theory, iterative selection of new participants/events to pursue emerging categories and relationships, guided by what the developing analysis needs next. Continue until theoretical saturation (no new properties of the core categories); this is for theory development, not statistical representativeness.

Thurstone scale A panel of judges rates statements for favourability; each item receives a scale value and is selected to span the continuum evenly. Respondents mark agree/disagree, and their score is the mean/median of the scale values of endorsed items (assumes interval-like spacing).

Time trade-off (TTO) Utility elicitation method: a respondent chooses between t years in health state H versus x years in full health; at indifference, the utility of H is $u(H) = x / t$ (anchored 1 = full health, 0 = death). Used to derive QALY weights; results are sensitive to the time horizon and to time preferences (e.g. discounting) and may use lead/lag-time variants for states worse than death.

Time series graph Plot of a variable indexed by time with observations ordered (and often connected) to reveal level, trend, seasonality, and variability. Use an appropriate timescale, label units, and annotate key events; for monitoring change, consider run or control charts.

Treatment policy estimator (TPE) Targets the effect of initial treatment assignment regardless of post-randomization events (e.g. non-adherence, discontinuation, switching, rescue therapy). Typically operationalized with intention-to-treat analyses that include all randomized participants as allocated and use observed outcomes irrespective of adherence.

Treemap Nested rectangles show hierarchical part-to-whole structure; area encodes magnitude and nesting reflects levels (e.g. category → subcategory). Good for many categories when pie/bar charts become crowded.

Triangulation (qualitative) Using multiple methods, data sources, or researchers to enhance credibility. Convergence of evidence supports trustworthiness.

Trim and fill method A funnel plot-based approach to assess and adjust for publication bias in meta-analysis. It imputes hypothetical missing studies to restore symmetry.

Triple-blind trial Participants, investigators, and analysts are all unaware of allocations.

***t*-Test** A statistical test used to compare the means of two groups. Assumes approximate normality and homoscedasticity; consider non-parametric alternatives if violated.

Tukey's HSD A post hoc test controlling family-wise error while comparing all pairs of means after ANOVA. It balances type I error control and power.

Type I error (α) False positive: rejecting a true null hypothesis. The type I error rate equals α (e.g. 0.05) and is set by the significance threshold; with multiple tests it inflates unless controlled (e.g. Bonferroni, Holm).

Type II error (β) False negative: failing to reject a false null hypothesis. Statistical power = $1 - \beta$ and depends on effect size, variance, α, sample size, and design; reduce β by increasing n, improving measurement, or (with trade-offs) using a larger α.

U

UK GDPR and Data Protection Act 2018 UK legislation governing lawful, fair, and transparent processing of personal data, including research uses. It mandates minimization, security, and rights for data subjects.

UK Research Integrity Office (UKRIO) An independent body offering guidance and support on good research practice and integrity. It assists institutions in handling misconduct issues.

Unadjusted vs adjusted analysis Unadjusted analyses ignore covariates, while adjusted analyses control for confounders via stratification or regression. Adjustment improves causal interpretation in observational studies.

University Research Ethics Committees (UREC) University-level committees reviewing non-NHS and academic research ethics.

V

Validity (construct, internal, external) Construct validity asks whether a measure reflects the intended concept; internal validity concerns causal inference; external validity addresses generalizability. Each can be threatened by bias.

Value-stream mapping Adds times, queues, and waste to a process map to reveal bottlenecks and non-value steps; prioritize changes with biggest patient/value impact.

Variance The average squared deviation from the mean; SD is its square root. Variance underlies many statistical models and tests.

Variation ratio (VR) A dispersion index for categorical data defined as 1 – (mode proportion). Higher values indicate greater heterogeneity across categories.

Verification (work-up) bias Occurs when not all patients receive the reference standard (often depending on test result); can inflate sensitivity/specificity if positives are over-verified.

Visual analogue scale (VAS) A 10 cm (0–100 mm) horizontal line anchored by contrasting statements (e.g. 'no pain' to 'worst pain imaginable'). The respondent marks a point reflecting their perception; the score is the distance in millimetres from the 'zero' anchor (treated as continuous).

W

Willingness to pay (WTP) An individual/population valuation concept: how much someone would pay for a specified health gain/risk reduction. Used in cost–benefit analyses.

Willingness-to-pay (WTP) threshold Policy benchmark for the maximum acceptable cost per unit of health gain (e.g. per QALY) used by a payer to judge cost-effectiveness; thresholds are setting-specific and guide ICER decisions. See also *Willingness to pay (WTP)*.

WinBUGS Bayesian MCMC engine (BUGS language) for hierarchical/NMA models with flexible priors; frequently called from R scripts for custom models.

Within-subjects design A design where the same participants receive multiple conditions. It controls for between-person variability but may suffer from carryover effects.

Y

Yates' continuity correction An adjustment to the chi-square test for 2 × 2 tables to better approximate exact probabilities with small samples. It can be conservative.

Youden index (J) A single statistic summarizing diagnostic test performance: J = sensitivity + specificity − 1. The cut-off maximizing J balances false positives and false negatives.

Z

Z-test Hypothesis test that uses the standard normal distribution. Appropriate when the population standard deviation is known or the sample is large enough for a reliable normal approximation (e.g. tests of a mean, a single proportion, or difference in proportions with large n). Assumes independent observations and approximate normality of the test statistic.

***z*-Value (*z*-score; standard score)** Number of standard deviations an observation or statistic lies from its mean. For a value x: $z = (x - \mu) / \sigma$ (population parameters). For a sample mean $\bar{x}$: $z = (\bar{x} - \mu) / (\sigma / n)$ when σ is known. Enables use of standard normal tables and comparison across different scales.

Index

Page numbers in "*Italics*" refer to figures; page numbers in "**bold**" refer to tables

2×2 contingency table, **35–6**, 107
  calculating treatment effects, **108**
  diagnostic test evaluation and, 42–50
  dyslexia screening, **60**
  for evaluating diagnostic test accuracy, **35**
  home glucose tolerance test, **52**
  interpretation of, 41–2, **42**
  new adult ASD screening test, **53**, **58**
  odds ratio of mortality, **114**
  positive predictive value (PPV) calculation of, 36
  randomized controlled trials and, 98
  raw counts, **46**
  structure for diagnostic test interpretation, **43**

absolute risk, 24
academic and non-NHS research, 294
accuracy, 35–6, 49
acute health events, 79
adaptive randomization, 93 *See also* randomization
AGREE (Appraisal of Guidelines for Research and Evaluation), 298
agreement between raters, 49
alternative hypothesis, 186
ambispective cohort studies, 66, 71
analyses, types of, 96–7
analytic cohort studies, 70–1
  design, 66–7, 71
analytical epidemiological studies, 1
analytical studies, 1–2
ANOVA (analysis of variance), 191, **193**, 210
antagonism, 22
  examples of, 22
area under the curve (AUC), 44
association
  measure of, 78
  measuring the strength of, 67–9, 71, 107
  strength of, 83
auditing process, 269

bar chart, example of a, *159*
bar graph vs histogram, *160*
bathtub model, prevalence, *2*, 12
Bayes' Theorem, 40, 216, 220, 222
Bayesian hypothesis testing, 186
Bayesian statistical analysis, 216, 219–20
  advantages and disadvantages of, 217
  components of, 217
  concepts in, 216–17
  steps in Bayesian analysis, 217
bias. *See* individual types of biases
biases, 17
  assessing publication bias, 119, **121**
  assessing the risk of, 119
  case-control studies and, 19, 26–7
  cross-sectional studies and, 8
  in diagnostic studies, 45, *47*, 51
  inclusion/exclusion (selection) bias, *18*, 19, 27
  information bias, 20
  lead time bias, 46
  lead time bias vs length bias, **47**
  length bias, 47
  observer bias, 257
  prevention of, 95
  purity bias vs spectrum bias, **46**
  recall bias, 12, 20
  selection bias, 12
  selection bias by researchers and participants, 19
  spectrum bias, 45
  statistical tests for publication bias, 120–1
  techniques to reduce biases in qualitative research, 269, **270**
binary (dichotomous) data, tests for, *230*
birth cohort, 70
blinding, 26, 95, 101
  challenges and solutions in psychotherapy trials, **95**
block randomization, 92 *See also* randomization
bootstrapping, 152, 172
  bootstrapped standard error, 172
  process flow diagram, *174*
  worked example, 173
box (and whisker) plots, *160*
bracketing technique, 264, 267
Bradford Hill criteria, 83–4, 86
  Austin Bradford Hill, 83–4
  criteria for cause and effect, **86**
  Susser endorsement of, 85
brain network analysis, 154

case studies, 260, 273
case – control studies, 1, 10, 17, 27
  biases in, *18*, 19, 27
  confounding in, 20–1
  critical appraisal of, 26–7
  data collection and, 19
  design of, 17–19
  differences with cohort studies, 26, 66
  illustration of confounding in, *21*
  information bias in, 19, 20
  minimizing bias, 19
  outcomes and risk factors, 18
  pitfalls of, 27

relative risk and, 25
reverse causality in, 24
selecting cases and controls, 18
strength of association and, 24
strengths and limitations of, 25
structure of, *17*, *27*
categorical data, 195
comparison of, 194
degree of heterogeneity in, 175
measures of dispersion for, 172–8
causal pies model, Rothman's, 84
causal web, the, 85
causation, comparison of approaches to, **86–8**
cause-specific death rate, 12
censoring, 211
central symptoms, identifying, 153
central tendency
for data types, 166–7
measures of, 166
centrality measures
network analysis, 151
chance, 17
Chi-square (χ^2) test, **194**
clinical audit, 281, 287
comparison with quality improvement, **287**
cycle, *281*
methodology for doing, 281
and research differences, **282**
vs research, *282*
clinical trials, 103–6, 294, 298
stages of, 108
cluster randomization, 93–4
clustering and community detection
network analysis, 151
Cochrane Risk of Bias Tool, 135
cognitive networks, 154
cohort, 70
definition of, 64
cohort studies, 1, 10, 64, 70 *See also* retrospective cohort studies
2×2 table for calculating relative risk, **68**
advantages of, 71–2
advantages of retrospective vs prospective cohort studies, 66
ambispective, 66, 71
analytic, 65, 70–1
analytic cohort study design, 71
analytic design, 66–7
comparison with case–control, 26
critical appraisal, 69
descriptive, 64, 70
with external control, 65
with internal control, 65
pitfalls and appraisals of, 72
prospective (classical), 65, 70
relative risk in, 67–8
retrospective, 71
strength of association in, 67–9
strengths and limitations of, **69**
types of, 70–1
types of based on timing, 65–6
comorbidity networks, 153
comparisons, 132–3
complete case analysis, 97
concurrent validity, 48
confidence intervals, 25, 171, 184
for ordinal data, 175
Confidentiality Advisory Group (CAG), 294
confounders, 27
controlling, 21
data analysis and controlling for, 21
definition of, 20
identifying, 21
confounding, 8, 17, 27
by indication, 23
case – control studies and, 20–1, *21*, 26–7
independent effects and, *22*
confounding factors, 11, 12
cross-sectional studies and, 8
connections. *See* edges
consent, informed, 259
consistency, internal, 49
Consolidated Standards of Reporting Trials (CONSORT), 297
constant comparative method, 265, **266**, 269
constant comparison. *See* constant comparative method
construct validity, 48, 51
content analysis, 262–3
content validity, 48, 51
contingency table. *See* 2×2 contingency table
contingency table cells. *See* 2×2 contingency table
contingent valuation, monetary values and, 237
control group, randomized controlled trials and, 95
convenience sampling, 252, 271
convergent validity, 48, 51
COREQ (Consolidated Criteria for Reporting Qualitative Research), 298
correlation analysis, 10, 218
correlation coefficient, *196*, 198
comparison of coefficients, *203*, 222
logistic regression, 204
multiple regression, 205
ordinal regression, 206
phi coefficient, 202
point-biserial correlation coefficient, 202
polynomial regression, 205–6
simple linear regression, 203
types of relationships and, 198–200
cost – benefit analysis, 236
steps in conducting, 236–9
cost – consequence analysis, 243, 244
advantages of, 243
limitations, 243
when to use, 243
cost – effectiveness acceptability curve (CEAC), *246*
cost – effectiveness analysis, 239
conducting a, 239–40
cost – effectiveness ratio, 243
calculating, 240
cost-minimization analysis, 236
cost-utility analysis, 240, 244
steps in conducting, 240–2
covert observation, 258

Cox proportional hazards regression, *215*, 219
Cramér's V, *203*, 218
criterion sampling, 253, 272
criterion validity, 48, 51
Cronbach's Alpha (α), 49
crossover trials, 100
  advantages and limitations of, **100–1**
cross-sectional studies, 1, 10
  crude and cause-specific death rates, 12
  definition of, 8, 11
  methodology of, 8–9, 11
  strengths and limitations of, 9, 12
  types of, 8
crude death rate, 3, 12
cut-off point, 44
  best, 51
  considerations when selecting, 51
  selecting, 43, *45*

data
  central tendency for data types, 166–7
  displaying, 158, 177
  displaying, graphical methods for, 158, **163**
  distribution of, 166–7, 177
  extraction table, **118**
  handling missing, 96–7, 107
  non-parametric, 171
  skewed numerical, 167–71
  tests for various data types, 189–95
  types of, **162**, 163, **164**, 177
data analysis, 10
  case – control studies and, 27
  controlling for confounders, 21
  methods of, 262, **266**, 272
data collection, 19
  cyclical process of, 264
data collection methods, **266**
  in qualitative research/studies, **254**, 256, 272
databases, studies listed in, 117
death rate
  cause-specific, 3, 12
  crude, 3, 12
deception, research and, 296
Declaration of Helsinki, 296
deductive reasoning, 185
degrees of freedom, 168–9, 183
depression management, cognitive behavioural therapy (CBT), and medication – comparison of outcomes, **243**
descriptive analysis, 10
descriptive statistics, 158, 176
diagnostic studies, biases in, 45, *47*, 51
diagnostic test
  deciding on cut-off point, 43
  evaluating the accuracy of, **35**
  negative predictive value (NPV), 36
  positive predictive value, 36
  predictive values of, 36
  rule in and rule out concept, 36–7
  selecting a cut-off point, 43, *45*
diagnostic test evaluation
  formulae for, 42–50
diagnostic tests, 34
  accuracy of, 35–6
  receiver operating characteristic (ROC) curve and, 43
diary methods, 259, 273
dichotomous data, 177
  standard error and confidence interval for, 175
direct costs, 233, 236–7, 243
direct standardization, 4
discounting, 234–5
  discount rate, 235
  future costs and benefits, 238
  how to apply, 235
discourse analysis, 263
discriminant validity, 48, 52
disease prevalence, effect on predictive values, 37–50
dispersion
  for categorical data, 172–8
  for dichotomous data, 174
  for skewed numerical data, 167–71
  measures for dispersion, 177
  measures of, 167–71, 176, 177
  measures of dispersion for skewed data, 171
display methods, data types, **162**
distributions, 164–5
divergent validity (discriminant validity), 48, 52
document analysis, 259, 260, 273

ecological studies, 2, 12
  definition, 10
  ecology, 10
  elements of, 10
  measuring association in, 10
  strengths and limitations of, 10
economic analysis
  direct costs in healthcare and, 233
  in medicine, 233
  indirect costs, 233
  intangible costs, 234
  opportunity cost, 234
economic evaluation methods, 236
  in healthcare, 243–4
economic evaluation metrics, calculating, 238
economic evaluation studies
  types of costs in, **234**
edges (connections/lines), 132, 147–8
effect modification, 22–3
  exercise and heart disease, *23*
  smoking as an effect modifier, *23*
effect size, 210
elastic net regression, 207
epidemiological studies
  causation in, 83, 86
  classification of, 1–2
  epidemiological measurements in, 12
  finding control groups, 79
  measurements in, 2–4
  what they are, 1
epidemiological study designs, key difference, 1
errors, 205, 219
  systematic, 27
  type II error (false negative), 210
ethical research
  approval process in the UK, 295
  research misconduct, 295
ethics. *See* research ethics
ethnography, 260, **261**, 273

experimental studies (interventional studies), 1, 2
exposure, 18
exposure cohort, 70

F ratio, 192
F statistic, **191**
face validity, 48, 51
fail-safe *N*, 121
false negative rate, 37
false positive rate, 37
false positives
  vs false negatives, clinical consequences of, 43, 51
falsification principle, 186
field notes, 258
field trials, 103, 108
focus groups, 256–7, 273
forest plot, *136*, *137*
  how to read, *126*
  visual inspection of, **124**
framework analysis, 264
Framingham Heart Study, The, 64
frequentist hypothesis testing, 186
  using single group research for, 186–7
  using two groups, 187–8
Friedman's test, 193
future costs and benefits, discounting, 238

Galbraith plot (radial plot), 122–3
GRADE framework, 127
grounded theory analysis, 262, 264, 265, 273
Guttman scale, 271, 274

harm, minimizing, 259
Hawthorne effect, 257
hazard ratio, 68–9
health and social care research, 296
health evaluation, and health-related quality of life, 235
Health Research Authority (HRA), 296
health status
  standard gamble and, 235
  time trade-off and, 235–6
healthcare interventions, analysing, 236
health-related quality of life, 235
heterogeneity
  assessing, 121, **124**
  methods to assess, 124
  testing heterogeneity in systematic reviews, **123**
  types of, 122
histogram, example, *159*
homogeneous sampling, 253, 272
human capital approach, monetary values and, 237
Human Tissue Act 2004, 296
hypothesis
  Bayesian hypothesis testing, 186
  comparing two groups, 187–8
  frequentist hypothesis testing, 186
  process of testing null hypothesis, 188–9
  single group research in testing, 186–7
  testing methods, 185–6

immersive research approach, 260
imputation, mean/median, 97
inception cohort, 70
incidence, 2
incidence rate ratio (IRR), 78
inclusion/exclusion (selection) bias, 19, 27
incremental cost – utility ratio, 241–2
independent effects, 22
  confounding and, *22*
indirect costs, 233, 237, 243
indirect questioning techniques, 269, **270**
inductive approach, 264
inductive reasoning, 185
inferential statistics, 185
information bias, 19, 26, 27
  case-control studies in, 20
  observers and, 20
  participants and, 20
informed consent, 259
Institute for Healthcare Improvement (IHI) model, 285, 288
intangible costs, 234, 237, 244
intention-to-treat (ITT) analysis, 96–7, 107
internal consistency, 49
International Standard Randomised Controlled Trial Number (ISRCTN), 298
interpretation, 68
interpretative phenomenological analysis, 265
interquartile range, 171
inter-rater reliability, 49
interviews, 272
  types of, 255–6
inverse probability weighting, 97
iterative approach, 261, 273

judgement sampling, 253

Kaplan-Meier Estimator (KM curve), 213, 219
Kaplan – Meier survival curves (KM curve)
  with log-rank test, *214*
Kendall's correlation coefficient, 200
Koch's postulates, 84, 86, 89
  criteria for cause and effect, **86**
  limitations of, 84
  Robert Koch, 84
Kruskal – Wallis ANOVA, 193
kurtosis, 165

last observation carried forward (LOCF), 96, 107
lead time bias, 46
  vs length bias, **47**
lean, quality improvement method, 285
length bias, 47
leptokurtic distributions, 165
life, health-related quality of, 235
likelihood ratios (LRs), 50
  of commonly used medical tests, 39
  negative test (LR–), 50
  of psychiatric rating scales, **39**
  positive tests, 50
Likert scale, 271, 274
linear relationship, 198
logistic regression, 9, 204

Mann – Whitney U test, 193
masking. *See* blinding
matching, 21
matrix-based approach, 264
mean/median imputation, 97
measurement bias, 20
measurement, reliability and, 52
median survival time, 213
mediating factor, 22
medical diagnostic tests. *See also* diagnostic tests
  likelihood ratio of negative tests (LR–), 50
  likelihood ratio of positive tests (LR+), 50
  likelihood ratios of common, **39**
medicine, economic analysis in, 233
Medicines and Healthcare Products Regulatory Agency (MHRA), 294
member checking technique, 268
Mental Capacity Act 2005, 296
mental disorders
  as network symptoms, 153
  comorbidity of, 153
mental health
  cognitive networks in, 154
  cost – consequence analysis, 243
  network analysis, 153–4
mesokurtic distributions, 165
meta-analyses, in sensitivity analysis, 128, **129**
meta-analysis, definition of, 117
meta-regression analysis, 127–8
minimization, 93
minimizing bias, 19
missing data, handling, 96–7
mixed models, 96, 107
modularity analysis, 152
monetary values, cost-benefit analysis and, 237
monotonic relationship, 198
mortality
  measurement of, 12
  standardized mortality rate (SMR), 4
multicollinearity, 206
multi-group analysis, and single-group analysis, 218
multiple imputation, 96, 107
multiple regression, 205
multivariable analysis (regression adjustment), 21
multivariate analysis, 27

narrative analysis, 263
narrative inquiry, 260, 273
National Child Development Study, The, 65
National Health Service Research Ethics Committees (NHS REC), 294
negative predictive value, 36, 37, 50
net present value, 238
network analysis, 147
  building blocks of, 147–51
  centrality in, 148–51
  in mental health, 153–4
  sample of, *150*
  steps for conducting, 151
  strengths and weaknesses of, 154
  treatment response, 153
network density and connectivity
  network analysis, 152
network meta-analysis, 129, 131
  limitations of, 135
  network diagram, 131, 3
  steps in performing, 133–4
  summary steps for conducting, **135**
  uses of, 134
network visualization, network analysis, 152
neurobiological and cognitive networks, 154
neutral questioning techniques, 269, **270**
Newcastle – Ottawa Scale, 135
node sizes, 132
nodes, 147
N-of-1 trials, 101–2, 108
  advantages and disadvantages of, **102**
Nolan Model for Improvement, 285
non-parametric data, 171
  confidence interval of, 171–3
non-parametric tests, **193**
  adjusting for small sample sizes in, 194
non-participant observation, 257
normal (Gaussian) distribution, *165*
normal distribution curve, *169*
normality, tests of, **191**
normally distributed data
  dispersion of, 177
  measures for, 177
null hypothesis, 186
  process for testing for statistical significance, 188–9
  type I error, 208
numerical data, 195
  test for numerical continuous data for, **189**
  tests for, 189

observation, 273
  challenges in qualitative research, 257–9
  methods of data collection in, 258
  in qualitative research, 257
  types of, 257–8
observational research
  ethical considerations in, 259
observational studies, 1–2
  design of self-controlled case series (SCCS) and, 79
observations. *See* observation
observed association, 17
observer bias, 257
odds ratio (OR), 24
  association and, 83
  interpretation of, 25
  vs relative risk, 25
one- and two-tailed tests, 195, *196*
opportunity cost, 234, 244
ordinal data
  confidence intervals for, 175
  measures of dispersion for, 172–8
  for pain severity, 176
  tests for, 230
original dataset, 173
outcome, 18
overt observation, 257

parallel-forms reliability, 49
participant observation, 257
participant validation, 268

p-curve analysis, 121
Pearson's correlation
coefficient, 200
peer debriefing, 268
percentile-based confidence
intervals, 172
permutation tests, 153
per-protocol analysis, 96
personal data, using for
research, 296
personalized interventions, 153
phenomenological analysis,
263–4
phi coefficient, 202
pie chart, example, *159*
Plan - Do - Study - Act
(PDSA) cycle, 284
platykurtic distributions, 165
point-biserial correlation
coefficient, 202
Poisson distribution, 207
Poisson regression, 207
polynomial regression, 205–6
pooled Mantel–Haenszel
estimate, 21
Popper, Karl, 186
population
determining population at
risk, *77*, 79
prevalence of disease in, 55
positive predictive value, 36, 50
post-hoc tests, summary
of, **193**
post-test probability, *41*
calculation of, 50–1
power calculation, 210–11,
219
pragmatic clinical trials,
99–100
pre- and post-test probabilities,
40, 50–1
concepts in, 40
predictive validity, 48
predictive values, effect of
disease prevalence on,
37–50
present value, 238
pre-test odds
converting from pre-test
probabilities, 40
pre-test probability vs post-test
probability, 50–1
prevalence, 2, 43
disease in the population,
55
high-prevalence
population, **37**
low-prevalence
population, **37**
prevalence bathtub model,
2, 12
PRISMA (Preferred Reporting
Items for Systematic
Reviews and Meta-
Analyses), 297
guidelines, 118
PRISMA flow diagram, 118
privacy and confidentiality,
ethical consideration
and, 259
probabilities
converting pre-test
probability, 40
pre- and post-test, 40
pre- and post-test
probabilities concepts, 40
proportion, 174
prospective (classical) cohort
studies, 65, 70
PROSPERO (International
Prospective Register of
Systematic Reviews), 297
psychiatric rating scales
likelihood ratios (LRs) of, **39**
publication bias, 119, **121**
assessing, **121**
funnel plots showing, *120*
methods of testing for, 121
statistical tests for, 120–1
purity bias, 46, 51
vs spectrum bias, **46**
purity diagnostic bias. *See*
purity bias
purposive (judgement)
sampling, 253, 272
p-value, 186

qualitative data
collection methods, **261**, **266**
framework analysis and, 264
scaling techniques for
quantifying, 270–1, 274
qualitative research
challenges of observation in,
257–9
distinction between
reflexivity and bracketing
technique, **280**
sampling techniques in,
271–2
strategies to enhance the
rigour of, 266–9
strategies to enhance
trustworthiness of, 266–9
techniques to reduce bias in,
269–70
qualitative studies, 252
data collection methods in,
254, 256
focus groups and, 256–7
sampling techniques in,
252, **254**
quality-adjusted life years, 244
quality improvement, 282, 287
benefits of, 286, **287**, 288
methodology for, 283, 288
principles of, 283
tools and techniques used
in, 285
types of methodologies used,
284–5
Quality of Reporting of Meta-
Analyses
(QUOROM), 297
questioning techniques,
269, **270**
quota sampling, 253, 272

radial plot (Galbraith plot),
122–3
random error, 20
randomization, 21, 95
comparison of types of, **94**
types of, 106–7
randomized controlled
trials, 106
2×2 contingency table
and, 98–9
analytical approaches in,
107
comparison of, **103–5**
control groups and, 95
definition of, 95
ethical considerations of, 99
features of, 95
missing data and, 97
rate, 3
raters, agreement between, 49
reasoning
by comparison, 84
deductive, 185
inductive, 185
inductive vs deductive, 217
theoretical, 51
recall bias, 12, 20

receiver operating characteristic (ROC) curve, 43, *44*, *45*, 55
for cholesterol – area under the curve (AUC), *45*
reflexivity, 266–7
distinction to bracketing technique, **280**
regression analysis, *203*, 218–19
comparison of, **128**
comparison of regression models, **207–8**
regression adjustment, 21
regularized regression techniques, 206
relationships
linear relationship, 198
monotonic relationship, 198
non-monotonic relationship, 227
types, 198–200
relative risk, 67–8
association and, 83
case–control studies and, 25
vs odds ratio (OR), 25
reliability, 49
types of, 52
research ethics
and ethical approval process in the UK, 293–9
key legislation and guidelines, 296
principles of, 293–4
regulating bodies in the UK, 294–5
reporting standards, 299
research misconduct, 295
special considerations for, 296
what it is, 293
research studies, guidelines for, 299
response-adaptive randomization, 93 *See also* randomization
restriction, 21
retrospective cohort studies, 65–6, 71
revealed preference approach, monetary values and, 237
reverse causality, 27
case – control studies, 24
ridge and lasso regression (regularized regression), 206
risk, 2
and rates of diseases, 12
population at, *77*, 79
relative risk, 67–8
role-play, 259, 273
Rothman, Kenneth, 84
criteria for cause and effect, **86**
Rothman's causal pies model, 84, 86, 89
rule-in concept, diagnostic tests, 36–7, 50
rule-out concept, diagnostic tests, 36–7, 50

sample sizes, 219
adjustments for small, 194
estimation of, 210–11
sampling techniques, 271–2
in qualitative studies, 252, **254**
scaling techniques, 270–1
scatterplot, example, 161
screen studies, 118
selection bias, 12, *18*, 19, 26
participants and, 19
researchers and, 19
self-controlled case series (SCCS) studies, 79, *82*
design components of, 77–8
measure of association, 78
of population at risk, *77*, 79
when to use, *77*, 78
sensitivity, 49
and specificity at different MMSE cut-off scores, **45**
diagnostic tests, 34
sensitivity analysis, **128**, 238
conduct, 242
network analysis, 152
systematic reviews and, 128, **129**
short-term exposure, 79
simple randomization, 92 *See also* randomization
single-group analysis/research and multi-group analysis, 218
frequentist hypothesis testing, 186–7
Six Sigma, 285
skewness
negative and positive, *166*
skewed data and measures of dispersion of, 178
skewed numerical data and measures of dispersion, 167–71
snowball sampling, 254, 272
Social Care Research Ethics Committee (SCREC), 294
social network analysis, 155
in mental health, 154
Spearman's rank correlation coefficient, 200
specificity, 36, 37, 49
diagnostic tests, 35
spectrum bias, 45
comparison with purity bias, **46**
split-half reliability test, 49
SRQR (Standards for Reporting Qualitative Research), 298
stability over time, 49
standard age group, 4
standard deviation, 169, 177
standard error
and confidence interval of non-parametric data, 171–3
for dichotomous data, 175
t statistic, 190–95
standard error of the mean (SEM), 169, **170**, 183
vs standard error of sample means, **170**
standard gamble, 235
standardized (adjusted) rates, 4
cross-sectional studies and, 12
direct standardization, 4
standardized mortality rate (SMR), 4
standardized rates, 4
Standards for Reporting Diagnostic Accuracy Studies (STARD), 298
statistical formulas, 171
statistical hypothesis testing, 195
statistical significance, 25
statistical tests, 10
choosing, 163–5
to quantify heterogeneity, 123, **124**
statistical validation, network analysis, 152
statistical validity, 27, 48, 51

statistics
analytic, 185
descriptive, 158, 176
inferential, 185
stratified analysis, 21, 27, 194
stratified randomization, 92 *See also* randomization
comparison of, **94**
STROBE (Strengthening the Reporting of Observational Studies in Epidemiology), 298
structured observation, 258
subgroup analysis, 127, **128**
survival analysis, 211, 219
features of survival data, 211–13, 219
methods, 213–14, 219
statistical tests in, 214, 219
survival probability, 213
Susser, Mervyn
criteria for cause and effect, **86**
criteria for cause and effect relationships, 85–6
Susser's causal web model, 89
symptom network analysis, 153
synergism
example of, 22
independent effects of, 22
systematic errors, 20, 27
bias and, 19
systematic review, 117
assessing bias risk, 119
assessing heterogeneity in, 121, **123**, **124**
comparison of regression analysis in, **128**
definition of, 117
developing the protocol, 117
extracting the data, 118
formulating the research question, 117
interpreting the findings of, 125, **129**
reporting and publishing the findings, 129
screen studies, 118
searching for appropriate studies, 117
sections of the report, 118
sensitivity analysis in, 128, **129**
steps in. *See* individual steps
summary of workflow, **129**
synthesizing the findings, 125

t statistic, 190–95
temporal ambiguity, 12
test/tests. *See also* diagnostic test
tests
comparing for categorical data, 194
consistency within the, 49
non-parametric tests, **193**
test – retest reliability, 49
thematic analysis, 262
theoretical sampling, 254, 272
therapy effectiveness, 155
assessing, 154
Thurstone scale, 271, 274
time trade-off, 235–6
time-consuming process, 257
time-to-event (survival time), 211
treatment
blinding, 101
clinical decision, 102
cycles, 101
data analysis, 102
outcome measurement, 102
patient identification, 101
randomization, 101
selection, 101
treatment policy estimator, 96, 107
washout periods, 102
treatment response, network analysis and, 153
trial registries, and grey literature, 121
trials. *See also* clinical trials
alternative trial designs, 99
crossover, 100–1
field, 103
N-of-1, 101–2
pragmatic clinical, 99–100
triangulation, 268
trim-and-fill method, 121
true negative rate, 35, 49
true positive rate, 34, 49
two- and one-tailed tests, 195, *196*
type I error
(false positive), 219
null hypothesis, 208
type II error (false negative), 210, 219

UK General Data Protection Regulation (UK GDPR), 296
UK Policy Framework for Health and Social Care Research (HRA), 296
UK Research Integrity Office (UKRIO), 294
University Research Ethics Committees (URECs), 294
unstructured observation, 258

validity, **47**, 51
construct, 51
convergent, 51
discriminant, 52
divergent, 52
logical, 48, 51
statistical, 51
variance, 167–8, 177
variation ratio, 174, 175
visual analogue scale, 271, 274
for pain measurement, *271*
vulnerable populations, 296

Wilcoxon matched pairs signed test, 193
Wilcoxon signed-rank test, 193
willingness-to-pay method, monetary values and, 237
worst-case scenario analysis, 97

Youden Index, 45
optimal cut-off point for dementia diagnosis, **45**

For EU product safety concerns, contact us at Calle de José Abascal, 56–1°,
28003 Madrid, Spain or eugpsr@cambridge.org.

www.ingramcontent.com/pod-product-compliance
Ingram Content Group UK Ltd.
Pitfield, Milton Keynes, MK11 3LW, UK
UKHW021918220726
473566UK00009B/335

* 9 7 8 1 0 0 9 1 8 2 5 2 2 *